HypnoBirthing

HypnoBirthing

For a safer, easier, more comfortable birth

Marie Mongan

SOUVENIR
PRESS

This fourth and expanded edition first published in Great Britain
in 2016 by Souvenir Press Ltd, an imprint of
Profile Books Ltd
29 Cloth Fair
London EC1A 7JQ
www.profilebooks.co.uk

First published in the USA by Health Communications, Inc.

First published in Great Britain in 2007 by Souvenir Press Ltd.

Copyright © 1992, 1998, 2005, 2015 by Marie F. Mongan

*Inside book design by Lawna Patterson Oldfield
Illustrations by Paul Svancara
Typeset by M Rules*

3 5 7 9 10 8 6 4

Printed and bound in Great Britain by
Clays Ltd, Elcograf S.p.A.

A CIP catalogue record for this book
is available from the British Library.

ISBN 978 1 78816 6225
eISBN 978 0 28564 3369

FSC
www.fsc.org
MIX
Paper from
responsible sources
FSC® C018072

This Fourth Edition of HypnoBirthing,
the Mongan Method, is dedicated to those many
genuinely caring birth professionals—doctors, nurses, nurse
midwives, Certified Professional Midwives, childbirth educators,
and doulas—who have witnessed the beauty of HypnoBirthing
and who have seen it with open eyes, open minds, and open
hearts, and who have then moved forward to bring calm
and gentle birthing into the lives of the parents they serve
and the colleagues with whom they work.

"Women have access to an unstoppable energy that transcends fear and negativity. Women who tap into that energy have the power not only to achieve their own life purpose and goals; but using their personal stories as a template, they inspire other women to do the same—to go beyond what they ever thought was possible."

—**Patricia Jocelyn**
Author, Journalist, Spiritual Lecturer

Contents

Foreword

Marie Mongan is a woman who has devoted her entire life to working with women of all ages and in all walks of life. Through her book and the HypnoBirthing Method, she shares the conviction of her own personal birthing experience and her sensitivity to the emotional and spiritual needs of birthing women. The message about the normality of birth that this book delivers is an essential one for all families who believe in and care about birthing their babies in safety, calm, and peace.

This book, and the HypnoBirthing program itself, has provided me, and other doctors who share a belief in normal birth, a framework within which to practise obstetrics in the manner in which our education has qualified us and in the direction in which our hearts have led us. It has changed the way many of us practise obstetrics.

I began "delivering" babies in 1983. I believed in the use of drugs to manage obstetrical pain. In spite of my best efforts to use good sound medical judgment, I saw lots of complications, including babies with compromised breathing. I believed that epidurals were a medical blessing for labouring mothers. I had a 25 percent C-section rate.

Many patients demanded natural births. I then performed hundreds of deliveries using pushing and blowing while holding off analgesics until the mother could no longer take the pain. I saw babies that were no longer respiratorily compromised, but both mother and baby were exhausted. Quite often there was a need for respiratory support with oxygen. But my C-section rate had fallen to 5 percent.

Next, I used visualisation and guided imagery with patients to manage pain. On occasion, I still had to use narcotics and a rare epidural. I continued to see exhausted babies who were not fully able to bond. I still had a C-section rate of 5 percent.

Eventually, I began using hypnosis to manage pain during birth. The results were okay. Babies were less often compromised and very rarely needed oxygen; but mothers still experienced painful births. My C-section rate remained at 5 percent.

A few years ago, I made the transition to HypnoBirthing, and I now truly believe that normal birthing does not have to involve pain. I have attended over 200 births of women who prepared for birth by learning and using the techniques and philosophy of HypnoBirthing—"The Mongan Method." All of the families have left their birthings excited about the birth event. I see support people meaningfully involved with the mother and assisting in many different ways. I have had no complications. No babies have needed oxygen or any support other than warming by mother's body. My C-section count is three—in as many years. I have given absolutely no analgesic drugs since I began using HypnoBirthing with mothers.

Over the years, I have come to realise that during a birthing, I no longer perform "deliveries"; I attend and observe as mothers birth their babies in calm and comfort, and birthing companions receive the babies as they emerge. It is as if my new role is to be present to witness the miracle of HypnoBirthing.

Now I enthusiastically lecture to medical groups on a regular basis about the merits of HypnoBirthing as a means of achieving easier, more comfortable births for labouring mothers. I am more than happy to talk to health-care professionals (or anyone else) about my experiences with truly natural birthing. I have a large number of happy HypnoBirthing families—mothers and fathers—who love to talk about their own birthing experiences.

In my position as a faculty member of the Atlanta Family Medicine Residency Program in Atlanta, Georgia, I trained medical residents to use HypnoBirthing as an option for the families they will serve.

I heartily recommend this book, and the well-thought-out program that it accompanies, for its contribution toward making the birth of our children a positive and gentle step on the way to a better world.

Lorne R. Campbell, Sr., M.D.
Clinical Professor, Family Medicine

Looking Back Over 25 Years

When the publisher of the third edition of our HypnoBirthing textbook invited me to write a revision of the book for our 25th anniversary, it opened up a flood of memories and thoughts about the journey that has brought HypnoBirthing to where it is today. Mongan Method HypnoBirthing is the leader and most comprehensive natural and instinctive birth education programme that exists. It has, from the very beginning, reached beyond simple relaxation and introduced many advanced hypnosis techniques into the birthing classroom. The coincidence of this being our 25th anniversary year called back thoughts of experiences that bubbled over in my mind and could not be quieted. Where have we been and where have we gone in a whole quarter century?

At this time 25 years ago, Maura, my daughter for whom the programme was developed, had just given birth to our grandbaby Kyle. The other two women who also prepared for their births with HypnoBirthing were due to birth at any moment. The success of Maura's birthing had the hospital staff talking about that woman in Room 201, who had no epidural, had soft music playing, and the room dimmed all through her labour. One of the nurses on duty that day, Pat, who was also pregnant, made it a point to step into Maura's room quite regularly. Each time she just stood by the door with a quizzical look on her face and stared at Maura. On one visit, she spoke, "And she hasn't had anything for pain? Really?"

I remember leaving the room briefly to get a tuna fish sandwich (usually a poor choice with a birthing mother); and when I returned, I found a midwife on her knees writing the name of the artist on the tape that was in the tape player that I had placed obscurely on the floor behind a chair.

When Maura's birth was complete, Nurse Pat came back into the room and asked for an appointment with me. As she left, she told the other nurses, "Hey, girls, this is the way I'm having my baby." My excitement doubled.

I went home that afternoon, and with my notes taken during Maura's pregnancy and her birth, I began to set down the philosophy of birth that had been waiting all these many years since I was a child. One by one, I started to expand on the chapters of the coil-bound book I had prepared for my first three pioneer mums. I knew that I needed to put these feelings and observations down so that they could be shared with others. Writing that book was the easiest thing I've ever done. My enthusiasm was at peak, and my mind just wouldn't shut down for anything.

With the other two births happening on the heels of the first, and followed by Nurse Pat's birth, HypnoBirthing became a buzzword in that hospital. Soon a number of curious hypnotherapists, who heard about what was happening in Concord, New Hampshire, called to ask, "Will you teach me what you taught Maura about birthing with hypnosis?" In no time, there were a number of hypnotherapists meeting with eager couples. The National Guild of Hypnotists invited me to present the programme at their annual educational convention, and then we were on our way. Simply by word of mouth, we had HypnoBirthings occurring all over the country.

A Paradigm Shift Began

There we were. I began to receive so many calls that I started to teach classes. Pregnant mothers and their birth companions filled the parent classes, and hypnotherapists, nurses, and doulas came to become practitioners.

I had no idea of how urgently pregnant women were craving a better way to birth than the standard births that were offered by hospitals. They were hungry for a programme that would allow them to forego anaesthesia, but at the same time, make it possible for them to birth gently and in comfort. Since most hospital personnel themselves did not believe that birth could be free of fear and pain, there was only the home birth route, which also bore the burden of lack of public recognition and a lot of misinformation.

I found out quickly when NBC's TV show *Dateline* presented a full-hour feature on birthing with hypnosis. At the end of the show, hundreds of people called or wrote to producers to tell them that they had neglected to tell the public that the programme is HypnoBirthing. The following morning there was a front-page article on the MSNBC website about HypnoBirthing, stating that it was I who founded the programme. They gave a link directly to our HypnoBirthing website. Without a bit of exaggeration, I can honestly say that we received almost 5,000 calls and emails over the next few weeks.

HypnoBirthing took on a life of its own, and in a very short time, it took over my life as well. All of a sudden we needed staff to be able to give referrals from a referral system we didn't even have as yet. We needed a second telephone and another person to receive the calls. We stepped beyond the realm of a passion and into the realm of business. A business we hadn't planned for.

It looked as though the change in the way birth was viewed by the general public, and care providers as well, would come easily. With the impetus of that NBC show behind us, we saw a large number of pregnant families flocking to our classes. It became increasingly obvious, however, that not many care providers were impressed.

When I first started teaching and accompanying birthing families into the hospital those many years ago, I remember naively thinking that surely doctors and midwives would be pulling me out of birthing rooms to inquire how they could replicate those beautiful scenes. I was sure that once they witnessed a few HypnoBirthing mothers breathing their babies down to crowning in deep relaxation, they would insist on having all of their mums know how to achieve this phenomenon. I waited. The nurses were enthusiastic, and several midwives joined our ranks. Doctors regularly commented on how "remarkable" the births were, but except for a few, they showed no curiosity as to how these results were achieved. Even though they saw it happening time and time again, they seemed to dismiss the birthings as flukes.

In looking back now, I must admit—the acceptance of HypnoBirthing didn't come the way I thought it would. It was a very steep uphill climb. A few times a doctor would inquire, "What did you say this is?" Many saw, and frequently complimented, the birth mother on her beautiful labour. Most had no questions, however, and were not interested in knowing how more of the mothers they were caring for could birth in this way.

They quickly dismissed what they had just proclaimed "really remarkable." They were content to move on to the next room and suggest a membranes rupture or even a Pitocin drip if the mother was not progressing in line with the Friedman Curve. Pitocin was usually the order of the day if the doctor's shift was to end in a few hours. So often a beautiful calm birthing was given over to manipulation, with little thought to the dramatic change in the mother's comfort level.

Once in a while, a doctor would ask me how I could prove that what we teach in HypnoBirthing classes resulted in what we were seeing. I was always amused by that question. It reminded me of the trial scene from the movie *Chicago*, when the defence attorney is asked for evidence of something he had just brilliantly illustrated. The defence attorney replied, "And what is it that you are seeing that you need evidence of?"

Though our success didn't happen overnight, as I reflect on those years, I realise that we gradually made some significant changes just from our requests. In the hospital in Concord, New Hampshire, where HypnoBirthing first "caught on," as a mother was settling into her birthing room, her nurse would pull a chair over to the side of the bed and ask to spend a few minutes with the family so that, ". . . I can be sure that I understand exactly what you mean by some of your birth preferences."

Over time, we would find that there was already a birth ball in the room, and the nurse would remind the mother to ask when she was ready to use the tub. Someone cared enough to assure the mother that she was welcome and her requests would be honoured as far as possible. The nurses' overt support made up for the oblivion of some of the other care providers. Eventually, there were some doctors who displayed approval, but they were closet enthusiasts.

Soon I began to receive invitations from places all over the world to bring certification workshops to their countries. Canada was the first, but not far behind were the Virgin Islands, the UK, and Australia, and on and on. Over the years we have had the pleasure of training some of the finest people in the world—our teaching practitioners, without whom HypnoBirthing may have remained simply the talk of the Concord Hospital staff for a few short days; and then it would have just faded away. Those who shared our belief gravitated to our programme. It was they who truly catapulted HypnoBirthing to the position it holds today as the leader in the field of childbirth education with hypnosis.

Prior to that time, the midwives who were teaching instinctive birthing had no instructional programme or key techniques to build upon. Many of these women came in droves, as did many nurses who were discouraged with what they were seeing happening in hospitals. Nancy Wainer, midwife extraordinaire and author of two books on natural birthing, joined our ranks and declared, "HypnoBirthing is the missing link we have all been seeking for years." With so many birth advocates sharing the same vision, HypnoBirthing grew. It became exemplary of what gentle birth should look like and what it should feel like for the birthing mother and baby. In addition to seeing what HypnoBirthing could do for the families, these birth professionals also realised how it brought more ease and joy to their own work. Nurses who saw instinctive birthing and worked with HypnoBirthing families were instrumental in bringing HypnoBirthing to their hospitals' education programmes.

It was a good fit, in spite of those who found it difficult to believe that a baby could descend and emerge without his mother scrunching up her body, holding her breath, and forcefully pushing her baby out with all her might. Even now, a whole quarter of a century later, there are people who still subscribe to "purple pushing." It's what is portrayed in movies and on television. The general public watches and accepts, and pregnant mothers cringe.

For a long time some birthing professionals tenaciously clung to almost gymnastic-like moves that had the mum pulling on a rolled sheet or hanging over a squat bar for endless periods of time. Some facilities had women hanging upright from a huge knot in a rope "to use the benefit of gravity." Eventually that all went by the wayside with only a few continuing to preach the inevitability of severe pain. Those few sometimes even felt the need to advise the birthing mother that HypnoBirthing may work at the beginning, but not later when the pain is more severe. They were oblivious to the fact that every word they spoke instilled more fear into the minds of vulnerable mothers.

The many positive features and benefits of this shift in birthing paradigm continued to draw the attention of health-care providers. We began to see more standard health-care providers supporting HypnoBirthing families with relaxed protocols and fewer unnecessary "precautions" being applied to women who are free of special circumstances.

The light shining upon HypnoBirthing became broader and brighter. Major television morning shows and leading publications printed feature articles. Local TV channels featured our birth stories on their evening news shows. Consumers were asking about natural, instinctive birthing. It was catching on among birthing parents.

Others came and trained, and intentionally copied, and imitated. They took our concept, our materials, and our trade name; and they started their own HypnoBirthing programmes. We knew then that we had a good thing, and that good thing continued to grow.

In so many places, over the years, we saw a sizeable shift away from traditional "standard" hospital birth scenes that had women tethered with epidurals, needles, IV poles, tubes, wires, and belts. These confining and frightening scenes began to be replaced with scenes of quiet and calm women, who were free to move about or just relax. The only wires that were anywhere near were those of the earphones that mothers used to listen to soothing birthing music and scripts. In some places, women requesting calm birth were no longer restricted from eating. Care providers came to see and recognise that when endorphins are present and the constrictor hormone catecholamine is not, digestion is not arrested because the mother's body is not in the state of alarm.

HypnoBirthing gained more attention. Requests for speaking engagements and interviews poured in, along with invitations to conduct training workshops for practitioners. The HypnoBirthing way of birth was catching on.

Working on this book revision has made me realise how successful natural birth advocates have been in bringing about substantial improvements in the birthing experiences of thousands of happy birthing families, most of whom chose HypnoBirthing to prepare for their babies' births. The concept of instinctive birth also attracted the attention of some of the kindest and most caring birth professionals, nurses, doctors, and midwives who were at first curious but are today more willing to openly support instinctive birth.

When we look at trends in birthing over the past two-plus decades, we see that, truly, new life and birth are celebrated in many mainstream health-care facilities, as well as in complementary settings. This shift also points to a vast increase in the number of birth centres that have opened their doors to couples seeking natural birth but wanting a homelike atmosphere. Home births are regularly considered an option by families of all kinds of life styles—from several Hollywood movie stars and well-known entertainers and sports celebrities to families in small towns and farmlands. Many hospitals are accommodating families who are seeking an environment where they can birth naturally yet have the comfort of medical staff on hand.

Throughout the world, birth is seen as the important transformational human experience that it is. It is far more than the "process" of getting baby born and just moving on. It is recognised and celebrated in various ways. I'm told there is a large hospital in Southern California that has an entire fourth floor devoted to ABC—"A Better Childbirth."

I visited a hospital outside of Detroit that has furnished their natural birth rooms with queen beds and a homelike atmosphere with soft light and soft music—no frightening apparatus visible.

In a hospital in Minnesota, the carpeting leading into the birthing centre has inlaid appliques of dragonflies, bees, lily pads, frogs, and flowers. The rooms look like five-star hotel rooms, and there is not a visible piece of equipment in the room that shouts "Be warned!" and "Be afraid!!" I asked where some of the usual machinery and equipment is. I was told, "Right around the corner, concealed, where it belongs unless we need it, when it takes only a couple of seconds to get it." Outside is a lovely walking path lined with flowers (in the summer) and benches for couples who want to spend some of their labour time outdoors in nature. (The surgical unit has a similar "healing garden.") When a baby is born in this hospital, strains of Brahms' Lullaby filters through the sound system, and patients and visitors alike honour the new life that has just come into the world.

I once attended a birth with a mother who was the first HypnoBirthing mother at that hospital. I met a doctor by the name of Dr. Care. When he left the room, I commented to the nurse, "What a fantastic name for a person who attends births." Shortly after a young doctor walked in and the nurse said to him, "When Dr. Care was here, Mrs. Mongan commented that she thought the name Care was a perfect name for an obstetrician." The doctor extended his hand and said, "I'm happy to see my first HypnoBirthing. By the way, my name is Dr. Luti, and in Italian it means 'care.'" We all laughed. After the baby was born, the mother was told that the nurse had to take the baby away to put the bands on. The doctor looked up and said, "Bring the bands to the baby." And the mother continued to hold her newborn baby in her arms. I am sure you can guess that this mother's birth story was a beautiful one. That is all it took to start a new trend in that hospital.

Fifteen years ago, I was invited to bring the first HypnoBirthing Certification Workshop to London to train practitioners. I taught the class at St. Thomas Hospital, Florence Nightingale's hospital. This gave me the opportunity to observe and learn much about the midwifery model—an extremely mother-baby friendly model of birthing. What I saw was a birth model that is strikingly different from what I was accustomed to in the States. I liked what I saw; and I learned a great deal about this exemplary birth model that is among the most common of approaches to maternity care in the world. And a trend was begun at the hospital.

With the help of a few midwives who became HypnoBirthing practitioners early on, we were able to blend the two philosophies into the book that is now used by practitioners in the UK. The birthing unit at St. Thomas is staffed by a group of midwives whose enthusiasm for natural birth matches their gentle and friendly manner.

In a hospital in New Hampshire where a large number of Hypno-Birthing families choose to birth, the family is treated to a beautiful dinner delivered to their room on a dinner cart as elegant as one would find with room service in an upscale hotel. This hospital also has tubs in a separate room. Post-partum rooms are furnished with a trundle bed for a sibling and a queen bed for the new parents. Their infant not only rooms in, but sleeps with his parents in a family bed with a special little bed frame for the baby to safely sleep.

For healthy mothers who present minimal risk, routine practices, protocols, and procedures are being relaxed. As more couples are requesting natural birthing, more hospitals are feeding their mums.

In some places where low-risk mothers are active and mobile, they have shed the dull, ill-fitting patient gowns for attractive labour gowns for this special event. The gown is especially designed to be hospital friendly, with a halter top that ties or snaps at the back of the neck for ease of breastfeeding and strategically placed openings in the front of the gown to allow for easy access when checking baby's well-being or for birth. These facilities are but a few of the places where the shift is taking place. There are many more, and more will follow. As parents begin to make their wishes known and are willing to seek out the right environment and the right birth professionals, they are able to achieve the kind of birth that leaves them feeling fulfilled and joyful.

These hospitals are only a few of the medical facilities where the shift has taken place; and birthing families are treated as if they and their births matter. There are many more where staff has seen gentle births, and they are welcoming parents wishing this birth style. Hospitals are adjusting, and it is clear that their services are not only for the birthing families whose pregnancies are at risk. There is much hope for those parents who want natural birth but also feel more comfortable in a hospital environment.

An Opposite Paradigm Shift Appears

During these same years while natural birth advocates were basking in the growing success of an increased awareness of natural instinctive birth, a second paradigm from within the medical community appeared to be going unequivocally in a direction that is opposite from calm, gentle birthing.

This shift supports an increasing number of inductions, often scheduled ahead of the estimated delivery date (EDD) for nothing more than the chronology of the matter. Many women are being told, not advised or given a suggestion, that if they have not gone into labour before their estimated date, they will be induced on that date. This is all in spite of the fact that the EDD is just that—an estimated date. Statistics show that first-time mums average 41.3 weeks of gestation. There is little or no room within this shift for consideration of a normal, natural birth. This model feeds on suspicions and fear of "impending danger." Very early on mothers are being told of some possible danger and advised that they should expect an early induction or a C-section. Parental wishes, emotions, and expectations are swept under the rug in favour of chemical, chronological, and technological factors.

In recent years, we are hearing of exceptionally large numbers of women who are suspected of having "dangerous complications." These possible complications will necessitate regimented and strict protocols. Labour usually will call for frequent interruptions and examinations. Overuse of technology and apparatus make it almost impossible to experience normal birth. The natural rhythm and flow of labour is destroyed, and, as a result, labour can often go awry, along with the parent's dream and excitement. There seems to be a disregard for the relevance of parental input. Advocates of this shift appear to have a disregard for the sanctity of birth and do not view birth as one of the most important of our human life rituals.

These unnecessary distractions that are part of this other birth paradigm are puzzling and quite discouraging to natural birth advocates.

Their existence speaks volumes about the need to move away from the one-size-fits-all approach to birthing. It points out a screaming need for birth professionals to take a good look at the people they serve. In this way, they can begin to see and to meet birthing mothers as whole people who are experiencing a once-in-a-lifetime family event that is unlike any other. Birth touches the emotions, the spirit, and the psyche of all involved. It calls for birth professionals who are kind, caring, and sensitive. One doctor in California describes the ideal birth attendant as one who loves babies, loves birthing women, and loves birth.

As we approach the end of this first 25-year period, it becomes clear that birthing parents who choose to learn and become prepared to experience a relaxed, natural birth must become informed about the philosophy of their intended care provider. They also need to be prepared as to what is routine and "standard protocol" for the facility in which they intend to birth. The time to make these decisions is before the birthing day, not when you are in labour.

My focus for the past quarter century has been to bring relaxed natural birthing to the attention of birth professionals. I hoped that they would see and understand that all birth need not be approached with fearful anticipation and preparation, for sudden complication.

I am now placing my hopes on the most relevant players in this transformational and human experience—the birthing families.

Most parents hear only of "standard care" or "routine protocol or practice." These two phrases do not always mean that what the birthing mother will experience is only evidence-based treatment or that it is the best path to take. In their innocence and lack of information, parents approach their births with resigned submission. It's not that they don't care; it's that they don't know what they don't know.

Today I am optimistic that there will be a full shift in the direction of natural birthing that will show more sensitivity to the simple needs of the low-risk and no-risk majority of mothers who need little "standard" or "routine" care. I feel, though, that I will not see that happen in my lifetime.

I'm convinced now that this awakening has to occur first within the mind-set of the consumer families. They are not asking for more, or for special, treatment. They are asking for less. Parents are simply asking that if everything gives reasonable indication of normality, they be given the opportunity to birth calmly and gently as Nature intended, without drugs and other procedures intended to "give labour a jump-start" or "move it along."

It is they who are most transformed. It is they who must step up and accept the importance of educating themselves and actively seeking the birth professionals who will respect their work.

Hopefully, we will soon see that parents do not need to ask the same questions that families have been asking for the last 25 years. They won't feel the need to make a case for gentle treatment and kinder birthings. With education, they will recognise that they have the power to find and choose the care provider and the birthing environment that will make the difference in their lives and the lives of their babies.

The First HypnoBirthing Story

When I looked into my baby's eyes
for the first time, I knew at that moment
what real love actually is.

MAURA GEDDES

I left home at about 5:30 that January morning in 1990. As I slipped into my car, I felt the shock of the cold leather seats. The air was exceptionally cold and crisp, even for an early January morning in Concord, New Hampshire. Ordinarily, I would never venture out at that time of the morning in the peak of winter; but this was a very special day and time.

I knew there was no real rush, but I found myself hurrying out of my driveway and out onto the road to the city. The main road was deserted and dark, and it was mine for the taking. I was eager to reach Maura's house to learn how she was feeling, and to help her gather her things to bring to the hospital.

The city was quiet, but the still-prevalent holiday lights added to my excitement and feeling of celebration. This was the day that we had all been waiting nine long months for. It was finally here. The first HypnoBirthing baby was soon to arrive.

Just before I reached Maura's house, I had to slow down as I caught sight of a police cruiser neatly tucked away, with lights off, at the entrance of a local cemetery. I slowly drove past him, smiled, and rehearsed what I would say when he pulled me over on our way to the hospital after I had picked Maura up. I fully planned to fly past him and get his attention. I chuckled, picturing the drama of our arriving at the hospital with a police escort. Not! The cruiser was gone when we made that return trip around 7:30. Even in a perfectly scripted scene, I couldn't interject that drama into our first HypnoBirthing.

When I arrived at Maura's house, I found a perfectly relaxed woman, who had an obvious "ready-to-go" air about her. I was both pleased and relieved to see that she was in a light mood, smiling and conversant. We talked as she moved about, tidying and checking her house before we left. I saw no indication of fright or nervousness.

There were two friends who had also studied HypnoBirthing at the same time that Maura did. All three were expecting their babies around the same time, and I prayed that Maura would be the first to birth. I so wanted my grandbaby to be the first HypnoBirthing baby. I wondered how each of these three trusting pioneers would meet the start of labour. I also wondered how the hospital staff would meet their determination to have their babies naturally. Maura was the epitome of calm, and I knew that she was prepared. I was encouraged that the other two "first HypnoBirthers" would experience that same confidence.

When we arrived at the hospital, Maura was brought directly to triage and then admitted, even though the attending nurse found her to be in less than what is considered "active labour." Maura assured the nurse that she was experiencing regular surges. It was only then that Maura was told that her midwife was not available and that she would be attended by a midwife whom she didn't know. Once more I wondered how she would handle that bit of information. True to a very important affirmation in HypnoBirthing—"I will accept whatever turn my birthing takes"—the news did not stress or upset her.

She remained at that same level of opening for almost four hours. I know now that this is not uncommon for HypnoBirthing mums. Their labours very often do not conform to routine numbers on progress charts. Their bodies labour, but there is little change in their appearance. It is also not uncommon for them to very suddenly register a greater degree of opening in a much shorter time. Concerned that her labour was not progressing sufficiently to match the prescribed expectation, at about 10:30 in the morning her nurse suggested that she ". . . get up and get those muscles moving. It will speed up your labour." Maura was helped into a suggested squatting position, but with no preparation for squatting, she decided very quickly that she didn't care for the squat. She then began to walk, but got as far as the door, and said, "No thank you. I need to go back to relaxing now." She was tuned into her body and realised that the pace of her labour was stepping up. She needed to relax into her birthing body as she experienced active labour.

We heard little from Maura from that point on, except after she had listened to a woman in the next room scream steadily for a couple hours and beg for help from above. Maura opened her eyes and looked at me and asked, "Am I going to get to that stage?" The nurse answered, "Heavens no. You are way beyond that stage." Things were good.

Shortly after 1:00 P.M., Maura was completely opened and was advised to begin to forcefully push, while her midwife strenuously "stretched" her perineum, sometimes with both hands. Maura was obviously in pain through this episode, and called out to me to have the midwife stop tugging with her fingers. The midwife continued; and after some time, she performed an extensive episiotomy, saying, "This will help the baby come out faster." Thankfully, an episiotomy is seldom performed in most hospitals today. Birth attendants have learned that the folds of the perineum open by themselves and that the majority of cases call for patience to allow the natural expulsive reflex to move the baby down to crowning.

At 3:30 P.M. that afternoon, Kyle Patrick Geddes, the first Hypno-Birthing baby, was born. We were ecstatic. HypnoBirthing Baby #1 had arrived. We had no idea that there would be thousands—and even hundreds of thousands—to follow or that we would have representation in over 48 countries around the world. What a landmark day. We were simply happy in the knowledge that babies can come into the world with kindness, gentility, and respect for both mother and baby. Birth is, indeed, the greatest Celebration of Life.

We had gone full circle—from Maura, the first intended natural-birth baby in that county, to Kyle, the first HypnoBirthing baby. I can't even begin to express how moving this experience was for me.

Maura, without realising it at the time, had blazed a trail; and she did it without having the encouragement of many mothers before her who birthed naturally. Additionally, while her regular midwife encouraged her to have a natural birth, when it came time for her birthing, her midwife of choice was not there. I believe that on some deeper level Maura remembered her own birth and that allowed her to trust that her body, and her baby knew how to birth instinctively. The trail this woman blazed continues to widen today, for her foot-steps have been followed by so many happy HypnoBirthing mums, who wanted gentle birthing but lacked a programme that would give them that choice.

We know that this is not the story of the first natural birth, nor was it the only natural birth. Women have been birthing naturally for centuries, but this was the first HypnoBirthing at a pivotal time. It proved that relaxed birthing that is free of stress and fear for all involved can be achieved routinely if the birthing mother is properly prepared and genuinely supported by her caring providers. It was significant at this time because some of the practices of Active Management of Labour, already with a foothold in other countries, were creeping into American births almost without notice. Hospital births were far from natural. Women who birthed in hospitals routinely expected to be medicated. In their apprehension, they demanded it. Today, we simply ask, is it not possible to acquiesce to the requests of the women who want less or none as it is to the women who demand more?

I chose to include this story not because it is the birth story of my daughter and grandbaby, but because it is a happy, positive birth story, and birth stories are important. Whether a birth story is a happy birth story or a not-so-happy birth story, it reveals the importance of parents taking the responsibility for knowing how they want to experience the arrival of their babies, whether their birthing takes place in a hospital, a birthing centre, or in a home.

This first HypnoBirthing mother, without the advantage of having watched many natural births on the Internet and in films and without the benefit of many happy birth stories, knew she wanted things to go differently; and they did. If this could happen for her, most certainly with the education, preparation, and choices that are available to you today, it could easily happen for you.

A Russian Mother's Comments
about HypnoBirthing

*I recall it now, and I would say my
son's birth is one of the best moments in my life.
My doctor was shocked. She said she had never seen
anyone being so calm and relaxed during the labour.
My HypnoBirthing experience made me realise how wrong
our childhood attitudes are toward birth.*

Anastasia Ivanova, Moscow, Russia

Mongan Method of HypnoBirthing—Its Roots

I think I always knew and believed that birthing should be simple, instinctive, and even joyful for mothers, babies, and birth partners. I think I came here with that knowing, because from a very early age, I held a fascination for babies. I thought that babies should come onto this earth plane gently—in keeping with the beings that they are. I had heard people speak of babies as gifts from heaven, and I was thoroughly convinced that meant that babies are angels. Everywhere I looked; there was proof of it: Greeting cards at Christmas, pictures at church, comments from adults referring to a baby as "a little angel." For me, it all led to the same conclusion. Babies are angels.

As soon as I was old enough to make my wishes known to Santa, I asked for a "real baby doll." My pleas were heard, because I did receive a baby doll that was so nearly real that she could drink water and then expel the liquid instantly onto her diaper and her blankets. She was a little small, but so was I.

The following year when all my neighbourhood friends were asking for Shirley Temple dolls, I again asked for a baby doll; but this time I wanted a doll that was the size of a real baby. Once more, my wish came true; and I found a life-sized baby doll under the Christmas tree.

I didn't put her aside for weeks—her eyes closed when I laid her down, and they opened when I picked her up. She was perfect.

I wasn't much older when Mrs. Burrell, our next-door neighbor, brought her newly born baby home from the hospital. She very kindly tolerated my curiosity and let me spend time at her house just watching the baby sleep and watching Mrs. Burrell bathe her and care for her. The baby affirmed my belief. She looked exactly like the angels I had seen pictures of. I didn't even notice that she didn't have wings.

I was still very young—almost five—when I first heard a birth story. My mother and a group of her friends used to gather regularly at one home or another in the neighbourhood. They often brought their babies with them. I used to hide just outside the living room door when they met at our house. I would sit quietly and listen because sooner or later—mostly sooner—their conversation would focus on their babies.

One day one of the women talked about what she had experienced when she "delivered" her second baby. As I listened, I know that my jaw must have dropped to my chest. Everything that she was saying was not at all how I had pictured angels being born.

Her story was terrible. The entire story was punctuated with the words, "danger," "afraid," and "miserable." She told of her journey by ship from New York to California by way of the Panama Canal, just weeks before she was due to have her baby. She was afraid of water, but taking the longer boat trip was cheaper than going by train across the country. She was violently seasick from the very beginning of the trip, and it continued throughout the journey. Her doctor on the ship was afraid that her baby would not be able to tolerate the constant retching, and he was afraid that she would be thrown into labour prematurely. She was dangerously dehydrated and was experiencing terrible cramping. He was not at all encouraging about the danger she and her baby were facing if it continued.

When she arrived in California, she was taken to the hospital, "just in the nick of time." She continued to describe her labour that followed. This part of her story was even more frightening than what she had previously been telling the group.

She spoke of a long, hard, and horribly painful labour that led to foetal distress. The situation finally required forceps to pull the baby down through the birth canal. When she awakened from anaesthesia, she was informed that her baby had damaged her pelvic region so badly that it was unlikely that she would ever be able to have more children.

I couldn't believe what I was hearing. I felt sick. I asked myself why she would say those things. Angels are not born that way. God would never have let that happen. I ran to my room in tears.

I cried many more times over that story, and it wasn't the last time I was to hear it, because the woman who told the story was my mother, and I was the baby who damaged her body so badly.

I felt a tremendous guilt throughout my growing up years. My guilt eventually turned into resentment every time I heard the story. I hated the thought of it. It was all so wrong.

As I grew older, I began to really listen and hear the repeated messages of what I looked upon as the "war stories." Birth is scary and dangerous. The more I heard, the more I sensed that I was growing up in a family and a society of women whose thoughts were very much occupied with the trials of being a woman and the perils of giving birth. It almost seemed that every woman who had experienced birth felt somehow compelled and delighted to tell her birth story, and it was always bad and filled with anguish.

I remember very clearly the day my sister had her first menstrual period. It was as though my younger aunts were welcoming her into a sorority of female victims. They told me, "Your sister is a woman now. She has 'the curse.'" I really didn't know what they meant by "the curse," but I quickly caught on that being a woman and having "the curse" was a free pass to spending at least one day a month languishing emotionally and physically and being excused from any chores that were strenuous. This curse wasn't all that bad, I thought.

It would have been very easy for me, as a child, to get pulled into this abyss of victimisation—to succumb to the fear-filled discussion and become so fearful of birthing that I may have chosen to avoid birthing all together, as many women have done for many years. Or, I may have chosen to seek a surgical birth out of fear and a lack of good information.

I honestly think that my mother's birth story made me the strong advocate for instinctive and natural birthing that I am today. Instead of developing a fear of birth, I searched and developed a philosophy of birth. Her story served as a catalyst for me. It challenged me later to reflect on what I had been feeling all those years and ultimately to seek a more balanced, natural, reasonable, and logical view of birth.

In talking with birth advocates in recent years, I find that I am not alone in having been led to natural birthing because of a friend or family member who for years repeatedly told a horrific birth story to anyone who would listen. Others said that they, too, chose to become involved in natural birthing because of these kinds of stories and felt the need to try to change the view of birth for that same reason.

The real tipping point came when I was in high school. Our English class was assigned to write a research paper. This provided me with an immediate and high incentive to really dig into books on birth and to find what I was looking for. I chose as my topic "Achieving Safe and Gentle Childbirth." I thought it would be easy. I was so wrong.

I found mostly thick medical textbooks, so heavy that I could hardly carry more than one at a time. These books were also heavily laden with the discussion of dangers, risks, abnormalities, and cautions that doctors in training would likely encounter in their practices. In spite of the fact that only a small percentage of women presented with these abnormalities, especially back then, the books I found were solely devoted to "what ifs" and subsequent procedures to remediate the problems.

There is no arguing the point that this training and knowledge is essential and that these well-honed skills and techniques have saved the lives of many women and babies over the years. However, I was struck by the absence of discussion on normal birth. I was also amused when I read an interesting caution in one of the leading medical texts of the time. The book suggested that the physician should exercise caution when working with the educated, sophisticated woman who may harbour a notion that she knows how to bring a baby into the world. There it was—in print—an identified enemy of birth, rather than the giver of birth.

I felt that the absence of discussion on natural/normal birth left a serious void in obstetric education and could, over time, have influenced the manner in which some doctors interact with their birthing families. From everything I could find, I came away with the feeling that the people writing the books considered only the human body and not the emotional and spiritual human elements that accompany the person they will be working with, probably more intimately than any person other than a mate. There was no mention of the privilege doctors enjoy in being invited to assist at one of the most transformational events in a woman's lifetime.

It was, indeed, straight forward, didactic discourse with an obvious breach between the psyche and the soma. These writings shed light on a possible reason for why such a large number of doctors, even today, may seem so uncomfortable with requests for their support of families who present low-risk or no-risk, when the parents are looking for natural birth in a hospital setting.

Years later when I was living in Arizona, I was invited on three occasions to speak about HypnoBirthing before the OB/GYN club of a medical school. Each time, I asked the students, who were about to graduate in a few weeks, how many of them had witnessed a natural birth. I explained "natural" as opposed to "normal." Not one hand was raised. I explained further, and still not a single hand was raised. This, too, may explain why so many doctors are reluctant to give their support to natural birth. It's uncharted territory to them.

The most significant piece of writing that I stumbled upon came, not in the form of a medical text, but within the pages of an issue of *Life Magazine*. This particular issue came onto newsstands on January 30, 1950, the very time that I was gathering notes for my paper.

On the cover was a young mother holding her newborn baby. She was radiant and had a soft smile of satisfaction on her face. The title on the cover read, "Childbirth without Fear." Inside it read, "A Young Mother Gives Birth to Her Baby with No Fear, Little Pain."

It told of a programme at Grace New Haven Hospital in Connecticut that was adopting the theories of Grantly Dick-Read, an English obstetrician, who staunchly fought for acceptance and recognition of the proven fact that there is no need for severe, lingering pain in normal, uncomplicated birthing. That magazine and the Dick-Read book that I subsequently bought changed my life.

I knew I had found the "Grail." The book was quite philosophical, though not largely instructional or even methodical. I was ecstatic that I had finally found something that was in line with all the thoughts I had been clinging to for years. It even explained *why* it is that there doesn't need to be pain in birthing in the absence of special circumstances. It was so simple and so scientifically logical—the Fight or Flight response within the Autonomic System. The logic was "hiding in plain sight." It showed me once more that normal birthing is more a philosophy and a belief than it is a technique or a method.

As I read *Childbirth Without Fear*, I was amazed to learn that Dick-Read had been putting these theories forward before medical boards and medical associations since the late 1920s and the early '30s. I found it hard to believe that he was silenced and grossly ridiculed. One paper after another that he forwarded was arbitrarily dismissed, without being read. When he persisted, his medical license was threatened.

Years later when I first became pregnant, I turned to that book and practically memorised every word. The main premise of the theory is that when the body is relaxed, the firing of neuropeptides in the brain are slowed, and, therefore, pain is lessened and often non-existent. The stress-free body is then able to function as it was created to function—without the self-defeating tension that can cause birthing muscles to shut down.

I fully accepted that fear is the enemy of the birthing room. I knew little of hypnosis at that time, and I didn't realise that self-hypnosis was what I was learning. I absorbed the logic like a sponge and relaxed daily. Soon I could bring myself into a deepened relaxed state within seconds. I faithfully carved out a portion of my life to relax every day. My body was so in sync with the whole idea. There was not a doubt in my mind.

I talked with my doctor and explained that I would be having the baby naturally. One must remember that this was at a time when all women were systematically anaesthetised during the birthing phase, and their babies were pulled out with forceps.

He smiled and agreed that he saw no harm in that. I truly don't think that he believed I was serious. Not being aware of how I was preparing for my birth, I think he merely humored me.

I laboured for a little under two hours in absolutely pain-free labour. My baby's descent was hardly noticeable to anyone but me—I did nothing to alert staff that my baby was moving to crowning. The baby easily moved down and crowned. I informed the staff that I was crowning, and then there was chaos. The doctor was not there. I was quickly transferred to a trolley and whisked down the hall to the delivery room. My legs were held together, and I was told to pant so that the baby wouldn't come out. The doctor still was not there.

In spite of my protestations that I wasn't supposed to have anaesthesia, my legs were strapped four feet into the air onto what looked like a series of rain gutters. My wrists were held with leather straps at the side of the table, my head was held, and the ether cone was forced onto my face. That was the last thing I remembered.

When I came out of anaesthesia, I was dreadfully sick and was told that I would see my baby in the morning, but I was not to mind the bruises on the side of his head from the forceps. I was upset, but said nothing to my doctor. I knew that I had had my natural labour, but felt cheated out of my completely natural birth. Just a couple more surges would have done it, but it would have to wait until "the next time."

The birth of my second son went the same sad way for all the same reasons. The labour was a little shorter and beautiful. But, once again, even though I reminded him of my intention for a natural birth, my doctor was not there; and he left no instructions for the nurses. They refused to allow me to simply let my baby be born. So as before, I awakened to an upset stomach and was sick most of the night. Again

I was told that I had a son and would be able to see him and hold him in the morning. I vowed, "Never again!"

When I became pregnant the third time, I promptly greeted my doctor on my first office visit with, "Dr. Massey, we've got to talk."

He looked at me and asked, "What do we have to talk about, Mickey? This is your third pregnancy. You know how it's done."

I smiled back and said, "Yes, but you don't. Twice you assured me that I could have my natural birth, and twice, I never saw you. I felt betrayed and let down. My babies were almost born when I was forced to take anaesthesia. I need to know that I can trust you to be there; to support me. If you don't feel comfortable doing that, I understand, but I'm going to have to walk." He repeated, "Walk?"

I continued, "I'll have to go somewhere else to find a doctor who will support me in this. I've lost two opportunities to have my natural birth, and I don't want to take a chance on losing another."

He paused for a moment, picked up his pen and began to write. He wrote down and recited all the things I had asked for. When he finished, he said, "There! Are you happy now?"

I spoke very quickly, and through a smile said, "I'm not finished. I also want my husband by my side in the labour room and the delivery room." To understand how outlandish this request was, you have to realise that in the late fifties, husbands were not allowed beyond the lobby of most hospitals. Most were sent home to wait for the call that would tell them, "It's all over."

He threw his pen down and said, "Oh, come on. You can't ask me to stick my neck out that far."

I again smiled and repeated. "I'm not asking you to go out on a limb. If you don't feel comfortable with this, I'll understand but I'll have to get another doctor."

He picked up his pen again and said, "Why not?" It was a very amiable conversation, and I knew that this time we were in sync. I could feel it.

He swore me to secrecy because we both knew that if word got out in that small town, the birth I was planning would never have occurred. My daughter was born in an hour and a half in the most beautiful birth that I could have imagined. My husband was not allowed to stay long after the birth, but I held her in my arms for more than an hour, and later walked down to the nursery to watch as they bathed her. Another first, since as mothers we were not allowed to be out of bed for a full day after giving birth. The next morning when they brought Maura to my room, the nurse commented that the whole hospital was talking about her birth and how fantastic it was. She then added, "But she's only 6 pounds, 3 ounces. I guess anyone could birth a baby that small without too much trouble."

My son Shawn was born two years later, weighing in at 8 pounds, 6 ounces, with only a little over an hour of labour and birth. There was no comment then about weight. His birth was as spectacular as Maura's was. I thought I had opened the door for all other women, at least in that community. My doctor's only comment was that he was amazed that anyone could endure that much pain without showing it. It was a very long time before there was another intentional natural birth in that hospital.

Soon the Lamaze Programme came into birthing rooms, and many of the births were natural (no drugs), if not altogether calm and relaxed. Women were awake, but often exhausted.

I believe that the Lamaze Programme could have worked and lingered, but many of the people who taught it felt obliged to lead discussions on how to cope with pain and moved away from the value of eliminating it.

Since women were no longer routinely anaesthetised, the concept of pushing the baby out came in, loudly and clearly. Many of the nursing staff, and doctors themselves, accustomed to seeing forceps as the major tool to bringing babies into the world, didn't believe that babies would come out their own.

I would cringe when I listened to women describe their births, but I found very quickly that women who have not experienced a calm and gentle birth were not too likely to applaud those who were doing it. I began to refrain from joining these conversations, knowing that few would believe me anyway. They didn't want to hear it. Surprisingly, that attitude sometimes exists today with both parents and birth professional alike.

It wasn't until years later when Maura became pregnant that the compulsion to set all of these thoughts down could no longer be ignored. The fervour began to build within me again. The teacher within me forced me to make up a small book for Maura and our two friends. With Maura's birth story and the success of the others, HypnoBirthing became an entity unto itself. The mission was well established.

In looking back on all of these years, I have to admit achieving the widespread acceptance that HypnoBirthing now enjoys has been an unbelievably steep uphill climb, mostly because of the reluctance of main-stream health care providers to acknowledge what is right before their eyes.

In making the journey, I've been fortunate in coming to know many very admirable birthing professionals—doctors and nurses and mid-wives, both Certified Nurse Midwives and Certified Professional Mid-wives—who are truly in birthing to serve the families they work with.

I look for the day when all birth attendants will become more sensitive to the emotional and spiritual human aspects of birth. I think that if doctors and other birthing staff would give natural birthing a chance, even for only a few births, they would also benefit from the relief and release of assisting at births that are joyful. As a licensed counsellor, I know how working with repeated war stories and human despair and disappointment can drain one's spirit. Doctors should be required to study instinctive birth, if for no reason other than the rejuvenation of their own spirit.

Thankfully, there are doctors and midwives and nurses—many of whom are now HypnoBirthing practitioners—who are able to see past that rigidity, and they view the mothers who are birthing as whole, healthy persons engaged in a wholesome, healthy human experience. These are the people who should be on the frontline of birthing, rather than practising joyful birthing one birthing at a time, as their patients request it.

Consumer families themselves are the answer to better birthing. We can only help them to be aware of the dream and to see themselves as the answer to achieving it. When that happens, most babies will enjoy the respectful, gentle, and calm birth of angels.

In HypnoBirthing you will be exposed to all sides of birthing so that you can make educated decisions. We don't make decisions for you. We do emphasise that it is important that no matter where you choose to birth, or with whom you choose to birth, just be sure that you feel confident that your decisions and your options are a good fit with your preferences about the manner in which your birth experience plays out.

The HypnoBirthing Philosophy

*Just as a woman's heart knows how and when to
pump her lungs to inhale, her hand to pull back from fire,
so she knows when and how to give birth.*

VIRGINIA D'ORIO

Our Mission Statement

The HypnoBirthing Mission Statement reflects an important part of our philosophy and purpose.

The administration, faculty, and teaching practitioners of the HypnoBirthing Institute are dedicated to providing birthing women and their partners a tried and proven method of birth education that guides and assists them as they prepare to experience birth in a peaceful and extraordinarily beautiful manner. It is a programme that considers the psychological and spiritual, as well as the physical, well-being of the mother, her birth partner, and the newborn infant, independent of context, whether that be in a home, a hospital, or a birth centre.

Mongan Method HypnoBirthing is built upon an educational framework of self-understanding, special breathing techniques, relaxation, visualisation, meditative practise, and attention to nutrition, positive body toning, and healthful family living. Most importantly, it fosters an air of mutual respect for the birthing family, as well as the health-care provider in a traditional health-care system or a complementary setting.

HypnoBirthing's philosophy and educational programme offers women an opportunity to explore birthing possibilities that are available to them and, in the absence of special circumstances, to step into a birthing experience that most nearly matches their birth vision.

The HypnoBirthing philosophy is based on the following premise:

- In the absence of a special medical circumstance, a woman's body should not be forced to do what it already knows how to do.

- Women's bodies and their babies know how to birth. The design is perfect and needs to be respected and unimpaired.

- Mothers and their babies should be treated according to the status of their own health, and not that of other women who may have special needs.

- Birth is a natural human experience. Each needlessly imposed procedure, test, exam, and interruption can upset the natural rhythm and flow and may cause the birthing to go askew.

- Each labour has its own time schedule. It may rest, or it may accelerate. The event should not be externally manipulated or managed if there is no special circumstance requiring it.

- Women's bodies are as sacrosanct during birthing as they are at any other time or in any other setting.

HypnoBirthing remains more a philosophy of the manner in which babies should be welcomed into the world than it is a "method" or technique for birthing. The basic tenet of the HypnoBirthing philosophy is that the birthing of your baby is a celebration of the most basic human experience of your lives. As such, birth and you, the family who is involved in this event, should be honoured and respected as the most relevant participants. The birthing should be experienced calmly, gently, joyfully, and peacefully, as well as comfortably.

When the suggestion to add "The Mongan Method" to the Hypno-Birthing title was first proposed, I fought it. I am convinced that when birthing families prepare for their own births with a conscious curiosity, they begin to understand the many medical and media myths surrounding birth. They educate themselves and they see these myths as just that—unfounded myths. They then approach the births as informed consumers.

The basic tenet of the programme is that childbirth is a normal, natural, and healthy human experience for the vast majority of women. When you are informed, you realise that when it comes time to birth your baby, the confidence that you develop in HypnoBirthing helps you to know that your birthing does not need to be accompanied by fear or severe pain and anguish. If you are healthy; if the baby you are carrying is healthy; and if you have had a healthy pregnancy, chances are in your favour that you will be able to anticipate and experience the labour of your choice, along with the other 90 to 95 percent of birthing women.

The HypnoBirthing view of birth is that it is a natural extension of the sexuality of a man and women; and, for that reason, we believe that birth is about them. It is about family fulfilment. It's about helping men to let go and free themselves from century-old programming that has eroded their role in birth and made them onlookers in one of the greatest and most important experiences of their lives.

It is about the manner in which they welcome a new little person in their family and into their lives, and it's about accepting responsibility for achieving the safest and most comfortable birth for their baby. Birth is not about science, although it is founded on science and supported by scientific evidence. More studies are supporting a natural approach to birth than ever before.

Families embracing the belief that birth is about them and the wonderful life-changing transition they are making into parenthood don't really need to be taught how to birth. They simply need to learn about birth. They come to understand that when the mind is free of stress and fear that cause the body to respond with pain, nature is free to process birth in the same well-designed manner that it does for all other normal physiological functions.

In spite of the fact that most births take place in hospitals, Hypno-Birthing does not believe birth is a medical incident. Healthy pregnant women are not diseased, nor are they ill.

The programme philosophy does not preclude the introduction of medical intervention, per se. It precludes the introduction of routine, arbitrary, unnecessary intervention.

Just as the animal mothers in Nature do not need a "medical lesson" to be able to bring their young into the world, human mothers also do not need extensive details of artificially fragmented stages of labour to instinctively bring their babies to birth. The bodies of healthy pregnant women instinctively know how to birth, just as their bodies instinctively know how to conceive and how to nurture the development of the babies they are carrying.

No matter how many children are born to a family, each child will experience birth only this once. He does not get a chance to do a retake. Emerging and just-born infants need to know that this is a place where respect, gentility, and love are practised. Especially at the beginning of life, they need to feel protected. In those first few moments of life, a baby can learn love, respect, and protection, or he can learn indifference.

The insidious growth of the second paradigm and the unexplainable blind acceptance of it by birthing parents tells me that no matter how many gains we make toward natural, instinctive birthing, it is not enough if there are still birthing experiences that are marked by indifference to the mother and baby's emotional and physical well-being. We have to somehow get the attention of those who, perhaps, don't even know that they are indifferent to what's right before their eyes.

HypnoBirthing guides mothers as they align with their own innate capacity to be able to give birth gently, comfortably, powerfully and joyfully. HypnoBirthing does not profess to offer preparation for births that are totally free of pain, discomfort, or unanticipated incidents. We do offer women an opportunity to explore the possibility of stepping into their birthing without fear or stress. Our experience over the past twenty-five years has allowed us to see these kinds of births repeatedly, and we've been sensitive to the way in which the couples leave their births touched with remarkable joy, fulfilment, and empowerment. We read it in their birth stories, and we hear it in their voices when they call or visit.

The HypnoBirthing philosophy will help you to learn to embrace your body's instinctual knowledge by relaxing into your birthing experience, and trusting in the many birthing gifts of nature that are already in place. You will want to let this experience unfold easily and gradually without interruption. You will gain confidence by rehearsing the birthing event. It is this confidence that will eliminate fear and fatigue and shorten your birthing time. The result of your preparation is a truly rewarding and satisfying birth that you and your partner and your baby are all a part of.

You will come to learn that women have been giving birth naturally and without intervention and instruments since the beginning of time. These are by no means new concepts. But the possibility of natural birth has been dismissed and even overridden for too many years. Even now, beliefs and the proof that support them are ignored by many.

In recent years women have been calling for their right to reclaim their birthing power. Women knew they had this capability from the beginning of time. It never occurred to the earliest of women that they didn't know how to birth. But through the years they have been taught to birth, and in such a manner that was actually contrary to their natural instinct. HypnoBirthing is helping women reclaim their ability to birth naturally.

Hippocrates and Aristotle were, perhaps, the first to extol a philosophy commending the efficacy of instinctive birthing. Birth was looked upon as a beautifully orchestrated natural human experience, designed to ensure the survival of the human race. There are many women who are clamouring for the return of gentle, instinctive birth, as evidenced by the many thousands of families who have sought natural birthing in the years since the inception of HypnoBirthing.

There have been many men in medicine down through the ages who have shared a philosophy of a simple and natural approach to birthing. These truly caring providers have supported birthing women and encouraged them to call upon their natural birthing instincts whenever possible. There are many doctors who have lent their respect and encouragement to birthing families when requested to do so.

One such doctor was Jonathan Dye of Buffalo, New York, who in 1891 wrote a book entitled *Easier Childbirth*. Dr. Dye pointed to the logic and scientifically back theory of natural birth when he wrote:

According to physiological law,
all natural, functions of the body are achieved
without peril or pain. Birth is a natural, normal
physiological function for normal, healthy women and
their healthy babies. It can, therefore, be inferred
that healthy women, carrying healthy babies,
can safely birth without peril or pain.

Dr. Jonathan Dye

More currently, Dr. Michel Odent, world-renowned advocate of gentle birthing, points out, "One cannot help a physiological process. The point is not to hinder it." He advises that birth attendants keep their hands in their pockets when they are by the side of a birthing mother so that the natural process can play out.

The late Dr. Gregory White, a supporter of natural birth, offers his view of the simplicity of birth in this excerpt from his book, *Emergency Childbirth*, a book written for the police and fire departments of Chicago.

"The most important thing for the lay assistant to know is that labour and the delivery of a child are normal functions, which Nature always tends to complete successfully.

"The women who deliver in taxicabs, ambulances, and police squad cars (or, unexpectedly at home) are usually those with short labours, and these are nearly always easy, normal deliveries. Since the babies in these circumstances are not suffering from the effect of anesthetics, or pain-relieving drugs given to the mother, they rarely require resuscitation.

"Generally speaking, mechanical assistance is rarely needed, but psychological or emotional support to the mother is almost always in order. This is usually given by means of a calm and confident manner and the frequent assurance that all is going well. Such moral support is given to the mother, not just because she is a fellow human being undergoing a trying experience—worthy as that reason is—but because calmness on her part and confidence in Nature, in herself, and in her attendant make it possible for her to do her part of the job better. Giving birth, at its best, is something a mother does, not merely something which happens to her (or is done to her).

"Reassurance and moral support are actually the major contribution of the attendant in most cases. This point should be stressed. (Complications) must be considered here (in the manual) because they sometimes occur in emergency childbirths. But they are rare—very rare. In over 95 percent of the cases of emergency childbirth, the emergency attendant will be overwhelmed with gratitude and widely praised as a hero or heroine, and he or she can smile at the knowledge that their simple task could have been performed by any bright eight year old."

When some people think of birthing, they associate it only with the physical aspect of its being the end of pregnancy and achieving the task of "getting baby out." While the baby's descent and emergence into the world are actually the end result of the physiological function of birthing, at HypnoBirthing we take a different and much broader view of this life-changing event.

We at HypnoBirthing see birth as deeply touching many facets of our human life, not just the physiological. With the birth of every baby, your personal life and responsibilities change.

The HypnoBirthing philosophy extends beyond birth into that adjustment period after birth. This is the time when you experience a phenomenal opportunity to assist your baby as he establishes a foundation of social and emotional responses that will last throughout his life.

As parents you will begin, if you haven't already, to assume the responsibility for seeing that your baby's womb life is calm, happy, and wholesome. His nutritional needs will become your nutritional needs; you'll become sensitive to his emotional needs, as well. You'll become sensitive to his need for safety, emotional well-being, and health. You'll also want to be sure that baby knows that he is welcome and that his actual reception into this world—birth—is equally as safe, calm, and gentle as possible.

This first birthday is also the most important birthday for your baby. How you look back on the birthing day experience is vital. It is said that there is no other single event that lingers longer in the mind of a woman than that of her birthing day. Deeper yet is the indelible imprint that the day of birth can leave in the mind of your baby.

It used to be thought that a baby is incapable of remembering events that occur when he is within the womb or at the time of his birth. Research conducted by the late Dr. David Chamberlain, author of

Babies Remember Birth, reveals quite a different story. According to Chamberlain, children, as well as adults, are able to recall, sometimes very vividly, the events of their lives within the womb, and they are able to act out events surrounding their births.

Preparing to welcome a baby is a life-changing experience, not just through pregnancy and birth, but long after. HypnoBirthing offers a remarkably simple, relaxed approach to this most important transition, as you step into your role as parent and become a family.

The philosophy is designed especially to serve the 95 percent of families whose pregnancies fall into the normal, low-risk, or no-risk categories. If you are part of this vast majority, HypnoBirthing will help you to experience this exciting time in your life with calm confidence as you look forward to your birthing day.

If, for some reason, your pregnancy and upcoming birth require special considerations, you will find that your HypnoBirthing techniques will beautifully complement whatever path your birthing will take, and it will help you remain calm, confident, and stress free. Additionally, the lessons you've learned in HypnoBirthing can help you to achieve a gentler, easier birth, regardless of any turn your birthing may take. Many women with special circumstances and even those who required surgical births have enjoyed happier and easier births as a result of their HypnoBirthing preparation. The gentle HypnoBirthing style also offered many benefits to mothers who had planned Vaginal Birth After Caesarean birthings.

If you have already embraced the concept of normal, natural birth as your choice, this book will provide an opportunity for you to explore its theories and learn more about how developing a calm approach to pregnancy and birth will enable you to prepare for a safer, easier, more comfortable and more joyful birthing.

Understanding the origin of many of the beliefs and myths surrounding birth that we, as a culture, have come to accept can assist you in making some of the decisions you will face in preparing for this most important time in your lives. This book will introduce you to ways in which you can connect with your pre-born baby and build a better understanding of your baby as a conscious little person, who is fully able to interact with you, even before birth. You can learn how to prepare your mind and your body in such a way that you will be able to achieve a happier birthing regardless of your present intent.

This book outlines the philosophy and many of the techniques used by HypnoBirthing families. You will gain much information and insight from reading this book. However, the comprehensive instruction and discussions covering specific methods, scripts, and demonstrations provided by your HypnoBirthing practitioner during classes, and even during your birthing, will prove to be invaluable.

The content of this programme is not intended to replace the advice and care of a birth professional. You should always seek the advice of a qualified professional caregiver for all pregnancy-related matters.

For information on HypnoBirthing classes in your area or for practitioner certification workshops, please visit our website at *www.HypnoBirthing.com*.

All natural birth has a purpose and a plan.
Who would think of tearing open the chrysalis as the
butterfly emerges? Who would break the shell and
pull the chick out prematurely? Who would force these
birth processes that are so perfectly designed?

Birthing Tips
I Learned from My Cat

Being an early teen and deeply involved with schoolwork, drum lessons, scouting, and cheerleading, my time and my mind were quite occupied. It would not be an exaggeration, however, to say that from time to time the Universe dumped situations upon me to keep me grounded as far as my quest for birthing information.

It happened on a beautiful late April afternoon in my twelfth year. I was in our backyard getting ready to plant sweet pea seeds. As I knelt over the bed I had prepared for the flowers, I felt a nudging at my hip. I turned and was surprised to see a very scrawny young tiger cat that looked much the worse for the wear of having been out on the streets. There were cuts on the edges of her ears and scratches on her face and head.

She continued to rub against me more emphatically. I saw this as a plea for food, so I picked her up and took her into the house to get some food. My mother took one look at my new friend, and shouted, "Where did you get that cat?" I explained and asked if I could keep it. Again, in a much elevated tone, my mother bellowed, "Get it out of here before it drops fleas all over everything." I took that as a "No" and quickly removed the cat, but I later sneaked food out to it. I did this for several days to make sure that the cat would stay. And she did. The cat chose to cohabitate with chickens in a coop behind my grandmother's house next door. It was an unlikely pairing, but she had found a home. The cat and the chickens seemed mutually disinterested in each other. She settled into the coop and became one of the residents. I named her "Squatter."

I continued to sneak food to her, and eventually my mother gave in and said she could stay. I checked on her every morning. I was really never sure that she would be there when I went out to bring her food.

Shortly after, I realised that Squatter's weight gain was not entirely from the improved nutrition I was giving her. There was a small bulge in her tummy below her ribs. My grandmother gave a quick assessment. "That cat's going to have kittens." I was ecstatic. My cat was going to have kittens, and I would be her midwife.

There are several things that are worth noting about Squatter's choices in living style. She picked the very last nesting box at the far end of the coop where there was very little light. The box she chose was piled high with straw, as none of the chickens had used it. She seemed happy and looked like she was thriving.

I went out to feed Squatter one morning and noticed that something was different. Squatter usually slept curled up in a ball, but on this morning, she was lying flat on her side, with all four legs stretched forward. I knew she was in labour. I found a wooden milk crate and pulled it over to her nesting box. She was purring. I wanted her to know that I was there for her. I would be her midwife. I reached my hand out and patted her head and her neck. She abruptly shook her head and knocked my hand away. She settled in and began to purr again. I got the message. She wanted no interference. She let me know that she could do this herself without my assistance. I realised that I had interrupted her focus. She resumed a deep relaxation and continued to purr.

There was no change in Squatter's behaviour. She just lay there and purred. Soon I saw a ripple running along the side of her body. She remained still. The ripple finally reached her outlet, and a little head slipped easily out of her body. She raised her head to observe, and then leaned down to clean away the afterbirth. The little one crawled its way to the nipples, with Squatter just watching. Once the baby latched on, Squatter put her head back down and began to purr again. This first-time mum was in no way distressed. Her instincts were in full gear.

I sat there mentally saying "WOW! Yes! There it is. That's the way babies should be born." All that I had imagined—but with human mothers, of course—was there. I was witnessing it first-hand. What a beautiful gift I was given.

Soon there was another ripple that proceeded exactly as the first one had. There was still no change in Squatter's behaviour. She remained still and kept purring. Her second baby emerged as easily as the first had, and Squatter reacted in the same way. She had an almost cavalier manner about what she was experiencing. She began to clean this kitten.

Suddenly there was a raucous in the yard. Some dogs had come into the yard and were fighting. Squatter abruptly sat up. She paused and quickly took one of her kittens into her mouth, jumped out of her box, and disappeared through a hole in the back wall of the coop. I looked at the kitten that remained in the box and wondered, "What do I do now?" Squatter was gone, and I was left with a newborn kitten that kept crawling around the box, bobbing its head and looking for its mother.

I didn't need to worry for long. About fifteen minutes later, Squatter came running back through the hole in the coop, totally ignored me, and rescued her remaining kitten. I was relieved but also worried for the safety of Squatter and her family.

We didn't see Squatter for many days, but one morning my grand-mother called me to come to the chicken coop. There was Squatter in her nesting box and with four young kittens. Somewhere she had given birth to two more kittens. As I approached her and patted her, Squatter began to purr with pride and satisfaction. All was well in her world.

I thought for many long hours on that experience. It all made so much sense, but it also raised so many questions in my mind. Squatter's birthing reinforced many of my early convictions and gave me insights that were considerably broader than my simplistic rambling. "It shouldn't be that way." There was a comparison there that all women need to consider. The evidence that birth can be beautiful and simple may be a needlessly well-kept secret, but it's there. It's been there for decades, even longer, and its supporters have been voicing it.

The most important message to me was that Squatter was startled and afraid when the dogs came into the yard. Then she escaped. She instinctively shut down her labour and brought her babies to safety. Human birthing mothers aren't able to escape when they are afraid. Ironically, though, there are people who could effect a change in the level of fear that women experience as they approach their births. They are the caregivers who routinely witness birth as a joyful and calm experience. But who also choose to dismiss it when it is there, hiding in plain sight.

Hiding in Plain Sight

. . .Theories are developed from
observations at the bedside of labouring
mothers, not in a laboratory.

GRANTLY DICK-READ, M.D.

As I grew older, I searched for evidence that would support my premise that most births can be instinctive, physiological experiences if they are not needlessly managed and interrupted. I discovered that the biggest secret about birth is that there is NO SECRET. The truth that natural birth enthusiasts have been espousing for decades is clear and simple. My young cat Squatter knew instinctively what to look for when she prepared to birth; and when the time came, her body knew how to birth her babies.

Our animal mothers don't need to gather in groups and have explanations of why and how they should accomplish this natural function. No one teaches them the parts of their anatomy or the fractionalised stages of labour. More importantly, no one cheers them on to push their babies out.

There are many who would have us believe that the same rules of nature don't apply to human mothers. I once asked one of the medical students in my class how it is that animal mothers in nature can achieve quiet, peaceful births in a focused, relaxed state. The young man replied with stunning conviction. "The difference is that animal mothers are quadrupeds. Human mothers can't birth that way."

Parents today are becoming consciously aware that this kind of rationale will no longer suffice to quell sincere questions. Healthy, active, involved parents today are not content to listen while someone else describes their birth story and then directs the event in a manner so that it no longer is the birth story the parents envisioned. A healthy mother and a healthy baby are not the only things that matter in a birth summary. Parents want a birth that is fulfilling and respectful of the dignity of mother, baby, and the birthing experience.

Today's birthing family who is looking for a natural and calm birth is very much of the opinion that the manner in which the birth is handled definitely matters.

To this day, I reflect on those still "best-kept secrets" that my young cat knew. The message of Squatter's birth is blatantly clear—birth is simple, natural, normal, and healthy, if left undisturbed. It doesn't need to be manipulated, fixed, or managed.

The facts are obvious. The female body is created to conceive a baby; to nurture the development of that baby; and to birth the baby, gently and peacefully. The incomparable precision of the female reproductive system during pregnancy and birth, absent any unanticipated special circumstances, has been brilliantly provided by nature. And it is seen every day in many places.

It is absurd to think that we live in a world today in which so vast a number of families every day, with intent, give birth quietly, gently, calmly, and in comfort. At the same time, there are more women clamouring for these kinds of births for themselves and for their babies, and they are not being listened to or heard.

Every day many in the standard health care system see this happening; and, yet, they don't see it. Their eyes are open, but their minds are closed, and they choose to ignore it, marginalise it, and ultimately dismiss it; instead, opting to use procedures and protocols that are less beneficial, less gentle for both mother and baby, less effective, and less psychologically and emotionally sound.

It's been suggested that women be assessed to determine if they are possible candidates for postpartum depression. If the medical professionals who are well aware of gentle birth would open their hearts and minds and concern themselves with implementing birthing protocols that would make the birthing experience less traumatic, there would be far less need for remediating these conditions with pills.

HypnoBirthing mothers are so exuberant over their births that they feel they could take on any obstacle. If only someone would listen to their birth stories. The answer to avoiding birthing PTSD is hiding in plain sight.

The number of routine annoyances, interventions, and surgical births in some countries is rising to the point that it is out of control and will continue to reach astronomical levels until parents, the consumers of birth services, speak out and let their wishes be known. Birth professionals need to listen; to really see; and then consciously evaluate the birthing experiences that they attend. They need to consider the disparity between what parents are asking for and what they are receiving. Parents should not have to beg for what is readily evident. They should not have to resign themselves to the realisation that some doctors won't even discuss their requests. And so they end up in "resigned submission" doing what they say they don't want to do instead of seeking a different option.

A birth professional told me, "People who want those kinds of births should stay home." What? People who want to be treated kindly and with consideration and care can't get kindness and care in a hospital? Those were the words. Is that the message? Are they saying that if you want a normal birth, you don't belong in a hospital? Hospitals are only for people who don't care if they are not treated with kindness and care? Why are they indifferent and disinterested?

Parents need to be able to trust in their care providers, but in many metropolitan areas mothers don't even know the care provider who walks into the birth room to attend the birth. The results of the 2010 "Listening to Mothers" survey indicated that half of the responding birthing mothers met their care provider for the first time as he or she walked into their birthing room.

Decades ago, Dr. White, whom I quoted earlier in the HypnoBirthing philosophy section, was pointing out what he viewed was most needed in a routine, normal birth. Today, those same kind and encouraging words are still needed by the mother giving birth naturally and, even more so, by the mother who is experiencing a precarious birth and, perhaps, a bit of difficulty. If all birth attendants offered support, rather than brash words that exacerbate a mother's fear, births would progress so much faster. Care providers need to recognise that birth is much more than a physiological function. There is such an obvious need for providers to establish rapport and a mutual trust with birthing families. They need to step into their title.

The lack of rapport and wholesome communication is why birth is considered broken today. Ironically, it is being ignored by many of the very people who are at the heart of the dilemma—the parents themselves, the birth professionals whom the parents hire to attend their births, the attending staff at the facilities in which the parents choose to birth, and the general public. There has to be a change in thinking to bring this about.

Squatter's birth revealed some very important suggestions for how birthing mothers should be accommodated. The healthy mother who is seeking a natural, instinctive birthing is not asking more from those who provide her care, she is actually asking less. Here are some of the things a birthing mum may look for.

1. She needs to feel safe, secure, and comfortable. She wants to know that the people who are attending her birthing are kind and caring and respectful of her and the work she is doing. She needs to be free of unnecessary devices and apparatus that make her feel abnormal—raised bed rails that cage her in and wall out her partner, and machinery and equipment that is uncomfortable, cumbersome, and creates a sense of impending danger.

2. She knows it is not normal to have a needle or a heplock attached to her wrist so that she can remain hydrated. Her birth companion or doula is prepared to take care of her fluid intake and output.

3. She wants to be undisturbed in a quiet and calm environment so that she can focus on her birthing and connect with her baby as much as possible.

4. She would like her treatment to be kind, respectful, and caring, so that she can birth with dignity. She wants her care to be dispensed according to the status of her own health, and not on the basis of other birthing mothers' conditions.

5. She wants to be spared unnecessary comments that could cause needless apprehension and fear of what could come in later labour. She does not want to have her labour shut down out of fear.

6. She would like to be encouraged to adopt positions and activities based on her preferred comfort, unless doing so is not advisable for her. She enjoys the soft buoyancy of "nesting with pillows" to assist in relaxation.

7. She would like a minimum number of interruptions and would prefer them only when necessary or in the event of concern. Interruptions break the focus she has established and change the rhythm and flow of her labour.

8. She would like to be acknowledged as a responsible and aware person.

9. She wants to rely on her natural birthing instincts without prompts that may be contrary to the mindful programme that she is working with.

10. She wants to breathe her baby down through his descent and crowning with quiet prompts only from her birth companion. Her body, through the natural expulsive reflex, and her breathing will push for her. She wants to remain at ease without the stress of time constraints if the baby is tolerating labour well and shows no signs of distress. When the body is fully relaxed, advanced opening can occur gradually even when it appears to be sluggish.

11. She would like to be encouraged and accommodated in spending at least a whole hour or more in private, quiet family

bonding in the "afterglow" of the baby's birth to help baby adjust to the early period outside the womb. Visitors and staff should respect the need for baby to adjust to his surroundings and to the touch of only his immediate family.

Some families who are choosing natural, calm birth are welcomed into hospitals; many are welcomed into birth centres; some choose to birth in their own homes with a doctor in family practice or a certified midwife; some birth in birth centres. All women should have this opportunity, regardless of where they are birthing. But the facts are that some don't have any choices at all.

The people who are seeing this are to be commended for their concern and recognition of the need to do something about this horrific condition. But, along with this recognition, we need to see assessment of the birthing system. Why are so many mothers leaving their births overwhelmed with grief? They are mourning the loss of the vision they held for their birthing, because, in many cases, they have been denied their vision. Something must be done to make their birthing less traumatic.

Only when birth is looked upon as normal, and birthing mothers are looked upon as normal, whole beings, can one hope to have them leave their birthing beds feeling jubilant and anticipating their new role as a parent. Concern over a mother's post-natal mental health would be lessened.

If the medical system could just take a look at the faces and the stamina and attitude of mothers who are returning to natural, instinctive birthing, they would see an exuberance and spirit that nothing can parallel. HypnoBirthing mothers are so filled with joy and accomplishment over their births that they want to leave their birthing beds and shout it from the rooftops. We hear it in just those words all the time. It's not only the birthing mothers who feel fulfilled. Dads, too, tell us that the birthing experience has touched them so deeply in so many ways, and that they are closer as a couple then they have ever been.

A dad's eye view of birth that follows is typical of the birth stories we receive.

A Dad's-Eye View of Birth

Conny's water released at 5:30 A.M., but nothing else was happening. She told me to go to work. At 9 A.M., she said she was having surges, but nothing regular. I decided to come home, just in case. We pulled stuff together for the hospital and decided to go to my parents' house, since they live only ten minutes from the hospital.

By the time we got to their house, the surges had faded; and for the next few hours, Conny didn't have even one. She was getting a little worried because soon, it would be twelve hours from the time her water released; and if things didn't start, it could cause her to be induced at the hospital, which we didn't want.

After we ate, she lay down on the couch. We put on soft, instrumental music and started going through the relaxation scripts to put her at ease. Within ten minutes, she started having strong surges, five minutes apart. Within an hour, surges were about three to four minutes apart.

By the time we reached the hospital, Conny was having surges every two minutes. When she was assessed in the triage centre, she was already 7 to 8 centimeters open. She continued to do her slow balloon breathing through all of this, smiling and at ease in between the surges. It was unbelievable. It was just like we saw in the videos, but now it was so real.

We got into our birthing room at 6 P.M. The nurse set up the foetal monitor on her belly and then left us alone until Conny felt the need to start breathing the baby down. By 7:35 P.M., little Colin Emanuel Varga entered the world (only three and a half hours of labour)—no epidural, no episiotomy, no IV, no screaming baby, no pulling or pushing.

The doctor was absolutely fantastic. She was patient, understanding and encouraging, and used all the right terminology. Even the nursing staff was supportive. They were so surprised and impressed with this type of totally natural birth that we had a room full of nurses (between six to eight on a regular basis, and most of those were just there to watch). Everything went so well and so quick and so painlessly. As Conny put it: a lot of pressure, but no pain.

HypnoBirthing really works. We had such a wonderful experience, and Colin is alert, content, and happy. Best wishes to the rest of you, and Happy HypnoBirthing.

Mark & Conny & Colin, Canada

If only more birth professionals would look and listen to what is "hiding in plain sight."

From Celebration to Trepidation:
A History of Women and Birth

W hen one really thinks about the disparity between the way most animal mothers give birth and the way human mothers give birth, one cannot but wonder what happened. When mothers from other cultures are put into the mix, the questions become even more pressing. Where and why have human mothers in so many parts of the world abandoned their human instincts? What kind of strange quirk of nature brought this about? Why have women chosen to stray from nature? The answer—they had no choice.

The truth of the matter is that women today are just as capable as their counterparts in nature to call upon their natural birthing instincts, but those instincts have been blocked. **Women have been taught to birth.** They have been taught to birth in a way that is contrary to their very nature.

To truly understand the events that led up to our present-day thinking, where women birth the way they were taught to birth, we need to look back as far as 3000 B.C.

There is much evidence to support the belief that ancient women had their babies easily, with little discomfort or drama, unless, of course, there was complication. Historical records at the time of Jesus confirm that babies were regularly born in fewer than three hours. Hebrew women had their babies easily and comfortably within a short period of time. Naturally, of course.

Helen Wessels, founder of Appletree Ministries and author of *The Joy of Natural Childbirth: Natural Childbirth and the Christian Family,* offers us much research and study with Hebrew biblical scholars; and in her book, she emphatically says that there is no evidence to support the theory that women in ancient times considered childbirth a curse or that they suffered in childbirth. It was not uncommon for mothers to give birth away from their villages and unassisted. They then would return to their villages with their babies in their arms. We have only to look to the Nativity of Jesus to read of such a birth.

In other parts of the world—Spain, France, the British Isles, and old Europe—the lives of the people centred around their gods of Nature and motherhood. They honoured Mother Nature, Mother Earth, and their top deity, Mother Creator. Because women were able to naturally bring forth children, they were revered and considered to be connected to Mother Creator. Pictures of statues found in their ancient stone temples depicted women, fully rounded in pregnancy and with full breasts. Some statues even show a baby crowning or emerging from the vaginal outlet of their mothers.

These primal people regarded birth as the highest manifestation of nature. Ceremonies centring around the happy occasion of birthing were of high importance. When a woman was to give birth, people of the village would gather around the pregnant mother praying to their gods that the child would be healthy, wise, and strong. Birth was a holy rite and a "Celebration of Life." There was nothing that suggested that labour was the long, dreadful, and painful ordeal that it later was believed to be.

Women were nurturers and healers, developing herbal brews and administering healing medicines. All healing came at the hands of the healing spirit in women. They collaborated and exchanged learning, overseen by the wise women of the village. Men were the gatherers of the herbs, food, and building materials. Their roles were different, yet equal in their society.

Eventually, men took the lead in medicine. Even then, there was no change in attitude or approach to birth.

Both Hippocrates and Aristotle, leaders of the Grecian School of Medicine, were sensitive to the emotional and spiritual needs of women who were birthing. They both wrote that a woman's needs and her feelings should be accommodated during childbirth. Neither wrote anything about danger or pain and suffering in his notes. Are we to believe that the presence of pain in normal birth was not recognised and simply went unnoticed? I think not.

Hippocrates believed that birth is a natural experience and ". . . should not be interrupted with 'meddlesome interference.'" He established midwifery for the purpose of giving birthing women emotional support. He also believed that in birthing, Nature is the best physician.

In his notes, Aristotle wrote of the mind and body connection and emphasised the importance of deep relaxation during birthing to relieve any discomfort. In the event of a complication, he also recommended relaxation so that the complication could be treated and resolved.

They both advocated for a support person to be with a birthing woman (today's doula), and Hippocrates was the first to organise and present formal instruction for midwives. With this distinction, many other women moved more openly into the realm of healers. They regularly tended to the ill of the villages with their brews and tinctures.

During the last century before the birth of Jesus, another leader from the Grecian School, Soranus, a medical student, put the writings of Aristotle and Hippocrates into book form. Soranus emphasised the importance of listening to the needs and feelings of women who are giving birth. He also advocated using the power of the mind to achieve relaxation in order to bring about an easy birth. Like his predecessors, Soranus, too, made no mention of pain, except when he wrote about complicated, abnormal birth. If there were no complications, under the watchful eyes of Soranus, women were kindly and gently cared for in a normal birth. This attitude remained for several hundreds of years.

At the end of the second century, a new wave of political governance, strongly influenced by the church hierarchy in Rome, began to sweep through all of Europe, bringing with it decrees of contempt for anything related to the worship of nature. Their goal of abolishing all rites and ceremonies previously practised in honour of nature was carried out swiftly and completely. Birthing rites and ceremonies were forbidden by the new laws, and the iconic statues and stone temples were destroyed.

Because women were living symbols of the connection of women to a "Mother Creator," it was essential that they be controlled and restrained. Since only God could heal, the talents of the wise healers were discredited and used as proof that they drew their power from the devil. Witchcraft, a very honoured position within the early villages, was forbidden by law. They could no longer go out to tend to the ill and were forbidden to be with birthing mothers. Pregnant women were segregated and confined to their homes. But for the healers, midwives, and doulas who were at the core of the strong female presence, the price to pay was much higher. For them, the punishment was death, usually by public burning at a pyre in the centre of the village square.

The condemnation of women escalated as the authority for all medical practice lay in the hands of the local priests and monks. More laws decreed that doctors could minister only to those who were "deserving ill" and only then after seeking permission. Women were accused of being seductresses; and, therefore, the unborn babies they were carrying were conceived, not through a connection with a Holy Mother, but rather through a connection with the devil. Because they had conceived their babies in "carnal sin," were undeserving and were totally isolated during their births. Under fear of execution, no one could accompany a birthing mother. Doctors were forbidden to assist, even in the case of a complication.

The fervour of the war against women became so heated that at one point in time, a council meeting was called with the intent of declaring that women were not even human beings.

With midwifery having been abolished, the only person who could attend to a woman in the event of a complication was the goat gelder, who swiftly cut the baby from the mother, and she was left to die. The life and soul of her baby was considered saved, and therefore the incident was justified.

It was at this time that what was known as "The Curse of Eve" was embedded into the translations of the Bible by Clement, who was later sainted. Previously there had been no mention of a curse. Other church leaders became blatant in their dismissal of the treatment of women.

---

* Pope John Paul II many times during his long papacy, in letters and in speeches, offered an unprecedented public apology, asking for the forgiveness of the world for the sins of those acting in the name of the Catholic Church for the attacks upon Jews, women and minorities, victims of the Spanish Inquisition, Muslims killed during the Crusades, and other infractions. He cited the burning at the stake of woman, and the violation of women's rights, and other Church abuses over the past 2,000 years. ("Pope John Paul II." Wikipedia: The Free Encyclopedia. Wikimedia Foundation, Inc. August 17, 2015. Web. August 21, 2015. <*https://en.wikipedia.org/wiki/Pope_John_Paul_II*>).

In the years between the 2nd century and the 16th century, matters became much worse for women and birthing. Later other church leaders became blatantly dismissive of what was happening to women. One such leader in Germany was quoted as having said, ". . .if a woman suffers and dies in childbirth, so be it. That is what she is there for." Midwives who attended birthing women were called Wehmutters or "mothers of woe." It was still generally considered that birth was painful and dangerous.

In the 15th century, the lost books of Soranus were discovered, and the world began to take notice. The madness and chaos of the former period had subsided. The Reformation caused the Roman Church to examine many aspects of its policies, doctrines, decrees, and practises. Much was changed. The blatant mistreatment and executions of women were lessened; however, they were not entirely out from under the veil of abuse and subjugation. It was even worse for women who were not of higher social standing. The poorer women were shown no mercy.

In 1853 and 1857 when Queen Victoria of England insisted on having anaesthesia for her births, its use in obstetrics became firmly established and was widely used routinely. It became the choice of doctors for achieving the obstetrical goal of "getting baby out." Because it was too cumbersome to administer anaesthesia in a home setting, upper class mothers and their babies made their way into hospitals. Lower class women remained in the care of midwives.

In the mid-1900s, following the lead of Dr. Joseph DeLee, doctors began to view all births as problematic. It was decided that since normal births were rare in hospitals, interventions should be applied to all births to prevent the evils of labour. These preventions included all interventions utilised in modern obstetrics for highly complicated cases.

At about the same time, the English obstetrician Grantly Dick-Read introduced his theory that pain was not an inherent part of birthing. Based on his experience, as he said, ". . . at the bedside of birthing women," he forwarded what he called the Fear–Tension–Pain Syndrome, emphasising that when a mother is taut, her body is also taut. Dick-Read's papers were not accepted, and he became the object of ridicule.

Also in the mid-1900s, Dr. Fernand Lamaze brought into the birthing scene the first real approach to natural birthing that took hold. Dr. Lamaze advocated unmedicated, natural births. Women were to remain awake and use their power of focus and breathing to distract them from the pain of labour. It was then that women were taught how to birth. They learned that they were to push their babies to crowning.

After Dick-Read, one doctor—Robert Bradley—looked upon Grantly Dick-Read as a hero and patterned his birthing programme with relaxation, as recommended by Dick-Read.

When we look back upon these events with our modern knowledge, we understand more clearly how fear of complication and resulting death, not fear of birthing, caused women to look upon labour with horror. Extreme fear created extreme tension, and the tension, in turn, resulted in a taut cervix, unable to perform its natural function. Those who lived through the ordeal, as well as those who witnessed it, attested to the agony that was experienced in birthing.

Birth was still very low on the list of priorities among medical people. Maternity wards were filthy and staffed primarily with physicians who were inept or alcoholics.

As a result large numbers of women were dying, not from childbirth but from "child-bed fever." The remnants of this period have contributed enormously to a fear of dying in childbirth. Obviously, this is a fear that is no longer valid today. It wasn't until Florence Nightingale used her clout as an exemplary fundraiser that the maternity wards were cleaned up and the professional level of staff was improved.

The stories and the scripts were firmly set. Birth, once a major celebration, had been turned into something that was filled with dread and trepidation.

It is not difficult to understand why women to this day feel so much anxiety over the thought of birthing. However, as we understand the cause, we must also understand and realise that hundreds of years have passed since that bleak period of time in birthing history. We also can understand that there is no longer the need for women to harbour a dread of labour. These thoughts are no longer valid in today's birth settings.

Today's women have many choices in birthing. They have many opportunities to explore those choices. The first and most important choice being the selection of a childbirth preparation programme that will help them to seek, explore, and find the people and the environment that feels "right" to them.

HypnoBirthing's philosophy and educational programme gives women the opportunity to explore their choices; and in doing so they are able to create the possibility of stepping into the birth that they feel is a right fit for them. They can decide whether or not what has become routine for other women must be a part of their birthing. They can learn, look at what currently exists, and choose "What can be." That is their prerogative as they fulfill the single life human function that is theirs alone to experience.

Today, even with evidence to the contrary, an incredible number of people in maternal services, and even women themselves, continue to accept the myth that pain and problems are an inevitable part of birthing, and that birthing has to be a laborious ordeal that leaves both mother and baby exhausted. It is widely thought, even by the birthing mothers, that the best thing they can do for themselves is to turn the birth experience over to their care provider and attending staff and depend upon them to guide them through the experience. Why do these myths persist? Why do women's bodies, perfectly created to birth, shut down even before they start labour? Why do so many women require that their babies be extracted surgically—a procedure that forty years ago was so infrequent that it was regarded with surprise?

The answer can be found in one word: fear.

How Fear Affects Labour

To those who say it is just not possible to
birth naturally and without pain, I say,
"But what if we're right? Wouldn't it be wonderful?"

LORNE R. CAMPBELL SR., M.D.

I once met a vivacious young woman who was five months pregnant. She glowed as she talked about her pregnancy and how she had felt so wonderfully healthy. She spoke of all the things she was doing to prepare her body for birth—swimming, yoga, walking. In the middle of all of this happy conversation, she paused, clenched her fists, and said, "But I can't even think about THAT day. I have totally blocked out all thought about the birth. I can't bear the thought of what it will be like. I am so scared."

"Terrified" is the more appropriate word to describe what women are feeling as they approach what should be among the most exciting moments of their lives. This young woman, obviously very sophisticated and very much in control of the events of her life, took on an air of helplessness when it came to the thought of birthing. Sadly, she represents women in many parts of the world. It is a travesty that manufactured fear, leading to manufactured consent, casts such a cloud over the otherwise joyful excitement that couples should feel as they anticipate becoming parents.

The belief in pain surrounding childbirth is so strong that instead of questioning the validity of the concept, there have been many efforts to rationalise its importance and to attach some reason and higher purpose to it.

Some programmes teach methods that attempt to take your focus away from pain so that you will not be so aware of it. Others will tell you that pain is a very important signaling mechanism, a sort of biofeedback that alerts you to where you are in your labour. The theory is that if you can identify the degree of severity and the frequency of it, you will be better able to determine where you are in labour and what coping techniques you will employ to continue. Still others suggest that you look upon it as an unavoidable but useful friend that can be tolerated, worked with, and learned from. There are even those who revere pain in birthing and see it as a vehicle through which to achieve the empowerment of womanhood. It has been suggested that we learn to honour pain, as other societies do, for the strength it builds in our character.

These programmes feel that because pain has to serve some purpose, it must be rationalised and accommodated in some way. For most women, these are not convincing arguments. Pain is still a four-letter word. Accepting the belief that it is necessary creates the very situation they want to avoid.

For those who refuse to examine the theory that there is no physiological reason for pain in birthing, the way to accommodate it is to provide a plethora of drugs that the birthing mother can escape into. For the pregnant mothers looking forward to such relief, the drugs are offered, not as a last resort during labour, but rather as a menu, presented within the childbirth education class so that selections and decisions can be made early on. These mothers want to believe that the drugs won't cross the placenta and affect their babies. No one tells them that the placenta has no barrier. And so they go into their labours believing that their birthing bodies are inadequate, but they can be "delivered" by drugs and technology, even when these interventions take them further away from normal and gentle birth for their babies.

Occasionally one of the women in a HypnoBirthing class will ask, "Why don't we human beings have our babies the way cats and dogs and horses and other animals do? There's nothing wrong with their labours." My reply is always the same: "Yes, why don't we?"

Medical professionals have long stood by the argument that pain is considered the "watchdog of medicine." Pain, they tell us, sends a signal that something is wrong. If that is true, we must make an exception for all other mammals for which labour is a natural, normal function.

We know that horses and other "dumb" animals will delay the start of their labours or shut them down when they don't feel comfortable with their environment or they feel endangered—just as my cat Squatter shut down her labour when she was in fear of the dogs nearby. Is it not unreasonable to think that women's bodies have that same instinctual capacity? Why do we believe this of animal mothers, yet refuse to consider it for human mothers?

I am frequently asked to prove that HypnoBirthing works—that eliminating fear and other stressors and building trust in the birthing process results in a truly safe, healthy, happy-baby and happy-mother outcome. This, in my mind, is like asking me to take a finely tuned, precision instrument that has been broken and prove that it would work perfectly had it not been broken in the first place.

The concept of birth has been distorted. The spirit of women with respect to their innate birthing power has been broken. We can do nothing about the millions of broken births that have already taken place, but by seriously looking at the effect of fear—the powerful emotion that clouds our thinking and causes the birthing body to break down and deviate from its natural course—perhaps we can keep the finely tuned, precision bodies of women whole for future generations.

Your Marvelous Birthing Device: The Uterus

Your uterus is perfectly designed to assist you to birth your baby. When we understand the way in which the uterus functions naturally when unencumbered by fear, the concept of easier, more-comfortable childbirth immediately becomes obvious and, therefore, attainable. This very brief explanation and the illustrations are, indeed, the crux of our entire programme. It is exactly this process of your body that you will work with during labour. This is the way the birthing muscles are designed to work—in perfect harmony.

There are three layers of muscle in the uterus. The two layers with which we will be concerned are the outer layer, with muscles that are vertical (aligned up and down with your baby), and the inner layer, with muscles that are horizontally circular (surrounding the baby).

The circular muscles of the inner layer are found in the lower portion of the uterus. As the illustrations show, the circular muscles are thickest just above the opening, or neck, of the uterus, called the cervix. In order for the outlet of the uterus to open and permit the baby to easily move down, through, and out of the uterus into the birth path, these lower, thicker muscles have to relax and thin.

The Uterine Layers

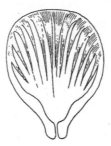

The outer longitudinal muscle fibres of the uterus

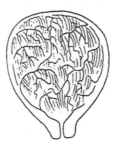

The middle muscle layers, interwoven with blood vessels

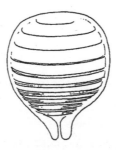

The inner circular muscle layers found mostly at the lower part of the uterus

The stronger muscles of the outer layer of the uterus are vertical fibres, with a stronger concentration at the top. They go up the back and over the top of the uterus. As these muscles tighten and draw up the relaxed circular muscles at the neck of the uterus, they cause the edges of the cervix to progressively thin and open. In an almost wave-like motion, the long muscle bands shorten and flex to nudge the baby down, through, and ultimately out of the uterus. It is this tightening motion that many HypnoBirthing mothers report as being the only sensation that they experience during the thinning and opening phase of labour.

When the labouring mother is in a comfortable state of relaxation, the two sets of muscles work in harmony as they were intended. The surge of the vertical muscles draws up, flexes, and expels; the circular muscles relax and draw back to allow this to happen. The cervix thins and opens. Birthing occurs smoothly and easily.

The Surge Breathing technique that you will learn and practise in your classes is designed to help you to work in concert with these birthing muscles. Combined with the relaxation practice you will do on a daily basis at home, this will help you learn to bring your body into a relaxed state that can make your surges more effective and substantially shorten your labour. You will learn to visualise the lower circular muscles as soft, blue satin ribbons, flexible and totally nonresistant to the draw of the upper muscles.

Fear: The Enemy of the Birthing Room

We have seen how the birthing muscles are beautifully orchestrated to work. Now let's look at what happens when the birthing mum is tense and fearful.

The effect of fear upon labour is not subtle, insidious, or complex. We see it in front of us in every uncomplicated birth with every labour that is slow to start or delayed or that later slows or rests. Yet this obvious emotion, one of the strongest and most debilitating that we know, is basically ignored. Instead of being helped to recognise the harmful effects of fear upon the body, mothers are asked to surrender themselves to drugs, technology, and manipulation to force their bodies to do what they are naturally capable of doing when left to their own means and when the circumstances are "right" for birthing.

The negative physical effect of fear on labour can be traced to the function of the body's Autonomic Nervous System (ANS). The ANS is the communication network within our bodies. Its main function is to interpret messages it receives, determine what action should be taken as a result of the message, and then immediately communicate that directive to the other systems of the body. The responses to impulses that are transmitted through the ANS are not subject to our conscious control and are, therefore, involuntary.

For the purpose of looking at the impact of stress upon birthing, as well as the beneficial effect of calm, we'll need to look at the two subsidiary systems within the ANS—the Sympathetic System and the Parasympathetic System. These systems control those responses that cause us to accelerate or slow our breathing, to blink our eyes, to step up or reduce our heartbeat, to arrest or maintain our digestive processes, and to carry out many other functions of the body.

The Sympathetic System is triggered when we are stressed, frightened, or startled. Therefore, I call this part of the system the "Emergency Room." It is the role of the Sympathetic System to act as the body's defence mechanism. It instantly creates the "fight, flight, or freeze" response within the body. When it is in motion, it causes the pupils in the eye to dilate, increases the speed and the force of the heart rate, and causes the body to startle and move defensively. It suspends activities such as digestion. Most importantly, it closes arteries going to organs that are not essential for defence. It prepares the body to deal with emergencies and danger. It is designed to save your life. The activities of the Emergency Room put you into a state of alert. For that reason, you should be spending no more than 2 to 5 percent of your life in the Emergency Room. It is like a "rainy day fund," and it shouldn't be tapped into on a regular basis.

On the other hand, the Parasympathetic System, which I call the "Healing Room," keeps the body and mind in a state of harmony and balance. It maintains the body functioning in a state of calm, slowing the heart rate, reducing stimulation, slowing the firing of harmful neuro-peptides, and, in general, keeping us in a state of well-being. The Healing Room restores and maintains the normal functions of our bodies. We should be living 95 to 98 percent of our lives in the Healing Room.

How does this relate to birthing? The Sympathetic part of the nervous system responds not just to actual threats, but to perceived threats. The mother does not need to meet the saber-tooth tiger face to face in order to feel fear. In other words, the negative messages that a mother constantly receives are processed as being real. Over time, these negative messages become part of her belief system and com-promise her body's chemical balance on a regular basis. They affect her emotional state and that of her pre-born baby.

When the mother approaches labour with unresolved fear and stress, her body is already on the defensive, and the stressor hormone cat-ccholamine is triggered. Her body is sent into the "fight, flight, or freeze" response. It is believed that catecholamine is secreted in large amounts prior to and during labour.

When circumstances are such that neither "fight" nor "flight" are appropriate, as in the case of labour, the body naturally chooses the third option: "freeze." Since the uterus has never been designated as part of the defence mechanism of the body, blood is directed away from it to the parts of the body involved in defence. This causes the arteries going to the uterus to tense and constrict, restricting the flow of blood and oxygen. Labour and birthing nurses and midwives have told me of seeing uteruses of frightened birthing women that are white from lack of blood, just as a person who is experiencing extreme fright often has the blood drain from his face.

With limited oxygen and blood, vital to the functioning of the muscles in the uterus, the lower circular fibres at the neck of the uterus tighten and constrict, instead of relaxing and opening as they should. The upper vertical muscles continue to attempt to draw the circular muscles up and back, but the lower muscles are resistant. The cervix remains taut and closed.

When these two sets of muscles work against each other, it causes considerable pain for the labouring mother. The situation can also have an adverse effect on the baby. The upper muscles push to expel, forcing the baby's head against the tightly closed lower muscles that refuse to budge. In addition to the pain that this causes for both mother and baby, labour can be drawn out, or it can even shut down. Thus, we hear from mothers whose labours end in a surgical birth lament, "I was told my uterus wouldn't open." Limited oxygen in the uterus also means that the supply of oxygen to the baby is compromised. Over a period of time, this can be a cause for concern. The situation often is labeled "failure to progress" (FTP), and it usually results in intervention. It is interesting to note that the very same initials, FTP, are used to abbreviate both Grantly Dick-Read's Fear–Tension–Pain Syndrome and the failure to progress that it causes. What labour needs is not more urgency or prompting to "move things along," but more awareness of the importance of calm, relaxation, gentle encouragement, and assurance that actually can move the labour along faster.

Regrettably, Dick-Read did not live long enough to see his theory buttressed with the discovery of endorphins. Still more regrettable is that, even with this knowledge in hand today, few medical caregivers are opening their minds to the relationship that exists between the birthing experience and the ANS, with its ability to secrete endorphins, the "feel-good" hormones that relax the muscles and allow the body to open, as well as the stressor hormone catecholamine.

Attempts to speed the birth of a baby only result in more pain for the mother and the baby, and frustration on the part of caregivers, as the baby's head pushes against muscles not yet relaxed and open enough to accommodate it. HypnoBirthing allows for the body to work at its own pace and facilitates easier birthing by using relaxation and visualisation to speed the release of endorphins and effect an even shorter labour.

You and your birthing companion will be taught how to identify emotional stress before and during labour and how to release it. You will learn how to bring yourself into a deepened relaxation. When you are free of fear, you can achieve a relaxed state from the very onset of labour. Verbal and physical cues that you and your partner have practised will help you to maintain a state of calm from the very start, as constricting hormones are overridden by your body's natural relaxants.

Learning to understand the benefits of living in the Healing Room—and avoiding people and situations that place you in the Emergency Room—is a skill that will infuse calm into your everyday life. It will greatly enhance your relationship as a family, as well as ensure a calm and gentle birth.

Releasing Fear

Preparing women for birthing by educating them in the true physiology of their birthing muscles, and the need for the mother to be free of tension, was the backbone of Dick-Read's work. This concept appealed to the intellect of many women in the middle of the last century, and it was enough to inspire them to break with traditional attitudes and bring their children into the world unmedicated and alert.

Free of debilitating fear, those who subscribed to the philosophy of natural birth were free of anaesthesia, free of needless management of their birth, and, for the most part, free of the discomfort of labour.

Most births were attended by family doctors, a person who was known to the birthing mother probably from the time that she, herself, was a child. There was a long-standing trust established in the doctor/ mother relationship. Mothers did not expect labour to be a picnic, but their labours were not anticipated with the fear that exists today. Birth, actually, was rather simple. Standard birth consisted of mothers, who with a little Demerol were able to bring their babies to crowning with little fuss. At that time, they were totally anaesthetised in time for the doctor to arrive to extract their babies with the help of forceps.

If you are like most pregnant women, you will find that as you move through these days and months of pregnancy, you will be met with a whole new set of feelings, anxieties, doubts, questions, decisions, and tasks that you never had to consider before. Some of these will centre on your pregnancy, labour, and birthing; but there may be more that will cause you to look at the many transformational experiences that bringing a baby into your life will present. This is natural. As you prepare your mind and body for your baby's birth, you will want to be ready in this regard also—free of any fears, reservations, or limiting thoughts.

It's helpful for both you and your partner to be able to identify feelings, experiences, or recollections that may be painful or hurtful, thus limiting your ability to approach birthing free of harmful emotions. Take a look at those emotions that may foster a feeling of uneasiness, meet them head-on, and release any conflict you may be harbouring (consciously or subconsciously) because of them. Once you have been able to work through and resolve lingering emotions, limiting thoughts, experiences, or memories that could stand in the way of an easy birthing, you will have a better sense of your own ability to approach the birth of your baby with trust and confidence.

Thoroughly search your inner feelings to discover the areas that you feel very confident about and those that you need to work through so that you can resolve any fears or misgivings that you are holding. Brushing aside matters that concern you may help you to get through your pregnancy, but these concerns can easily surface as fears when you are in labour, and they can affect the course of your labour. You will want to take advantage of the opportunity to talk with your partner, your birthing companion, or a good friend who can help you explore and discuss any thoughts that could be troubling you.

Your HypnoBirthing practitioner will help you inventory and identify those areas of your life that could possibly serve as obstacles. The
practitioner will help you work with fear-release sessions in class. If
you still feel you need some assistance in releasing lingering fears after
you do the sessions in class and talk with your partner and friends, ask
your practitioner for a private session. If you are not able to work with
a trained practitioner, you may find it helpful to seek the counsel of
a hypnotherapist to do release work with you. A fear-release hypnotherapy session is truly one of the most effective ways of eliminating
toxic emotions.

Listed below are just a few areas of concern to pregnant women that
surfaced in the early nineties as a result of Dr. Louis Mehl-Madronna's
study on turning breech babies with hypnosis. Your own inventory may
reveal other issues that you would like to resolve.

- **Your own birth**—What stories have you heard about your own
  birth? Are they positive and encouraging, or negative and frightening? Do you feel that you will duplicate your mother's labour?
  If what you've been told is less than encouraging, you might
  want to work on establishing that you are not your mother, and
  this is not her pregnancy. You are an entirely different person at a
  different time and under different circumstances and are preparing for your birth differently.

- **Others' birth stories**—Have you been surrounded with stories
  of joyful birthing, or have family members impressed upon you
  "family patterns" of long labours, back labour, severe pain, and
  medical intervention? Again, you do not need to assume the
  experiences of the people who are relating these stories. There
  is no reason to believe that you will birth as they did. Work at

checking those kinds of thoughts so that you don't bring their past baggage into your birthing.

- **Previous labours**—Has your own experience with labour been easy and satisfying, or are you carrying recollections of an arduous ordeal? If you had a less-than-satisfying labour, take hope in the fact that you are better prepared for an easier birth this time, and you now can approach birthing with more knowledge and planning than you did before. Make your HypnoBirthing skills work for you, and get rid of the memories of the previous birth or births.

- **Parenting**—Did you learn positive attitudes toward parenting that you feel comfortable with? If not, do you feel less than adequate about your ability to be a good parent? Do you feel overwhelmed? Quite often people who did not grow up with good role models can learn a great deal from less-than-great models about what they wouldn't want to do in their own parenting. Turn it into a positive factor.

- **Support**—Do you feel secure with the support that your partner and/or family will provide? Is there someone who will share the responsibilities of caring for the baby? Sometimes just tackling the issue and letting people know you will want and need support will resolve the matter. In other circumstances, take advantage of the opportunity to see what strengths you must build to effectively provide your own best support.

- **Marriage/relationship**—Is your marriage/relationship secure, loving, and mutually nurturing? Are you confident that your relationship is strong and that it will weather the additional concerns of raising a child? Are there some agreements you need to work out? Have you really "talked"? Perhaps a confidence-building session can help you sort out your abilities. Working together in HypnoBirthing can bring about a stronger bond than you ever believed could exist.

- **Career**—Will you be able to continue to pursue your own goals with reorganising and planning? Will your plans need to be put on hold? Are you ambivalent about going back to work or staying home with your baby? Sorting through these questions can help you reconcile with what you really feel you want to do.

- **Housing**—Is there room in your home, as well as in your heart, for your new baby? Can accommodations be easily made? Can you make changes? If not, express those wishes; and you'll soon see how your circumstances can change.

- **Medical care**—Do you feel comfortable with your present medical care provider? Do you feel that he or she is supportive of your plans for your birthing? Are there lingering doubts? Have you discussed your preferences for a natural birth with this person and made your wishes known? Are your decisions fear-based or confidence-based?

- **Finances**—Do you see finances being "stretched" as a result of adding another person into your life? Ask your HypnoBirthing practitioner about some abundance work. The Law of Attraction can help in this regard: Remember, you get what you say and see.

- **Prior relationships**—Are you carrying around some unhappy memories of an earlier relationship or an experience that has left hurtful thoughts? It's time to eliminate those thoughts and let them go by having a release session.

• **Personal experience of abuse**—Are you harbouring unhappy
memories of an experience of physical or sexual abuse? Because
these experiences are so associated with your body, bitter or
hurtful memories can easily rise to the surface during birthing.
Birthing is one of the most profoundly physical experiences you
will know in your lifetime. Overwhelming feelings of helplessness, inadequacy, and fear have the ability to make your body
shut down or resist. It is important that you do release work with
a qualified hypnotherapist before you advance any further into
your pregnancy.

Please take this assessment seriously. Your mind and body work best
when both are in harmony so that you can approach your birthing as
free of limiting thoughts and emotions as possible.

The Power of the Mind

Every thought becomes a plan.
If you think a negative thought or vision, it becomes
a negative prediction; if you think a positive thought or
vision, it becomes a positive prediction and plan.

MARIE MONGAN

W e've just seen the power of the mind, specifically how fear can interrupt the body and the natural birth process. The good news is that the opposite is also true: Positive thought and relaxation can help the body and enhance its ability to birth freely, effectively, and with no ill effects. That is, after all, what HypnoBirthing is all about.

As far back as early Grecian times, relaxation, visualisation, and quiet recitations have been used by priests to aid people in ridding themselves of illnesses. Tribal Indian customs and "old wives" superstitions were used for centuries to bring about physical and emotional healing.

Now, many years later, we are coming to an awareness and acceptance of the ways in which self-hypnosis can physically and chemically affect your body's tissues and mentally reprogramme behaviours that can impede success.

Dr. Bruce Lipton, a well-known author, is in the forefront today with his work on the effect of the mind in changing tissues at the cellular level. Through studies of everything from memory to dreams to subtle eye movements, researchers are discovering that the mind and the images held within it can largely determine your success or failure in life. Motivational consultants, Olympic coaches and other sports trainers, as well as people in medicine, are realising that visualisation—the process of mentally producing pictures of a desired goal or result—is an important factor in the achievement of that goal, and they are routinely incorporating self-hypnosis and visualisation sessions into their programmes.

Educational psychologists have conducted visualisation studies suggesting that extrapolative learning—the method of mentally working through a physical process—can produce a response within muscles that is similar to what would occur if the routine were physically practised.

When in self-hypnosis you visualise your ideal birth scene, it becomes stronger than any of the birth stories and negative comments that you have heard. The brain and nervous system are saturated with a picture of a specific, ideal sensory vision that seems so real it becomes imprinted in the brain. This occurs exactly the way that real experiences become embedded within the memory of the inner-conscious. When a person is in a relaxed state, the mind more easily adapts to the imagery and accepts the suggested vision as being real. The assimilation of the repeated image causes the belief in the desired outcome.

Though neuroscientists are just beginning to understand how this occurs on a cellular level, sufficient study of this phenomenon has resulted in a very clearly defined set of Laws of the Mind. The concept of easier birthing through the positive application of these Laws is changing the view of birthing and is the basis of HypnoBirthing.

The Powerful Laws of the Mind

The application of four specific Laws of the Mind has a direct effect on changing the view of birthing, and these Laws are the basis for much of the work that we do in HypnoBirthing.

The Law of Psycho-Physical Response
The Law of Repetition
The Law of Harmonious Attraction
The Law of Motivation

The Law of Psycho-Physical Response: The Body Follows the Mind

The process of achieving desired results through application of the Laws of the Mind can be more clearly understood by examining the Robot Theory forwarded by Dr. Al Krazner in his book *The Wizard Within*. The Robot Theory is based on the Law of Psycho-Physical Response. This law states that for every suggestion, thought, or emotion one entertains, there is a corresponding physiological and chemical response within the body. This is the most important Law of the Mind in regard to birthing.

According to psychologist Candice Pert, the body is the action component of the mind. What is experienced in the body is determined in the mind. Therefore, what the mind chooses to accept or perceive as being real, the robot body, accordingly, responds to. The mind does not have the ability to act. Therefore, it sends messages to the body demanding action. The body, in turn, plays out the thought. Pavlov's experiment with the dogs that eventually became conditioned to salivate at the ringing of a bell in anticipation of receiving food is perhaps the most commonly recognised example of this mind-body connection.

We experience this law almost every day of our lives. I'm sure it would not be difficult for you to recall any number of incidents when a loud, sudden noise or the unexpected appearance of a person or an object in your path caused you to startle, duck, draw back, or involuntarily cry out.

A dad in one of my classes described experiencing an instant and noticeable physical response when seeing the flashing lights of a police car in his rearview mirror at a time when he was driving well beyond the speed limit. It was not until he pulled over to the side of the road and the policeman continued past him that he became aware of how strong a physiological effect his thoughts had created within his body. He could feel the accelerated pounding of his heart, the dampness accruing at his underarms, the white-knuckle grip he had on the steering wheel, and the long, continuous intake of breath, without exhaling. He was also hugely aware of the relief he felt as he exhaled and his shoulders receded back into the frame of his body. When the mind no longer perceived that he was being threatened, he relaxed back into a state of calm.

Of course, the most obvious example of the psycho-physical response is the one that has brought you to HypnoBirthing class to prepare for your baby's birth—sexual arousal.

When the mind entertains a sexual thought and a subsequent visualisation, the body responds by preparing for the sex act with the male experiencing penile erection and the female experiencing lubrication of the vaginal wall. This all comes naturally, with the robot body acting out the desires of the mind. It is part of the master plan for all reproduction.

Utilising this Law of the Mind so that it works with you and for you, and not against you, during your birthing is essential. If the mind is dwelling on fearful, negative images of birth, the body is thrown unintentionally into a defence mode. The physical response then becomes the antithesis to normal birthing—tension.

You will become skilled in using your own natural abilities to bring your mind and body into psycho-physical harmony so that the thoughts you use in practise are those that will condition your body and your mind to create endorphins—those neuropeptides that create a feeling of well-being. You will learn special deepening techniques that will help you to connect with your baby and work with your body to bring yourself even deeper as your labour advances.

The Law of Repetition

Since repetition is the key to conditioning, the Law of Repetition becomes an important aspect of your preparation. The more you take a single thought and express it mentally or out loud, the more deeply it becomes ingrained in your mind's eye and the more readily the mind accepts it as reality.

Had Pavlov rung the bell once or twice or only on occasion, the dog would not have been able to make the association of the ringing of the bell with receiving food or a treat, and he would not have salivated. Therefore, it is important that you routinely recite the birthing affirmations that your practitioner will provide you in your class and that are recorded on the Rainbow Relaxation CD or MP3 that can be purchased as an accompaniment to this book.

The Law of Harmonious Attraction: The Power of Language

Words and thoughts are powerful and profoundly affect our every-day experiences and beliefs. Equally significant is the harm that is created by the negative energy of the confusing, harsh, and frightening words of conventional birthing.

A second Law of the Mind, the Law of Harmonious Attraction, is very much in evidence here. This law states that what we put out in the way of thinking and speaking creates energy that comes back to us in the same form in subsequent experiences. This is what I call the "echo effect" or the "boomerang effect." Whatever thought or emotion you throw out to the world will come back to you exactly as you first proposed it. Applying this law on a daily basis is important. The best advice, according to Esther Hicks in the Abraham-Hicks Material, is, "If it's not what you're wanting, don't go there."

Words have energy, power, and vibrations that translate into action. Regardless of whether you are the person speaking or the person being spoken to, the sound and vibration of what is being said cause an emotional response within your mind and a physiological and chemical response within your mind-body. Over time, the frequency of that response becomes part of your belief system, strengthening itself each time a similar vibration is accepted. It then attracts more of the same.

Even when we silently engage in self-talk, our words have force. Each time we speak to ourselves in a less-than-complimentary way— "Are you stupid, or what?"—or use similar self-denigrating words, we leave an imprint of inadequacy upon our subconscious.

You can see this demonstrated as you listen to the people around you. Notice that healthy people rarely speak of becoming ill. However, people who are not healthy frequently punctuate their conversation with talk of their physical ailments. Think about the phrase, "The rich get richer, and the poor get poorer." Rich people don't often speak of being poor or not being able to afford goods. On the other hand, poor people, or people who "think poor," regularly end thoughts of spending with the phrase, "I can't afford it." They remain in that situation and go through life affording very little. It is therefore essential that you keep your thoughts and language focused on what you do want rather than creating wasted negative energy around circumstances that you don't want.

The little ditty that you may have heard on the playground when you were a child—"Sticks and stones may break my bones, but names will never hurt me"—may be a good comeback as a temporary defence against words that sting, but, physiologically, it is not true. Caustic, belittling, frightening, and abusive words do, indeed, hurt and can cause a lasting imprint. Tell a baby just learning to walk or beginning to accomplish tasks on his own that he is clumsy or a klutz, and after a while, the child begins to feel clumsy and moves in ways that are clumsy. Tell him that his everyday, normal bodily functions are "smelly and disgusting," and he begins to feel bad about his body and himself for having created a disgusting situation. The negative imprint takes hold, stays with him, and grows. The more potent the thought, the more potent the imprint.

Concepts that you are exposed to repeatedly in many places and from many sources become part of a conditioning that becomes embedded in your thoughts over time. The Law of Repetition governs that process. It is important for you to recognise that frequency does not necessarily equal fact.

The association of pain with childbirth is an example of a universally held conditioning, and it has become the source of needless suffering because of the myths that have grown up around it. By the same token, if you listen to affirmations of positive, gentle birth on a daily basis, it will contribute to positive conditioning.

Words and suggestions set off a chain of feelings, beliefs and reactions that can be uplifting, encouraging, and supportive—or totally debilitating. The following chart shows the flow of energy and the effect of words.

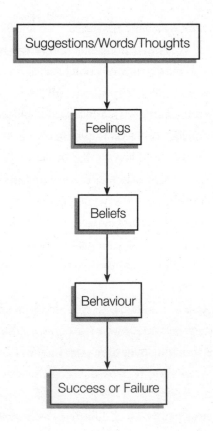

Words create thoughts and emotions; repeatedly entertaining the same thoughts conjures up feelings. Over time, these feelings become beliefs. We begin to act out those beliefs by our behaviour. Our behaviour shapes our experiences. Positive behaviour creates positive experiences; negative behaviour creates negative experiences. Hence, in HypnoBirthing, we focus only on the positive.

For all of these reasons, HypnoBirthing parents learn to use language that more nearly describes what is happening within the birthing mother's body during birth. This gentle language is more meaningful to parents than language that is couched in medical academicism— appropriate for the medical caregivers in communicating with each other, but frightening and potentially harmful to the birthing family.

The language you use and the language you hear from people around you, including caregivers and childbirth educators, keeps your mind in a state of calm, or conversely, triggers a state of unrest, stress, and fear. Learn to choose your words carefully and associate with people who reinforce your own positive thinking about birthing. If you are being bombarded by people who want to tell you birth horror stories, suggest that you wait until after you have your baby to exchange birth stories. Don't get pulled into those kinds of conversations.

This kind of thinking, speaking, and living, as well as the support that you give to each other, will help you to work together toward a positive birth experience. This calmness will be there for you during birthing, and it spills over into every aspect of your family life.

To truly embrace the concept of gentle, normal birth, learn to think and speak in the kinder, softer word substitutes that appear on the list that follows. As you become accustomed to this language, you will become aware of the importance of this mental transition.

HypnoBirthing Language	Medicalised Language
Use:	**Instead of:**
Uterine surge or waves	Contractions
Birth Companion	Coach
Receive the Baby	Catch the Baby
Birth/Birthing	Deliver/Delivery
Birthing Time/Month	Due Date
Pressure/Sensation Tightening	Pain or Contractions
Membranes Release	Water Breaking/Rupturing
Birth Path	Birth Canal
Birth Breathing	Pushing
Special Circumstances	Complications
Uterine Seal	Mucous Plug
Birth Show	Bloody Show
Near Completion/Nearly Complete	Transition
Thinning Opening	Effacing/Dilating
Pre-born/Unborn Baby	Foetus
First-/Second-Time Mum	Primip/Multip
Perineal Rim Unfolds	Perineal Rim Stretches
Parents	Clients/Patients
Pre-Labour Warm-ups	Braxton-Hicks
Pelvic Floor Exercises	Kegels
New Born	Neonate
Resting Labour	Stalled or Shut-down Labour
Practise Labour	False Labour

Birth-savvy Mothers, who value totally
unmedicated and intervention-free birthing,
have a new term for it—"Pure Birth."

William and Martha Sears, *The Birth Book*

It is this kind of birth that we refer to as instinctual.

The Law of Motivation: What You Want Is What You Get

The Law of Motivation also affects the physical body's capabilities. We have all read accounts of nearly impossible feats accomplished by people who risked their own lives to save the life of a child. When the mind is highly motivated, the body responds properly.

Consider the football player who sprains an ankle at the beginning of the last quarter of the game. Because his conscious attention and motivation is totally focused on playing the game and winning, he may feel the pressure of the swelling of the ankle but feels no pain. His mind has narrowed its focus and is accepting only the suggestion that he must remain in the game and play his hardest. His ankle does not accept the sharp twist as a source of pain because only the mind is able to think or react to pain stimuli. If there is no pain stimuli, he feels no pain. It is not until the game is over and the motivation to put all of his energy into winning the game is no longer necessary that his mind is directed: the message of the sprain is relayed to the mind, the mind interprets it, and sends it back, and he begins to feel the discomfort.

When we examine motivation to see how it affects the way in which a woman births, we need only to look at a story that received national news coverage several years ago. It involved a very pregnant young woman who was attending a prom when she went into labour. She excused herself, left the dance floor and went into the ladies' room where she proceeded to have her baby, quickly, quietly, and unbeknownst to anyone else. Her fear of being detected created a motivation far stronger than any fear she may have regarding the birth; and she was able to return to the prom activities after only a brief period of labour. Her mind never accepted, or even considered, that there would be any impediments to this birth or that she would experience the long, typical labour that our society has come to expect, especially for a woman having a first baby.

While it is difficult to believe, we sometimes see the reverse of the previous example. If motivation is accompanied by a "secondary benefit," a person can actually bring about what, for most people, would be an unwanted situation—an illness, a bad outcome, a hardship. Without consciously being aware of it, "victims" of the secondary benefit can create circumstances that allow them to accomplish what they consider is a better end, even though it means they endure less than optimal circumstances.

Could the need for attention create motivation for a high-maintenance pregnancy? It definitely can and occasionally does. If a pregnant woman wants and needs to be pampered, "waited upon," and coddled, and buys into the concept that pregnancy is an abnormal condition and she is "ill," the attention that she gains during a troublesome pregnancy and a difficult birthing can definitely make it all worthwhile in her mind. She barely tolerates her pregnancy and constantly proclaims her annoyance at all the aches, pains, and other pregnancy "disorders," while she uses body language that demonstrates her plight. Family members often contribute to this scenario by cautioning the woman that she must "give in" to her frailty during this precarious time of her life.

Several years ago, a mum came to my classes talking about the horrendously long and difficult births her mother and all of the women in her family experienced. This was the centrepiece of her conversation week after week. As I got to know her family, I saw that all the women in the family talked in "victim" language. In spite of the fact that their birth stories were horrific, they were delighted to tell all of the details, each one surpassing the other, and each rushing in to grab her opportunity to tell how bad her pregnancies and birthings were. The mum and dad appeared to embrace the HypnoBirthing philosophy, but I was not surprised that her birthing story was one that could easily match and top those of her family members. The drama surrounding the birth was incredible, and there was a gathering of family and friends invited in to observe the performance. It was more important for this young woman to be able to remain in good standing in the sorority of her family and friends than it was to remain outside the group and to birth her baby calmly and peacefully as she had prepared.

This is not to say that all labours that are drawn out and difficult have behind them some secondary benefit. Nevertheless, it is important to assess your own motivation and intent as you approach your birthing and consider, in light of all we've spoken of here, how you will apply these Laws of the Mind so that they work for you.

Motivation is closely tied to your intent and your self-image. It is said that a woman births pretty much the same way that she lives life. For that reason, it is imperative that you take the time to do an assessment of how you see yourself and whether this image is productive for you or counterproductive. Much of the determining aspects of how you will make important choices concerning your birthing are factored on how you regard birth and your own role in this experience.

Two models—the whole-person model and the dependent model—determine how you will approach your pregnancy and birthing. Review each model and evaluate which traits you want to strengthen and expand upon as you make important decisions regarding your baby and your birthing. The model you choose to follow will be invaluable to you as you continue your adventure into pregnancy, birthing, and lifelong parenting.

Dependent Model	Whole-Person Model
uninformed/unknowing	knowledgeable
submissive	powerful
passive onlooker	involved
conforming	forward thinking
reconciled	fulfilled
easily led	directing
vulnerable	trusting
helpless	self-sufficient
vacillating	decisive
threatened	confident
embarrassed	assertive
resigned	satisfied

Understanding Self-Hypnosis

There is a considerable amount of misinformation and a terrible lack of good information surrounding self-hypnosis. This is because the only exposure that many people have had to hypnosis, in general, is what they've seen as entertainment—stage hypnosis. Without going into detail, I will simply remind you that the people who are on the stage during a stage show are volunteers, there to have a good time. Since all hypnosis is self-hypnosis, it is easy for them to accept the roles that the hypnotist suggests to them. They're having fun.

Contrary to what is portrayed in movies and literature, it is impossible to cause someone to do something that is against his morals or his principles while he is participating in hypnosis. If a suggestion were to be made that is contrary to any value that a person holds, the person would immediately revert to an alert state and refuse to carry out the directive.

What many people may not know is that hypnosis is being used to benefit people in many medical, dental, and therapeutic applications. Hypnosis is widely used to help people release fears, overcome the discomfort of the effects of chemotherapy, prepare for surgery, stop stuttering, end nail-biting, and a host of other annoying habits. Hypnosis is so effective that it was recognised in 1957 by the American Medical Association as a beneficial therapy for many physical and emotional needs.

Hypnosis is a very natural state that most of us exist in during a large part of our day. When we become engrossed with our work and lose track of time or of what is going on around us, that is hypnosis. We are in a hypnotic state when we get caught up in daydreams or become so immersed in a movie or a television show that we emotionally react to what the actors are experiencing.

When you are in hypnosis during your labour, you'll be able to hear conversations and may or may not wish to join in. Though you will be totally relaxed, you will also be fully in control. To the person who is not familiar with self-hypnosis, you may even appear as though you've taken some kind of medication to put you into this profoundly relaxed state. During your birthing you will be aware of your uterine surges, but you will experience them comfortably and with the knowledge that you are very much in charge. You'll be able to interrupt your relaxation whenever you wish and resume it whenever you wish.

As your labour moves nearer to birth, you will most likely choose to go even deeper within to your birthing body and your baby so that together you can work in harmony through birth. Though you will not be able to visually experience it, you will be able to physically know that your baby is very much a birth partner in this adventure. When you are tuned into your body, you will sense and know exactly what you and your baby are doing.

You'll become skilled in using your own natural abilities to bring your mind and body into perfect harmony. You will gain an understanding of the physiology of labour that goes beyond what is usually taught in other classes. You will learn special relaxation conditioning and labour techniques that will enable you to connect with and work with your body and your baby as you experience labour. The repetitive practise of these techniques will make it possible for you to instantly achieve this relaxation and maintain it for as long as you wish through labour.

The value of self-hypnosis comes from learning to reach that level of mind where suggestions that you give yourself effectively influence your physiological experience. Your HypnoBirthing practitioner will help you learn to reach this level, where you focus only on calm and comfort. You will see, hear, and practise these techniques in class and will be given practise tapes or CDs that you will work with on a daily basis at home. Your birth companion will also be given scripts to use when you practise together two or three times a week.

There is no magic benefit that accrues from just coming to classes. You must be willing to apply the practice that is required to reach these levels of relaxation that will be there for you when you are in labour.

These skills will be applicable to many facets of your life, as well as for the birthing of your child. Many couples find that the months of preparation in relaxation benefit them in the way they deal with day-to-day situations and have a positive effect on how they interact with each other. A mother who was in one of my classes said, "I came to HypnoBirthing to learn how to have a baby, and I learned how to have a life." It's that powerful if you learn to utilise it.

Relaxation also has a calming effect upon the baby. "Mellow" is the word many parents use when describing their babies. We like to think they are "better natured."

Falling in Love with Your Baby

Leave it to a baby to turn your world
upside down, take your breath away and make you
fall in love again. With his toothless grin,
your baby sets your heart on fire.

JAN BLAUSTONE, *THE JOY OF PARENTHOOD*

We know that calm, soothing thoughts and emotions have a bearing on the way in which you bring your baby into the world. Love is one of the most important emotions in helping to build a positive anticipation—the love that you as parents feel for each other and the love that you actively share with the baby that you are carrying.

When is the best time for you to fall in love with your baby? If you haven't already fallen madly in love with your baby and are not playing and communicating with her on a daily basis, now is the time. Getting acquainted with your baby is a very magical experience, and you don't have to wait until she is born to enjoy making this connection.

Once your baby is born, you wouldn't think of going about your daily routine without making time for frequent breaks that are especially devoted to talking, playing, and loving her. Babies have a way of drawing that kind of attention from family members and strangers alike. No one can resist their magnetic charm—so compelling it can bring activities and conversation to a screeching halt.

You can begin to connect socially and emotionally with your unborn baby as soon as you know that you are pregnant. In addition to making your pregnancy so much more enjoyable and exciting, when you "tune in" to this little person who has become part of your life, you lay the foundation for a relationship that can last for the rest of your lives. Pre-birth parenting activities tell your baby that he is welcome and wanted.

The idea that both parents influence their pre-born baby is neither supposition nor superstition. The close bond that is built while the baby is still in the womb can be very real when it is time to connect with your baby during birthing.

Thanks to the relatively young study of foetology, advanced during the late seventies and early eighties by Dr. Thomas Verny in his book *The Secret Life of the Unborn Child,* we know that babies are cognizant during their time in the womb. All of baby's womb life is actually his first classroom. There he learns lessons and develops emotionally, physically, spiritually, and socially. Parents should do all they can to be sure that the baby's emotional development, his sense of well-being, and his esteem as a loved being are being fostered through caring and consistent pre-birth parenting.

The nine months that the baby spends in the womb are nine months of growth and development for parents as well. They learn the importance of evolving as a family, and mums learn the importance of planning and working, together with their babies, toward achieving the goal of a gentle birth for both baby and mother.

Dr. David Chamberlain, author of *Babies Remember Birth,* later published as *The Mind of Your Newborn Baby,* spent many years investigating the effects of birth trauma upon a baby. He states that babies are active participants in birth, and they do remember their birth experience. The imprint of that experience is carried throughout their lives. All one has to do is gaze into the alert, knowing eyes of a newborn who has not been drugged during her journey into being, and it is immediately evident that there is a lot of thought going on. Without saying a word, the baby transmits a message: "I know."

Pre- and perinatal psychology is a branch of research that focuses on the effects of environment upon the baby as he is developing within the womb and during the birthing experience. Ongoing study is attempting to determine the degree to which a baby in the uterus is affected by the environment in which he is living and the manner in which his parents interact with him and each other.

While we know that everything the mother puts into her body crosses the placenta and affects the baby, this is also true of emotions. When we offer the pre-born baby love, play, and music, we reinforce his positive feelings of security. On the negative side, it's been found that the pulse rate of the unborn baby rises abruptly when the baby is exposed to screaming, yelling, loud or disturbing noises, and emotional upsets. Be aware of the kind of environment and experiences you are providing for your unborn baby.

It is so important that dads get involved in nurturing both mother and baby and that mothers recognise the need for nurturing both dad and baby. Reciprocal nurturing of one parent for the other sends a strong message of security to their pre-born baby: This is a loving family.

As a result of Verny's studies, and those of his colleagues, it was found that babies in the womb react to stimuli outside of the uterus. Intentionally initiating certain kinds of interaction and love-play can result in positive prenatal, perinatal, and postnatal bonding.

Findings suggest that babies within the womb react to vibrations, stroking, tapping, rubbing, squeezing, conversation, voices, music, light, heat, cold, pressing to simulate the birth experience, teasing, loud noises, TV sounds, and humor.

Babies who were exposed to soft music and singing during their time in the womb were calmer, happier, and better adjusted to life outside of the womb. It is also believed that they are better sleepers. Babies love the sound of their parents' voices, especially when they are sung to. Some mothers report that while singing to their pre-born babies, the babies responded with a gentle moving action. Music has vibration that babies are sensitive to. If the vibration is gentle and calming, they have a feeling of well-being.

Dr. Michael Lazarev, a leading Russian paediatrician, emphasises the importance of helping the baby to become familiar with musical sounds. He concluded that if you listen to your unborn baby, he will let you know what activities and sounds he prefers.

In a study at the University of Salzburg, mothers who developed a real sense of being connected with their pre-born babies and who interacted with the babies in talk and play tended to view their bodies with an air of pride and fully accepted their increasing size as a natural part of the development of the baby. Fathers who were involved in bonding displayed the same kind of awe with respect to the shape of the mother's body and the development taking place inside. There was a respect for the life being carried in the womb. Overall, their pregnancies seemed to be easier, as were their birthings. They approached birthing with a relaxed confidence. Later, both parents seemed to adopt a softer, more balanced attitude toward caregiving. Parents displayed greater feelings of enjoyment, love, and respect for each other and for the baby.

The benefits to babies were also profound. There were fewer premature births and fewer low-birthweight babies. Reports showed a noticeable increase in the socialisation of the babies who experienced pre-birth parenting. Overall health and weight gain were very positive. HypnoBirthing parents tell us that their young babies hardly cry and are exceptionally alert.

I believe that one of the most important advantages of pre-birth parenting to the baby is that when parents truly connect in attitude as a family prior to the birth of the baby, they accept the responsibility for planning and directing their births. They are as committed to ensuring the safety and comfort of the baby during its journey into the world as they are when their baby is part of their family outside the womb. I also believe that pre-birth parenting helps them become practised in accepting the responsibility of parenting later.

Knowing that the baby is fully aware of its surroundings and the people who are his parents, it is only reasonable that the baby also thrives when there is interaction and socialisation with the people with whom he lives.

Recommendations for Pre-Birth Parenting

- Learn the suggested relaxation techniques and practise them daily—baby needs peace too. Since baby is aware, he is listening to the music and calming suggestions at the same time as his mum.

- Play with baby physically—sway, sway, sway; dance, dance, dance; rub, rub, rub; pat, pat, pat; squeeze, squeeze, squeeze; press, press, press (all done gently).

- Use guided imagery and visualisation. (See the Birth Companion's Reading and Rainbow Relaxation in this book, as well as the Pre-Birth Parenting CD.)

- Carry on conversations with baby—say affirmations, read stories with animation and imitation of animal sounds, play children's tapes.

- While relaxing in the tub, massage your belly with lukewarm water and sing or talk to your baby.

- Play soothing music—sounds of ocean, birds, wind, soft piano, guitar, madrigals, flute, harp, nature sounds, and animal sounds—so that baby develops a wider awareness of these things.

- Have family and friends greet and interact with baby.

- Put yourself in the baby's frame of reference—how wholesome are the surrounding noises, voices, attitudes, emotions, foods, temperatures, air, odours?

Prenatal Bonding Exercises

Important facets of the HypnoBirthing programme are the discussions and exercises for parents that help them to truly connect and fall in love with their pre-born baby. These activities help the parents develop a sensitivity to how the baby perceives his surroundings and often cause them to evaluate how their lifestyle, their emotional well-being, and their relationship with each other can impact the baby's emotional development and sense of feeling loved and secure.

The exercises on the HypnoBirthing Pre-Birth Parenting CD are valuable relaxation lessons and image-building tools for both parents. These activities help them develop a stronger sense of their own self-worth, as well as serve as meditations that will help them bond with their pre-born baby. The time spent with these guided images may prove to be among the most valuable gifts that you can give to yourself and your baby.

Another way to establish a connection with your baby and to explore his world is to take part in the following exercise. We call it "Be the Baby" because we ask you to imagine yourself in the role of the baby in the womb, experiencing what life is like for the baby.

As the practitioner leads you through this exercise, take advantage of the opportunity to think about how your unborn baby might respond to these questions and how you can begin to actively do things that will enhance the baby's feeling of being loved and wanted.

Be the Baby Exercise

What your baby perceives—what she accepts and embraces while in the uterus—becomes part of her essence and identity and forms the creation of a conscious ego that accepts, caresses, and acknowledges its own true self.

Imagine that you are the baby developing within your mother's womb, listening to conversations, experiencing your surroundings, absorbing emotions and moods of those around you. Reflect for a few minutes on how you feel as that child who will soon be born into your family.

- To what degree are your parents spending time in relaxation practise to help ensure a calm birth for you?

- How welcome do you feel? Do you already feel that you are part of the family?

- How loved do you feel? Do people talk to you with love each day?

- What kinds of messages are you receiving from things that are said about you?

- How do you feel about the way your parents interact with each other?

- What kind of pace do your parents keep? Do you feel sure there will be time purposely created for you as you're growing up?

- What kind of atmosphere will you come into? Peaceful? Loving? Caring? Happy?

- How confident are you that you will be raised with love and patience?

- How calm a world is being prepared for you?

- How kind and loving are the people you will be living with?

- Do you feel that your parents will do what is necessary to ensure your gentle entry into the world?

- Do your parents talk in gentle, loving ways?

- Is each motion that you make received with joy?

- What kinds of sounds/music/noises do you live with?

- Are you being provided with the best nourishing food to help you grow and develop in a strong, healthy way?

- How wholesome is the air that you are breathing? Will it foster good health for you?

- Is your environment and your body free of smoke, alcohol, and drugs?

- How certain are you that you will be helped and guided toward becoming a loved and loving human being?

- What kind of assurance do you have that your parents will give you understanding as you learn to adjust to your strange, new world?

- Are you confident that you will learn by guidance, not punishment?

Take a moment now to quietly connect with your baby. Ask your baby to tell you what it is that she might like to add to this list. Is there a message that your baby has for you? What would make her feel more loved, more secure?

Reflecting on your responses to these questions, are there some changes that you feel you can make in your baby's environment? Are there some resolutions that you, as parents, need to think about and adopt?

We recommend these activities for creating lasting expressions of welcome for your baby:

- Write letters to the baby or keep a journal expressing your delight that he will soon be here. Save letters to present to the child later.

- Take pregnancy photographs of mother, as well as mother and dad together.

- Record messages to your baby on a tape or CD in addition to letters.

- Videotape your birthing, complete with a birthing-day message given to the baby during labour.

- Videotape siblings talking and listening to the baby or telling the baby a story.

- Involve siblings in decorating baby's room and take pictures.

- Start a scrapbook and includes pictures that show how your body is changing as the baby develops, as well as special events like a visit from grandparents, trips to memorable places, a baby shower, a mother-baby luncheon, or a blessing way.

The Power and Art of Doing Nothing

This chapter on experiencing a beautiful, calm, and tranquil birth while doing absolutely nothing will pull together all of the facets of this programme that you have already studied with those parts of the programme, particularly the birth, which is yet to come. It includes the rationale behind the previous chapters—the educational component, philosophy, the breathing techniques, the history of how we got to where we are, the ways of preparing your body and your mind and relaxation with the parts of the programme that are yet to come, i.e., the actual birthing experience.

To understand the connection between birthing and "doing nothing" we must first address a topic that is more commonly related to animals in nature.

What we are talking about here is something that is not often attributed to human mothers, but is more commonly related when we speak of animal mothers in nature. What we are suggesting is that you look within the gifts that nature has already bestowed upon you—collectively called instinct.

Are You Out of Your Mind?

It is futile for you to attempt to direct your body. While we do spend time teaching you breathing styles that will assist you to relax to the point where you can quiet your mind, we do not attempt to teach you how to use your mind to keep your birthing on target. Just the opposite is true. We teach you how to keep your mind out of the way while you do nothing but allow yourself to completely relax. With the help of your natural instinct, the perfect physiological order and design of your reproductive system will carry you through your entire birthing. If your keep your mind clear of chatter filled with questions, doubts, instructions, and techniques intended to teach your body how to birth, it will happen on its own. Without this interference of your mind-talk, your natural instincts will take over for you. Not anything or anyone knows better than your own instinct.

Of course, we know that there are devices, apparatuses, and drugs that forcefully make your body do what it already knows how to do. But how dare we presume to attempt to improve upon what nature has perfectly orchestrated and validated over centuries?

Dr. Michel Odent, world-renowned birth professional states, "You cannot improve upon a natural function. The answer is not to hinder it."

In presenting your relaxation session, we suggest you give your body permission to take the lead, not the other way around.

If we examine the definition of instinct, we find that the words and phrasing related to instinct all suggest activity that occurs naturally without thought or initiation.

Here are some words and phrases related to instinct:

spontaneous impulse   action not self-initiated
inner sense   reflex
compulsion   predisposition
A knowing that it is not based on experience or learning
A natural, inherent tendency to make a complex and specific
    response to stimuli without involving reason

All these words indicate that the body is capable of functioning and reacting to situations without your conscious thought or consent or input. Some everyday situations that call for involuntary action would be:

- When you attempt to maintain balance.

- When you cower or use your hands to protect yourself from an object hurtling toward you.

- When you pull back your hand from an object that is burning hot.

- When you startle at a sudden loud noise.

When instinct is used to complete a natural body function, these occurrences are naturally set in place while "nothing" is needed to initiate them. Why then are birthing women asked to believe and accept that somehow the beasts in the animal kingdom are endowed with this gift of instinct, while human mothers are somehow overlooked?

You may not have given it a great deal of thought along the way, but you've been depending upon nature and instinct throughout your life, even before you were born. When you were in the womb, no one taught you that when your bladder was full, you needed to do something to release the urine that you were accumulating. Your bladder just released the urine into the amniotic sac. You did nothing to make it happen.

From the moment that you emerged, you took your first breath. Who taught you how to take that breath? You did absolutely nothing to make it happen. Had you been allowed and assisted, you would have instinctively made your way to your mother's breast to feed, as do all mammals. It is no accident that the scent of colostrum is the same as that of amniotic fluid.

Over time as you grew and developed, with nothing to tell you how or when, you used your own special form of communication to let your parents know that you were hungry or needed a little extra comforting. When you felt secure, you could fall asleep in your parent's loving arms. What did you do to learn to fall asleep or to awaken? That's right—nothing.

Fast-forward to when you were a teenager. Your body changed with nothing but internal hormonal secretions to act as catalysts—you became a woman. The Power of Nothing was, and has been, alive in your human experiences in so many ways, and it is ready to perform this magnificent task easily and adeptly. You found yourself in tune with your body and knew its signals.

Nothing had to teach you that you were experiencing your first love. You instinctively knew it and felt it. And when the time was right, you needed nothing to teach you how to express that love physically.

But here we are today, you are pregnant or planning to become pregnant, and all of a sudden it seems that you require advice and counseling from all directions. You are bombarded by well-intentioned friends and family who feel the need to tell their birth stories.

You learn from your care providers and all the experts and women who have birthed a baby that your body is flawed.

You learn that you must place your trust and power into the hands of others. Your previous trust and confidence in yourself as a vital healthy woman quickly crumbles. All of society views you as fragile, vulnerable, and hopelessly emotional.

Abraham Maslow (an American psychologist best known for his theory of a hierarchy of innate human needs) would argue that all these occurrences that pregnant women experience are necessary because human mothers have lost their ability to call upon their birthing instincts. How then do we explain the well-documented fact that since 2009 in the United States alone, seven women in complete comas have given birth to babies unassisted? Their instinct was alive and well and allowed them to birth, in some cases, without being noticed.

HypnoBirthing takes exception to the notion that human mothers have lost their power of instinct. Actually, human mothers have not lost their instinct but have in fact been taught how to birth within the standard medical system.

You will further learn that many of the protocols and procedures that now surround birth are totally contrary to natural, normal means of birthing. One has only to witness that period within a birth when it is time for the baby's descent down through the birth path to total emergence to see that there is little or no allowance for instinct.

It is at this point when care providers are telling mothers that they can now assist and help themselves to birth their babies when just the opposite is true. Complete opening and thinning of the cervix ushers in an entirely new approach. Additional staff are now introduced to the birthing room, the bed on which the mother has been calmly labour-ing in deep relaxation is "broken down," and mother is directed to "scooch her bottom" to the very end of the bed. Her legs are lifted onto grooved metal stirrups or her knees are held by her birth partner or an attendant up and back toward her shoulders. It's common for hospital staff to become genuinely enthusiastic when you near completion of this phase, as they anticipate your actively "pushing" your baby down to crowning.

From this position the mother is expected by most people in the room to begin to forcefully push her baby into the world, using what is known as the Valsalva manoeuvre, all the while with staff almost rhythmically coaching her with loud voices to, "Keep it comin, keep it comin, keep it comin," or "Push harrrrd!!!" This can continue for as long as two-plus hours while both mother and baby become exhausted. At some point the woman is asked to stop pushing because the baby's head has emerged and baby gets his first impression of his new world.

With a few more surges, baby's body usually emerges on its own. Frequently, however, the baby is pulled from his mother's vaginal outlet. Hardly a scene that reflects instincts associated with birthing.

Aside from all the lessons she is learning about how to birth her baby as directed, the birthing mother soon realises that in spite of all her preparation, she has lost the calm and gentle birth she envisioned. She also becomes aware that she has been stripped of her dignity.

Sadly, doctors, too, have been taught to birth in ways that totally exclude instinct. Many graduates go into practise never having seen a normal, instinctive, and unmedicated birth.

Even more regrettable is that some medical schools are advocating that birth can best be accomplished by removing the baby surgically from its mother. Not too many years ago, the local evening news in a metropolitan city featured interviews with medical students who were to graduate within a few days. One woman announced her specialty: obstetrics. When asked why she chose obstetrics, she replied, "Because

I always wanted to be a surgeon." One can only wonder how her statistics read today.

Why We Don't Push—
There's a Kinder Way

"Pushing your baby out" is a rude concept that has no place in gentle birthing; though there are occasions when it becomes necessary to move the birth along more quickly. Pushing is usually counterproductive and is actually a detriment, causing the vaginal sphincters to close ahead of the descending baby. It creates an atmosphere of stress for all involved. Very recent studies suggest that forced pushing over a long period of time can be harmful to a birthing mother and do damage to her pelvic floor. Because the mother is asked to hold her breath and push, the baby is then deprived of much-needed oxygen causing a change in baby's heart rate.

Completion of the opening phase doesn't need to mean the onslaught of a sudden flurry of activity, confusion, or additional staff on the scene. It is important that you avoid any attempt to force or rush this stage. The descent of your baby can be experienced as calmly as your first stage of labour. Many times, HypnoBirthing mums just allow this phase to begin almost unnoticed, as they remain in the position of their choice and just allow the birthing phase to play out, calmly and gently. Because there is no noticeable change in your behaviour, only the most trained eye will detect that you are birthing your baby.

The moves that fall into place at this time should follow the requests you expressed in your birth preferences. You don't want to find yourself caught up in procedures that are different from what you have anticipated or those that your natural instinct dictates.

The material in the chapter—The Law of Natural Birthing Physiology —will clearly show how relying only on nature's gifts, in total relaxation, will allow you to experience the calm and gentle birth of your vision by doing nothing more than what you normally do as you practise your breathing and deepening exercises.

So when it is suggested that you are out of your mind to attempt to birth naturally, you can confidently smile and reply, "Yes, isn't wonderful?"

The Law of
Natural Birthing Physiology

You've explored the Laws of the Mind, as well as the psycho-physical laws, and you've read how important it is to "empty your cup," so to speak, to release any and all fears and limiting thoughts. You've learned that negative thoughts can stand as obstacles to the confidence you've been building in your ability to birth your baby as nature intended. Only when your cup is empty can you make room for new positive thoughts and the real truth about giving birth instinctively. This chapter will discuss the gifts that nature has already provided to you to ensure a natural birth. It will tell you what happens without any effort on your part, but more important, you will learn the details of *how* and *why* birth can be accomplished instinctively. It will assure you that there is a precise design, and you are not on your own.

While relaxation, release, and positive affirmations are essential to your birth preparation, becoming familiar with nature's gifts and educating yourself to the ways in which your own body and your baby are fully capable of performing this magnificent task is equally important. Those nagging fears can be dismissed when you know that the precise design of nature has already taken care of those issues for you in many surprising ways.

The physical natural functions behind what is happening in labour are not generally discussed. Most women know only that "What happens next" includes the information that their babies will descend down the birth path, crown, and then emerge past the perineum. But they don't know what is in place to help that descent go smoothly and comfortably. They inhibit the journey by using activities that they've been mistakenly taught. The details of what is happening are glossed over. Some of these gifts for birth have occurred already along the way of your pregnancy as your baby was growing and developing. Others are specific to your labour and birth.

There is nothing that you have to do to activate the inner body workings of instinctive birthing. Nature has freely provided you and your baby with these incredible birthing gifts. Relax and learn how and why your birthing plays out smoothly and easily.

The Body Begins to Prepare for Birth at Conception—

Nature has provided for the calm and gentle birth of your baby in many ways that most pregnant women are not made aware of. These gifts are naturally well designed, in physiological ways in which your body and your baby work together to help make birthing easier. Several of these manifestations are subtle and start almost from the very beginning of your pregnancy. Some of them will continue after birth. Others occur at various times during pregnancy and labour, and still others come into play only during labour.

The most welcome of the gifts are those that come during the birthing phase of labour. Because of media portrayal of birth and the profusion of unpleasant birth stories, this phase is the one that birthing mothers seem to fear most. Becoming acquainted with these physiological gifts of nature will allay your fears and boost your confidence.

Formation of the Uterine Seal

After the mother's egg is fertilised and the egg cells begin to divide and develop, the egg makes its way through the fallopian tube down into the upper portion of the uterus. The egg sends out little pseudo pods, which attach the egg to the side of the endometrium. Now, here is the remarkable part. At the instant that the egg has successfully attached to the wall of the uterus, the uterine seal begins to form down at the cervix. At this point the cervix is long, thick, and closed and, along with the uterine seal, will remain that way until just before the start of labour. This seal protects the developing baby from exposure to any bacteria that could otherwise enter the uterus. The uterine seal remains intact until it releases at the beginning of labour.

Early Effects from Hormonal Changes

Almost from the beginning of pregnancy, hormones are secreted that change your cervix from a hard, cartilaginous substance into a substance that is loose, spongy, and pliable. The opening of the cervix is one of the processes of labour that women dread because they think it is a serious cause of pain. You can allay that fear and learn just how effective the hormonal change is by feeling the same cartilaginous stiffness at the end of your nose and then feeling the soft supple substance at the end of your earlobe. Over time, the same transformation happens to allow your cervix to open easily. When you are relaxed during the first phase of your labour and endorphins are flowing, your thinning and opening phase moves along more quickly.

Relaxation

Pregnant or not, your body takes its prompts from your mind. Through your pregnancy, you learn to prepare for your birthing by releasing, relaxing, and letting go. There is not much to learn. If all is going nicely, you actually are doing nothing. You will see from the other gifts that trusting the perfectly designed plan of nature will help you to release and relax. You cannot force relaxation, and only you can bring it on. The relaxation that you experience on a daily basis teaches you to become conditioned to instantly relax your body and to enjoy the euphoric comfort that endorphins provide. Relaxation is one of the most important ways to prepare for birth. This is especially true if you are using a programme with a birth companion or friend or reciting a script especially designed to educate you further about your birthing. Relaxation works because of the way in which your mind works. The mind doesn't know the difference between reality and fantasy. Like a child, your mind accepts a message it receives repeatedly; and, over time, it comes to accept that message as being true. It then works toward the goal. Here we see that Law of Repetition in play.

Endorphin Release

Relaxation is the safest and most effective comfort measure that you will use during birthing. The rapid release of endorphins is particularly prevalent if you have practised deep relaxation and deepening techniques on a daily basis.

Since the constrictor hormone—catecholamine—cannot co-exist with the "feel good hormones"—endorphins—the goal is to reach a state of relaxation from the very start of labour to preclude the secretion of catecholamine. After a while, this focused awareness of being able to reach these deeper levels brings on a feeling of being steeped in the almost buoyant state that is created when larger amounts of endor-phins are secreted. Endorphins multiply themselves, so the more you reach deeper levels of relaxation, the more your body will seek that level of relaxation, and you are able to attain it in a shorter amount of time. This natural state of euphoria will gradually become addictive, and you'll find yourself looking forward to each session.

Baby, too, experiences the benefits of daily calm and peace, and his temperament is affected in a positive way. When endorphins are present during labour, the secretion of catecholamine is inhibited; and your body releases the exact amount of oxytocin to cause the birthing muscles to function as they should. With this perfect formula in place, you are able to birth without discomfort, and so is your baby. Because there is no obstructing tension, your birth is able to move along easily and naturally and within a shorter time frame.

As you advance in your pregnancy, you are able to cultivate a deeper trust in instinctive birthing because you are accessing the knowledge of the already-functioning mechanism that is in place within your body. It is a lack of understanding and/or fear that causes constricted birthing muscles. With an ample supply of both knowledge and understanding, you can allow your mind to step aside as you follow, rather than try to lead, the rhythm and flow of your labour that makes all of this possible.

Parents regularly tell us that their babies are mellow and calm and easy to care for during those first few months when they are making the adjustment to life outside the womb. The vertex turn is an early indica-tion of the benefits of remaining stress free through your pregnancy.

Vertex Turn

Between the thirty-second and thirty-seventh week of your preg-nancy, your baby will most likely turn into the vertex position, with his head down in preparation for birthing. Because the brain is housed within the baby's skull, the head is the heaviest part of the body. And, therefore, it usually responds readily to the pull of gravity.

Engagement

As soon as the baby's body turns down, engagement can occur. The studies have shown that when you remain upbeat, rather than uptight, throughout your pregnancy and you teach yourself to avoid stress, your baby is also relaxed and upbeat. She is also developing a calm manner and is better able to respond to events and situations that will carry over into her life outside of the womb. Sometimes babies will not turn until well into that thirty-seventh week. There is no cause for alarm if this is the case. Don't allow yourself to be unnecessarily anxious, and don't start anticipating alternative birthing procedures. The vertex turn is an early indication of the benefits of remaining stress free through your pregnancy.

Two or three weeks before the baby is due to be born, he may move down to a point where the widest part of his head will be at the widest part of the midsection of the pelvis. When this occurs, the baby's head is said to be engaged. This is a good sign, though your walking pattern may change, and sitting may become a whole different experience.

Relaxin Release

The hormone relaxin is secreted during the latter part of pregnancy and contributes to normal birthing in a number of ways. It allows the walls of your vagina to become lubricated, to expand, and to become smooth. It assists in softening the lower segment of your uterus and the expansion of the pelvic region.

1. It causes ligaments within your baby's body to relax, and the baby's body becomes more flexible and supple for easier descent and emergence.

2. It weakens the amniotic membrane and allows it to release.

3. It loosens the mother's skeletal ligaments, allowing the front pubic bone (the pubis symphasis) to shift forward to facilitate an easier descent through the birth path to crowning. (This can also cause a change in your walking pattern that makes wearing sensible shoes a must to help avoid falls or sprains.)

Prostaglandins

When you are nearing your birthing time, you may experience a small amount of pre-labour opening. Many women do. In order for this to happen, your body secretes prostaglandins, which eventually trigger oxytocin, which initiates the start of labour. Oxytocin, in turn, causes uterine surges to begin, and it releases the uterine seal. The appearance of the birth show from the release of the seal is one more signal that the onset of labour is near.

Uterine Surge or Wave

Uterine surges or uterine waves are another result of the effects of the presence of oxytocin. During a surge, the longitudinal, or vertical muscles, in perfect precision, smoothly draw the lower horizontal muscles up and out of the way of the baby's head like an ocean wave. It draws back and then gently nudges the baby forward slightly until the cervix is short, thin, and open. The surges then propel the baby out of the cervix and into the birth path. As this happens, another gift of nature often sets in. Surges rest for a while, and mother and baby also rest. There is nothing to be alarmed about if your labour rests. Your labour has not "shut down." Your body is simply resting. If all is well with your baby, do not be pressured into beginning to "push to get things going." If you're not having surges, you should not be prompted to push. Rest and be thankful for the break. Your labour will start again when baby is ready.

Time Distortion

By being relaxed and focused you may lose track of time—this is another welcome feature for both the opening and thinning phase, as well as the birthing phase when baby is descending.

You may decide to doze during this period, which will help the effect of time distortion. Even if you are not asleep, you will look as though you are. This is where you call upon the deeper relaxation levels and use the Power of Nothing, where you go into your birthing body and let your body birth your baby. You may be aware of the downward motion of the baby, and you will experience a full, bulging feeling at the perineum when the baby is crowning. While the descent may seem to take a long time to onlookers, you will hardly be aware of the passing of time. In many cases the reason for that is that with instinctive birthing, nature often does her job more quickly.

Nature's Birth Journey

The journey that your baby takes down through the birth path to crowning and ultimately to emergence is one of the most feared and actually dreaded phases of birthing. This is unfortunate and needless. I say "needless" because fear of this phase is unwarranted. There is no pathological reason for pain in this second phase of birthing. The media has cast a shadow over the joy, excitement, and anticipation that a mother feels during her pregnancy, and it can affect her level of confidence during birthing.

Harbouring fear of this phase is truly unnecessary because it is precisely at the actual birthing time that nature steps in and takes over the course of your labour. You should remain doing nothing. Nature is in charge and assumes management, unless you are thwarted by other means of management from external sources. Of all of the gifts of birthing, the ones provided during the birthing itself are the most remarkable.

Nature's Gifts for the Birth Phase

The Amnesiac State

Toward the end of the thinning and opening phase of your birthing, just before you reach completion, you will sense a feeling of even deeper relaxation drift over you. Through this period you may even feel a deeper connection with your baby. You will forego conversation and just melt into your birthing body. Many women speak of being better able to connect with their babies' downward movement, and they experience a stronger connection with what is happening within them. In those brief moments as the baby nears birth, you may hear people around you, but you definitely will not care to engage in conversation or take part in any activity other than birthing with your baby. We would like to claim that this ultimate relaxation stems from something that you've learned in your HypnoBirthing classes, but this is purely nature's instinctive birthing. All we've done to assist you in this is to teach you how to easily slip into this ultimate state and provide you with the brief script to learn how to do it. So simple.

As your labour advances, you redirect your mind to your birthing body and go within to birth with your baby. It is a very comfortable state where you find you are so relaxed that you don't really care to speak. It will seem as though it takes too much effort to remain in contact with others. You will be able to hear what is happening and you can choose to listen in, or you can shut out noises or conversation entirely, or you can even drift in and out of this state. You can be selective in tuning out all but your birth companion's voice, as the companion prompts you to begin to relax even deeper.

Dr. Gregory White explodes the myth of chaos and pain in this period of descent. Dr. White says:

1. *"The Second Stage is easier: When the mouth of the womb is completely open, the baby begins to slide into the birth canal. The mother begins to feel heavy pressure on the rectum, as though she were about to have a large bowel movement. This is the phase in which there is no physiological reason for discomfort.*

2. *The mother appears to be markedly indifferent to and withdrawn from what is going on around her, although she is not unconscious; she hears everything that is said. Usually, the mother is calmer and more purposeful during the second stage."* (This is the amnesiac state that we in HypnoBirthing *refer to*.)

Fontanels

There have been many jokes and frightening comments made about the size of a baby's head posing a problem when moving past the pelvis and vaginal outlet. These have also caused an unwarranted fear surrounding birth in the minds of women.

Actually, it is very rare that a mother will carry and birth a child whose head is too large to make the birth journey. It can happen, but not often. Relax and release these fear-provoking thoughts. Here's how it all happens.

This news about fontanels is probably the best news that a pregnant mother can receive. Most people know about the "soft spot" that is evident on a newly born baby's head. Not commonly known is that the soft spot is not there to accommodate the growth of the baby's skull as she gets older. It is there to accommodate her smooth, easy descent through the birth path and her emergence. The process is appropriately called "moulding." The sutures of the baby's skull mould to the contours of your birth path, and they facilitate the turns that the baby makes as she descends.

Surrounding the bony frame of the baby's skull at the top and back of her head is a flexible membranous material called fontanels. This material, much like the texture of a heavy canvas fabric, allows the bones of the skull to "mould" and overlap each other. The usual procedure of the bones involves the lower back suture moving up and under the upper back sutures. Likewise, the front sutures move up and under the front of the upper sutures. All of this reduces the circumference of the baby's head. As the baby emerges, most often the overlapped top sutures can be seen briefly, but as the baby emerges fully, they move back into their normal positioning, leaving what is commonly called the "soft spot." Until the skull suture fully closes, which in some cases can take well over a year for the frontal suture, the soft spot is protected by the membranous fontanels.

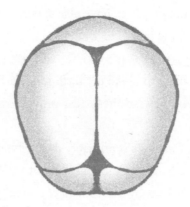

Bone Formation of Baby's Skull (Top View)

Natural Expulsive Reflex (NER)

When the baby is ready for his gradual descent to crowning and birth, your body's natural expulsive reflex (NER) will rhythmically move the baby down with natural pulsations, as you assist with soft gentle Birth Breathing during a surge. You may be aware of the downward motion of the baby, and you will feel a full, bulging feeling at your perineum when the baby is crowning.

You remain in a comfortable, relaxed state and just gently breathe your baby down as you've practised. There is no need for forced pushing.

On this subject, Dr. White further says:

"She feels the progress of the baby's moving, and she becomes more satisfied that she is accomplishing something. At this point, the mother may desire to help by bearing down and she should be allowed to, but (if there is no cause for concern) she should not be urged to do so. She should begin this work only when she feels she must, not because she or the attendant thinks it is a good idea. (Most babies do not require urgent pushing, though attendants may strongly encourage such activities because they do not trust the body's ability to expel the baby naturally.)"

This natural function of your body will assist in clearing your baby's lungs of mucous and may avoid the use of a suction bulb, which is a rude welcome afforded your baby, especially when suctioning is done on the rim of the perineum before your baby is fully born. The benefits and importance of the natural expulsive reflex cannot be over emphasised. When you avoid forced pushing, you maintain a flow of oxygen to your baby and avoid the foetal distress that often occurs in that late state of birthing. Your baby maintains a healthy heart rate. Both baby and mother birth without severe pain, though you may be aware of a bit of pressure. There is no physiological reason for forced pushing. As explained earlier, this is a conditioning that occurred when women were taught to birth. There should be no pain if you use calm breathing to avoid a spasm-like breath and don't force the baby against tissues that may not be ready to receive him.

Let's take a look at the pros and cons of both of the breathing styles used during the actual descent and birth of the baby.

Mother-Directed Birth Breathing	Staff-Directed Forced Pushing
Allows parents to maintain control over their birthing	Tires mother and reduces her effectiveness and participation in birthing experience
Conserves mother's energy	Closes and constricts vaginal passage ahead of baby
Provides continual supply of oxygen to the baby	Emergency intervention can result. Mother becomes exhausted; baby is distressed
Gently opens the birth path for smooth descent	Ruptures eye and facial blood vessels
Increases prospect of birthing over an intact perineum	Limits flow of oxygen to baby, often causing heart-rate deceleration
Perineal tissues unfold naturally for the gentle emergence of baby	Surrenders control of birthing to others
Baby maintains healthy heart rate during descent	Contributes to tearing or the need for episiotomy

On occasion, staff members may tell you that breathing down works for a while, but you need to switch to forced pushing at the end of the descent. If you are using the Power of Nothing, it will just be time that you are not expending a strong effort and you won't be exhausted. Many women find that it is actually faster. Birthing in water will add to your relaxation and to the suppleness of your perineum. You need to trust your natural expulsive reflex to do its job. Sometimes staff members become a bit impatient, but if you stick to your natural expulsive reflex you'll find that it will help your baby to emerge in less time and with less risk of distress. To optimise this gift, you will want to practise Birth Breathing daily on the toilet as you expel a bowel movement. The same expulsive muscle action is used in both situations. (See the section on Breathing Techniques)

Perineal Folds

Because the perineum is toned, the rim is supple and gently unfolds as the baby passes down and out of the vaginal outlet. You will feel some pressure as this happens, but pressure has its own numbing effect. We experience this happening when resting on an arm or a hand while sleeping or when we cross our legs for any length of time. So will the rim of the perineum numb when the baby passes through it. You will not have to deal with the myth of the burning ring, and most mothers don't need an episiotomy. This same pressure will kindly numb the area should you have a small tear.

As the baby emerges from the vaginal outlet past the rim of perineum, you will not experience the stretching of the perineum that most people speak of. The folds of the perineum will gently open. All of the folds are there, and they do not require the assistance of an attendant to pull or tug by "ironing the perineum," as it is sometimes called.

The fact that you will not be forcefully pushing your baby also enhances the gradual unfolding of the rim. It works. Just as the anal rim unfolds, so do the folds of the perineum. It does not need the assistance of a staff member if you have prepared with the perineal massage.

Umbilical Pulsations

When the baby is born, the cord is left unclamped and intact for optimum benefit to the baby. When the cord is left unclamped, the baby's blood supply continues to provide him with oxygen while he gradually becomes accustomed to breathing on his own. This is a very important adjustment that your baby is making, and he needs to be accommodated in this way. By allowing the baby to use his own blood, there is no sudden, sometimes painful, gasp for air. It is also not necessary for attendants to vigorously rub or poke or prod to start the baby breathing or urging him to cry, all of which create an abrupt and confusing experience for the baby. The placental blood remains to oxygenate the baby until his lungs are fully functioning. Umbilical pulsations also allow the baby to receive the blood that is rightfully his to increase his iron storage and ward off anaemia. The placenta will detach more easily when allowed to empty naturally.

There is no particular risk to a baby being born with the cord around its neck, contrary to all the drama that is used to describe this condition. More than a third of babies are born with the cord situated around their necks. The only true danger is when the cord is wrapped and compressed so that circulation is cut off.

Most care providers gently remove the cord by slipping it over the baby's neck at the time of emergence, and the baby continues to be born without incident.

Placental Release

After your baby is born, the cord will continue to pulse until the optimum amount of blood is returned to the baby. The baby will instinctually feel the need to crawl to your nipple for his first feeding. This should be allowed. The scent of colostrum will lure the baby to your nipple and set him in the right direction. This is in keeping with the instinct of all mammals. When the baby is sucking, more oxytocin is released, and this helps to release your placenta from the uterine wall. It also provides you with even more of that valuable "love hormone" that helps to make the mother-baby connection. It helps to allay your baby's fears and gives him a sense of security and safety. It makes the birth afterglow that much more special as you and your partner bond with the baby.

It is important that you learn the importance and significance of these perks of nature so that you can learn to trust that birthing is, indeed, intended to be natural and accomplished with ease.

Relaxation Routine

Muscles send messages to each other.
Clenched fists, a tight mouth, a furrowed brow,
all send signals to the birth-passage muscles, the very
ones that need to be loosened. Opening up to relax
these upper-body parts relaxes the lower ones.

WILLIAM SEARS AND MARTHA SEARS, *THE BIRTH BOOK*

Most athletes will readily advise that relaxation and visualisation are crucial to successful performance. Golfers quickly learn not to "press," but to release and let go. It is not uncommon to see Olympic athletes standing off to the side running visualisations of their perfect performance through their minds. Sports greats know that stress and tension in the mind equate to stress and tension in the body; the two cannot be separated. Conquering stress and fear is what allows sports figures to appear to perform so effortlessly. It's impressive.

There are six basic techniques that we will cover in this section. Each technique has several alternatives so you can choose the one (or more) that you find most effective and that you like best. Learning to use all six techniques so that they become second nature to you will prepare your body and mind for the birth process.

The Six Basic HypnoBirthing Component Techniques

Education	**Relaxation**
Breathing	**Visualisation**
Deepening	**Affirmations**

Taking the time to practise these techniques is an essential part of your daily routine. There is absolutely no substitute for the work you will do to condition your mind and body in preparation for birth. You cannot simply attend classes and hope that the conditioning will occur without your dedication to making it happen. Conditioning involves your mind and your body. A skier would never attempt to compete in a tournament unless his body was conditioned. A runner would never attempt to enter a marathon unless his body was conditioned.

While birthing should not be the exhausting, pushing-your-body-to-the-edge feat that athletes face, it nevertheless requires the same kind of discipline so that when the time comes, you are ready. Since you are conditioning your mind for ultimate relaxation, it is important that you form a pattern that your mind can automatically respond to when it comes time for your birthing. It is time well spent, and it can cut the time and the effort you will spend in your labour. As one who has been there, I can emphatically say that conditioning is a must. You can't slough it off and hope that you'll get lucky.

Your Relaxation Programme

By far one of the most effective ways of dealing with tension, stress, and discomfort without drugs is your own conditioned ability to slip into relaxation and visualisation quickly and at any given moment. In HypnoBirthing you will learn relaxation techniques and visualisations that will see you through your labour and quickly bring about a renewed state of energy following your birthing. It is important that you rehearse these techniques so that you can call them up readily when they are needed.

Establishing Your Routine

- When planning your relaxation, select a time when you won't be disturbed. Take the receiver off the phone or turn off the ringer and answering machine.

- Set aside the same time each day and dedicate yourself to that time.

- Choose a comfortable practice spot that has soft, dim light and make that the place you will use daily.

- Be sure that your bladder is empty.

- Warmth is essential to relieve tension so use a soft throw over your body. Wear clothes that are soft and not binding.

- Use HypnoBirthing CDs or MP3s. We recommend Stephen Halpern's *Comfort Zone* for consistency, as that is the background music used for the Rainbow Relaxation. This music contains tones and rhythms that the body responds to best.

Positions for Relaxation

Your body is the best source of information for the position you will assume when doing relaxation. The general rule is to use the position in which you feel most comfortable. The two recommended positions to follow are Nesting and Side Lying.

Early in your pregnancy, you will no doubt be comfortable on your back while you practise relaxation. Later in your pregnancy, you will want to elevate your upper body to accommodate the extra weight of the baby. Once you gain more weight, you may choose to use a different position. Avoid lying flat on your back, to ensure that the pressure from your growing baby does not obstruct the inferior vena cava, which is a main source of blood and oxygen to your baby.

Nesting

Nesting is one of the best ways of reaching a fully relaxed state quickly. To make your relaxation nest:

- Place one or two pillows under your head and shoulders.

- Allow your shoulders to drift downward and outward.

- Place one pillow under each arm. Allow your arms to gently rest on top of your side pillows with your elbows slightly bent.

- Fingers should be gently and softly cupped.

- Place pillows under the bend of each knee.

- Feet should be about six inches apart, turned outward, relaxed.

Lateral Position

The lateral position is chosen most often by birthing mothers during late labour and frequently for birthing their babies. It is also a position that is usually assumed for sleeping during pregnancy.

- Lie on your left side with the left shoulder, neck, and left side of the head resting on a pillow. The left arm should be placed loosely by your left side.

- With the elbow bent, rest the right arm to the side of the pillow.

- The left leg should be straight down, with the knee slightly bent.

- Bend the right leg up, placing the knee even with your abdomen, with one or two pillows under the knee for support.

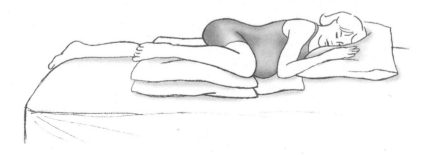

Lateral Position

As you continue to work with the exercises for relaxation, you'll find that each one gives you an explanation of the benefits of the exercise and a brief script that you can use in practise with your birth companion. As you practise these recommended exercises, you will naturally find the one or ones that feel most comfortable for you. It is not necessary that you work with all of them. It is more important that you work with the technique that works best for you.

Facial Relaxation

Achieving deep facial relaxation is most important, as it will set the tone for the rest of your body. The lower jaw area directly affects the vaginal opening. When your lower jaw is relaxed, the vaginal area will be relaxed also. Relax your mouth, just where your teeth meet your pallet. This will prevent your upper and lower teeth from becoming clenched. When you have mastered the art of facial relaxation, your jaws will be totally relaxed, with the lower jaw slightly receded. You will be able to bring yourself into a natural state of relaxation instantly.

Facial Relaxation Technique

Let your eyelids slowly close. Don't try to force them shut. Just let them gently meet. Place your awareness on the muscles in and around your eyes. As you feel a natural drooping of the eye muscles, sense relaxation spreading from your forehead, down across your eyelids, over your cheekbones and around your jaws. Let your lower jaw recede as your teeth part. Your eyelids will feel heavier as your cheeks and your jaw go limp. Bring the relaxation within your eyes to a level where it seems as though your eyelids just refuse to work. Place the tip of your tongue at your palate where your upper teeth and palate meet, bringing about a sense of peace and well-being as you connect with an energy orbit in your body. Feel your head making a dent into your pillow. As you practise this technique, you will feel your neck, shoulders, and elbows droop. Picture your shoulders opening outward and sinking down into the frame of your body as you go deeply into relaxation.

Relaxation Techniques

Once you have learned to bring your breathing into a smooth, rhythmic pace and you can ease yourself into relaxation effortlessly, you can then learn to bring your relaxation on instantly by using one of the methods included here. You do not need to master all of these techniques. You will naturally turn to the ones that are most effective for you and that you like best.

Progressive Relaxation

Sitting in a comfortable chair or sofa, associate each of the designated parts of your body from the top of your head to your toes with the number that corresponds to it on the illustration that follows. Take a deep breath, then as you exhale let it all instantly flow down through your body, causing your muscles to go totally limp. We refer to this state as "Lucy Limp" (Loosey Limp), the name of a soft doll that is like a Beanie Baby.

Eventually, you will be able to take one deep breath and rapidly count off the numbers as you exhale, bringing those parts of your body immediately into a limp state. The more rapidly you think the numbers, the more rapidly you will feel the effects. In using this practise, you should let your body go absolutely limp from the top of your head down to your toes. Let your head hang loose and forward, and let your arms and hands fall limp down by your side.

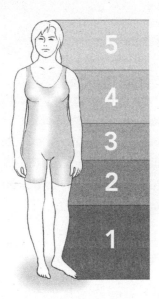

Disappearing Letters

A similar technique for bringing yourself into a deep level of relaxation is to use the Disappearing Letters exercise. It is perhaps the easiest of all the instant relaxation techniques that you will use. It is especially helpful if you feel stressed during the day at work or home or if you need some help falling asleep. When using this technique as an aid to falling asleep, you will actually feel your head creating a deeper indentation into your pillow as your neck muscles thoroughly relax.

With practice, you will find that by the time you reach the first or second "C," the rest of the letters of the alphabet will be erased from your mind. It will be too much effort to say or think the letters, and your body will be limp, as described earlier. This exercise is one of the fastest ways to bring yourself into a wonderful, comfortable state at any time. I recommend it especially to maintain a feeling of calm during that period of adjustment after your baby is born.

Disappearing Letters Technique

- Close your eyes.

- Take in a quick, deep breath—pause.

- Quickly visualise the letters rolling by or coming forward and mentally say to yourself quickly while you exhale:
  AAA—BBB—CCC—D . . . etc.

- Allow your head, neck, shoulders, and upper torso to instantly sink into the frame of your body. Give yourself permission to let your arms, hands, and legs hang loosely. This can be accomplished in seconds and will be very useful for you when you are birthing, as well as at other times.

Light Touch Massage

Birth companions are taught the art of applying Light Touch Massage, a technique developed by Constance Palinsky of Michigan after much research into pain management and the release of endorphins.

The theory of Light Touch is that the smooth muscle just below the surface of the skin, called erector pili, reacts by contracting when stimulated. When this occurs, the muscle pulls up the surface hair, which becomes erect and causes goose bumps. The goose bumps, in turn, help to create endorphins, those feel-good hormones that promote relaxation.

We use Light Touch Massage in birthing because when endorphins are secreted, catecholamine is not. The two cannot co-exist. So the goal of relaxation is to create the feel-good endorphins so that catecholamines cannot take hold. The technique is very simple, yet effective. It is a wonderful comfort measure that the birthing companion brings to the labour room and as a means of nurturing during pregnancy. It is a great way for couples to feel physically closer to each other in the later stages of pregnancy.

The creation of endorphins resulting from practising Light Touch Massage helps to keep our mums calm and comfortable, both prior to birthing and while in labour. If, while the birth companion is applying Light Touch, he extends his hands out and around the sides of the breasts and nipples to apply light nipple stimulation, not only are endorphins produced, but also the hormone oxytocin is created, which naturally enhances uterine surges. For that reason, until you are approaching the very end of your term, the birth companion should not massage the nipples when practising this technique.

Light Touch Massage can be applied while the mother is sitting on a birth ball leaning on pillows at the side of a bed. If the couple is in a hospital, they can request that the foot of the bed be adjusted to create a kneeler. Mothers can also have the head of the bed adjusted upright so that she can kneel on the centre of the bed and rest her arms and head at the top of the bed on a pillow. This is an excellent position to give her the advantage of being upright when baby is descending during birth. If birthing is taking place at home or in a birthing centre, the same effect can be achieved by kneeling on a pillow in front of a chair, a sofa, or at the side of a bed with pillows stacked upright for you to rest your arms and head on. Your birthing companion can kneel behind you while administering Light Touch Massage as illustrated or can also use a chair.

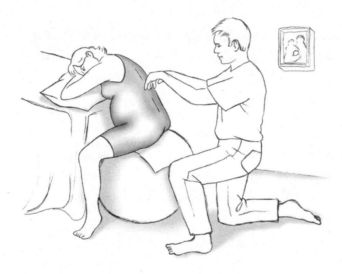

Birth Companion Applies Light Touch Massage

While children, as well as adults, enjoy Light Touch Massage, it should not be used with infants as their nervous system is not developed sufficiently to be able to experience the kind of stimulation that Light Tough offers. After three or four months, you can use Light Touch to calm a fretful child.

Light Touch Massage Technique

- The birth companion places the BACK side of his or her fingers so that they meet at the base of the tailbone. The fingers are then drawn up and out from the spine in a V-like motion. The pattern is gradually continued upward across the back until the base of the neck is reached. The hands are then brought around the neck and to the sides of the ears. The undersides of the arms and around the elbows are particularly effective areas for the massage.

• The second motion involves placing the BACK of the fingers at the base of the spine and then, as before, gradually working upward, forming a horizontal, figure-eight pattern that criss-crosses at the centre of the back.

• This technique is demonstrated in HypnoBirthing classes, and you will have the opportunity to practise it as well. It is an extremely important element in HypnoBirthing. When the birth companion does it right, the mother will be amazed at the results.

Anchors

In the practice of hypnosis, an anchor is a means of creating a lasting imprint or signal through an association with a gesture, sound, image, or touch. The thought or suggestion is said to be anchored into the memory of the subconscious. In HypnoBirthing, the birth companion will plant an anchor that is a signal to you to go more deeply into relaxation by placing his hand on your shoulder during your practise sessions. The birth companion instructs the mother that when she feels the hand being placed on her shoulder, with a gentle downward press, she will immediately relax twice as deeply as she is at the moment. You will be amazed at the power of this technique. I suggest that you make it a regular part of your practice together.

Anchors can be used in any number of ways for birthing and in other situations. One woman in a HypnoBirthing class kept forgetting to take her vitamins. She anchored a reminder that when she picked up her car keys to leave in the morning, she would remember to take her vitamins. She never missed a day after that.

Breathing Techniques

There are only three gentle breathing techniques used in Hypno-Birthing: Calm Breathing, Surge Breathing, and Birth Breathing.

Calm Breathing

Calm Breathing is simply what its name implies. This breath can easily be applied on a regular basis to many situations in your life when you are feeling tense, frightened, or fatigued. It is a breathing style designed to help you enter a calm, relaxed state so that you can continue with imagery and visualisation practice. You'll find it especially helpful after your baby is born when you just sit quietly with your baby and connect with her. It is the breath usually used at the beginning of a meditation or relaxation session.

Calm breathing maintains the sufficient, continual supply of oxygen to your baby during labour. This oxygen is the most important fuel for the working muscles in the uterus. That is why proper breathing is so important to your relaxation. The Calm Breathing technique is used at the beginning of each relaxation practice to help your body gradually slip into a comfortable state of relaxation. You will want to focus your awareness on this technique early in your programme.

Calm Breathing will help you to achieve relaxation when you are practising alone or with your birth companion. It is also one of the methods you will use to resume relaxation between uterine surges during birthing. This technique will help you to conserve energy during the thinning and opening phase of labour. To establish a proper breathing technique for Calm Breathing, practise the following exercise.

Calm Breathing Technique

- Relax and settle into the comfort of a chair or sofa and let pillows support your head and neck.

- Allow your head to gently lean forward toward your chest, or let it rest back onto pillows behind you.

- Let your eyelids gently meet without forcing them shut.

- Your mouth should be softly closed with your lips touching lightly.

- Place the tip of your tongue at your palate where your teeth and your palate meet and feel the wonderful sense of relaxation drifting throughout your body.

- Take in a short breath through your nose, to a count of four: mentally recite "In–2–3–4" on the intake. Feel your stomach rise as you draw the breath up and into the back of your throat. Pause.

- As you exhale, mentally recite "Out–2–3–4–5–6–7–8." Do not exhale through your mouth. As you breathe out very slowly through your nose, direct the energy of the breath down and inward toward the back of your throat, allowing your shoulders to droop into the frame of your body. Breathe your body down into relaxation. Release all tension and let go.

To determine if you are doing this exercise correctly, place your left hand on your stomach and your right hand on the lower part of your chest. As you inhale, you should feel your left hand rising as though your stomach were inflating like a balloon. As you exhale, you will feel your hands fold into each other as your chest and stomach create a crevice.

Calm Breathing is easy to master. You will use it regularly in your classes and in your home practice. You'll feel relaxation coming more easily and rapidly each time you do it. When you have mastered the concept, it will not be necessary for you to recite numbers or test with your hands to guide yourself into this state. After doing this only a few times, you will be able to bring your body into a deep state of relaxation in preparation for further deepening work.

Surge Breathing

The name of this breathing, Surge Breathing, suggests when it is used in labour. This breathing style is used throughout the entire period that your cervix is opening and thinning. Each time that you experience a uterine surge or wave, this breath helps you to work with your birthing body. It is actually assisting labour progress rather than resisting. It works in conjunction with the vertical muscles as they draw up the horizontal muscles to allow the cervix to open. HypnoBirthing mothers find that because of this feature, their surges last a shorter time than usual, and, therefore, the opening and thinning phase is shortened.

You will want to devote time to Surge Breathing, as it is this technique that will be with you until it is time to breathe your baby down to crowning.

The following exercise will take you through the steps of Surge Breathing.

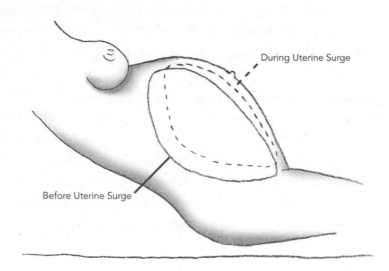

During Uterine Surge

Before Uterine Surge

The Uterus During Surge

Surge Breathing Technique

- In a lateral position, place a pillow under your back and shoulders.

- Place both hands across the top of your abdomen with your fingers loosely meshed between each other.

- Breathe down into your abdomen to clear your breath.

- Using only your abdominal muscles, take in a breath and let your abdomen expand into your cupped fingers. Do this several times and note the way your abdomen moves outward as it expands. Once more, expand the abdomen and note the motion and the way in which your fingers move outward. Repeat this several times to get the feeling of the expanding and receding abdomen.

- Now you are ready to practise the actual Surge Breathing.

- Again with your fingers slightly cupped, slowly inhale to a rapid count of 20 while you take in your breath and expand your abdomen as though it were a large colored balloon. Pause.

- With an equally slow pace, exhale down into your abdomen as it recedes.

You should begin to practise Surge Breathing as soon as you can. Continue to practise this exercise throughout your pregnancy until your body becomes conditioned to this expansion with each surge.

Birth Breathing

The third style of breathing is called Birth Breathing. It's the technique that you will use during birthing when you are breathing your baby down through the birth path to emergence during the birthing phase. You will begin to practise Birth Breathing immediately.

Like the other two breathing styles, Birth Breathing clearly describes when this breath is applied. Once your cervix has reached a degree of opening sufficient for the baby to pass down out of the cervix, Birth

Breathing will step in and will assist the natural expulsive reflex (NER) of your body to move your baby down to crowning and birth.

Birth Breathing. . . Don't Push Me, Mummy

Birth Breathing is used when you are breathing your baby down during the birthing phase of labour. It is intended to assist the natural expulsive reflex (NER) of your body to move your baby gently down to crowning and birth.

Birth Breathing is NOT pushing. Pushing can be counterproductive and actually slow down the birthing process. The concept of pushing your baby out is a rude and unnecessary one. This is one of the classic examples of how women, contrary to their natural birthing instincts, have been taught how to birth.

For hundreds of years, totally anaesthetised women had their babies extracted from their bodies with forceps. They were unable to immediately see their babies and sometimes did not see or hold their babies until the following day. As a result of this extraction and the other unnecessary procedures that resulted, women were confined to their beds for days following their births.

Few doctors had the opportunity to witness a baby being naturally born, as most natural births were still taking place at home with midwives.

Unanaesthetised birth came upon the birthing scene when Dr. Ferdinand Lamaze introduced his concept of easier birthing through focused attention that distracted mothers from the pain of birthing. The problem presented, however, was that so many birth professionals, accustomed only to seeing women giving birth with forceps, did not believe that the baby would descend and emerge on his own. (A belief that remains even today as HypnoBirthing mothers are told that their babies will not be born unless the mother is willing "to help yourself and push that baby out.")

It was then thought, however, that since there was no means of extracting the baby with instruments, the baby would have to be "pushed" down through the birth path and out past the vaginal outlet.

A technique was devised and readily accepted in birthing circles. Staff members "coached" the birthing mother in unison, while she held her breath and violently pushed, usually to the count of 10. They cheered her on while one staff member and a birth companion would draw her knees up to her shoulders with each surge. Another means was lifting the mother's head and shoulders forward, forming what was called a "C position," while other staff members counted 1 and 2 and 3, all the way up to 10. Because the mother's pushing caused the blood vessels in her face and eyes to bulge and become purple from the violent pushing, this was called "purple pushing."

Sadly, today this very scene still plays out in most hospital births. It has become the source of many attempts at humour. No one seems to question the indignity that the mother experiences during this time.

Forced pushing creates stress for the birthing mother, which is self-defeating in that it closes the sphincters of the vagina ahead of the descending baby. Any woman who attempts to simulate forced pushing will immediately verify that there is a tensing of the muscles in the lower birth path, not a release.

In spite of this, most birth professionals cling to the loud, chaotic means of "helping" the baby out.

There has been much written about the inefficiency of forced pushing and the possible damaging effect it has on the muscles of the birthing woman's pelvic floor.

While the woman who finds herself unable to push because she has been administered an epidural is allowed to "labour down" by letting her body naturally expel her baby, the woman in the next room who has deliberately planned for a natural birth is expected to forcefully "push her baby out." It is an unnecessary carry over, when we consider that women in comas have given birth undetected.

With Birth Breathing, there is no need for a lengthy period of hard, violent pushing during descent. Your baby's descent will be gradual, but it will not necessarily take longer. The natural pulsations of your body will move your baby down the birth path efficiently and gently. Many mothers report using only two or three Birth Breaths to bring their babies to full emergence. That's because the sphincters at the outlet are not tense and closed. The relaxed body will naturally open for you. Birth Breathing also gives your baby the advantage of a kinder, safer, and gentler birth.

Forced pushing can exhaust you and press your baby against a resistant passage that is not yet receptive to his journey. Stories of exhaustive pushing that extends over hours bear out the fact that the baby will descend when he and the birth path are ready. There is no need to rush. The natural birthing process has a purpose that must be respected and trusted.

Often women themselves will speak of an overwhelming urge to push taking over. If this is felt, it is also because of conditioning that stems from a deeply embedded notion that babies cannot descend on their own. We seem to be the only mammals who turn our birthings into what appears to be a gymnastic event, complete with "squat bars" and knotted ropes on which mothers can suspend themselves. This scene hardly holds a mirror up to nature. Our animal sisters elect to gently expel their babies.

A calm, gentle nudging breath can be recaptured by slowly establishing the same kind of relaxation that you used for your Calm Breathing practice. Even if you initially feel the conditioned "urge to push," surrendering to this impulse can totally turn your birthing around, as it limits the amount of oxygen going to your baby. This can cause concern on the part of caregivers, as your baby's heart rate can decelerate. It may lead to the very special circumstance that you've worked so hard to avoid. Let your baby and your body determine the pace. Breathe down into your body to relax the vaginal outlet and follow whatever lead your baby takes.

Birth Breathing is one of the most important of all the exercises you will practise. It is easily accomplished by using your body's natural expulsive reflex that occurs each and every time you use the toilet to expel your daily stool. It is the most natural function that the expulsive muscles use routinely.

When your cervix has reached completion, you should feel the urge now to breathe downward rather than upward. This will be a natural transition for you. Rather than allow your body to slip in a spasm-like surge, you will remain in whatever position is comfortable for you and simply allow Calm Breaths to guide you into breathing down.

Birth Breathing Technique

- Assume a comfortable position.

- Your body will feel the urge to breathe down, and you should only breathe down when in surge.

- Follow the lead of your body and your baby.

- Your mouth should be softly closed and not pursed; no breath should escape through the mouth.

- Breath is taken in and let out through the nose.

- You will remain in an amnesiac state as you and baby birth together.

- Use Calm Breathing to avoid pushing.

- Direct the energy of your breath to the lower back of your throat and allow that thrust of energy to move down through your back as it gently nudges your baby down and out through your vaginal outlet.

- Inhale again and direct that energy to the back of your throat and down your back all the way to the vaginal outlet.

- Keep the vaginal outlet and your anal passage open in between breaths so you will not lose the momentum.

The perfect place to practise this exercise is on the toilet as you are guiding the stool down and out of the anal passage. Make it a point to do this each and every time you are using the toilet in this way. You will find that you will accomplish the task easier and more quickly each time.

Visualisation Techniques

The breathing and relaxation exercises in the previous chapters are fundamental elements of HypnoBirthing and should be practised daily. The visualisation exercises are merely tools to help you during labour. You may find one or all of them useful to calm your mind and relax your body. Therefore, you should experiment to find the ones you like. These visualisation exercises, while helpful, do not need to be part of your daily routine. The exception is Rainbow Relaxation.

Rainbow Relaxation

Rainbow Relaxation is the cornerstone of our relaxation and visualisation programme. It incorporates the many colors that are associated with the energy centres of our body. The background music, "The Comfort Zone," is a composition by Steven Halpern, a world-renowned author, composer, and recording artist whose sounds are designed to bring your thoughts into harmony with the natural flow of energy within your body.

The following explanation of how the Rainbow Relaxation technique is used will give you an understanding of what to expect and how the important repeated practise with this recording is more effective than a scripted theme in effecting your ultimate conditioning for birthing. You should practise the entire Rainbow Relaxation every day. Your HypnoBirthing practitioner will provide you with the Rainbow Relaxation recording along with your textbook, both of which are included in your tuition.

During deep relaxation practice, the brain and the nervous system become saturated with the picture of your specific goals or ideals. The repetition of these images seems so real to the subconscious that the images become imprinted in your mind and embedded in your subconscious. The assimilation of these visions creates acceptance, belief, and confidence in achieving the desired outcome. In your case these images are easier, gentler birthing and a calm, peaceful life.

If there are any words or images on the CD that you don't feel comfortable with, just mentally substitute a word or a phrase that you feel better suits you and let that substitution bring you even deeper into relaxation. All hypnosis is self-hypnosis, and it's important to know that no one else brings you into this state except yourself. Hypnosis is a therapy of consent. If you are finding that you need help in reaching a deep level of relaxation, speak to your practitioner so that together you can get to the root of why this is happening.

Often mums will question if the time they are spending in practice is working for them. They find that after one or two practise sessions, they no longer are able to stay with the material because they drift off into their own thoughts or they fall into a deep sleep. Actually, nothing could be better. If this should happen to you, be aware that you are not actually asleep. You have successfully conditioned your mind to respond immediately by bringing yourself into a state that seems like sleep. If this happens regularly, just know that your subconscious is tuned in to your practise sessions and is processing them for you. That is part of the conditioning effect.

For the purpose of conditioning your mind to relax, Rainbow Relaxation does not have a sequence or "story" to it. The repetition of the wording is especially designed to help you tune out your surroundings and bring you to the level of relaxation that you want to reach quickly. As pleasant as it may be, visualising scenes in nature or spending an inordinate amount of time in progressive relaxation during your practice sessions is not necessary. Whether you mentally visualise the process, your birthing companion walks you through it, or you listen to the CD, you will easily master the art after the first week if you allow yourself to just go with it. If you are enjoying the process, you may obtain other discs from the Institute, but the Rainbow exercise will do the trick for you if you are conditioning your mind and body to respond with deep relaxation.

The birth companion is an active participant throughout the birthing experience. Rather than an onlooker who vacillates between feeling helpless and unknowledgeable, in HypnoBirthing the birth companion is actually the trained facilitator and primary support person for the birthing mother. The perinatal bonding that takes place among mother, baby, and the birthing companion during this wonderful interlude, combined with the mother's conditioned relaxation, is the whole key to achieving a satisfying birth for all of you. The baby becomes familiar with the birth companion's voice during these sessions, and all of this contributes to the important post-natal bonding and helps the newborn's adjustment.

As often as possible, the birthing companion should practise the Rainbow Relaxation with you, following the outline below. This practice is important so that you will be able to drift into a deep level of relaxation on hearing your birth companion's voice. When you practise with your birth companion, it is better to keep your sessions shorter, but more frequent. This will prevent your time together from becoming a lengthy chore that can be put off until you "can find more time."

While reciting the sequence of colours, the birth companion should stroke your hand and arm in a soft downward motion, simulating the flow of natural relaxation that will drift throughout your body while you are in the thinning and opening phase of labour.

The Birth Companion's Reading (to follow) provides a visualisation of moving through labour that can help you to envision a smooth, calm birth. This can be practised alternately with the Rainbow Relaxation. When you choose to use the Birth Companion's Reading, have the mother picture herself stepping into the happy scene of both of you holding and bonding with your baby seconds after birth. This is an important visualisation for creating an imprint of a positive, happy outcome.

The practice that you do together is intended to strengthen the conditioning that comes from your learning to respond to your birth companion's voice and touch. It will also strengthen the bond between you as you anticipate your upcoming birthing.

Rainbow Relaxation Technique

- Find a place where you both can be comfortable and where the lighting is soft. Mother should be sitting in a chair with her head resting on the back of the chair or on a sofa with pillows beneath

her head and shoulders so that the top of her body is elevated
slightly.

- Mother, gently bring yourself into a deep state of relaxation—the
kind you have been teaching yourself. Breathe in relaxation and
breathe down relaxation throughout your body, using the Calm
Breathing technique.

- Once you have brought yourself into this calm state of relaxation,
picture yourself gently resting on a bed of strawberry-coloured
mist that is about a foot and a half high. Picture the soft red mist
as a mist of natural relaxation flowing through and around your
body. Continue to relax until it seems that your body is almost
weightless and seems to meld into the mist. Feel the coloured
mist caressing your shoulders, midriff, buttocks, and legs. Allow
yourself to "let go" and feel as though you are floating on the
strawberry-coloured mist. Feel the gentle sway. See this soft mist
saturating your body as you go deeper into relaxation. Feel your
body growing numb, almost as though it were a piece of soft,
strawberry-coloured cloth. Allow yourself to feel the mist of deep
relaxation permeating your mind and body from the top of your
head to your toes. Feel the tingling of relaxation on the soles of
your feet. Imagine your own natural mist of relaxation swirling
over and around your body—mind and body at peace and tranquil.

- Now picture yourself resting on a bed of pale, orange-coloured
mist, while your body becomes even more comfortable. Follow
the same visualisation as you did for the soft strawberry colour.
Imagine the coloured mist sweeping across your body, starting at
the top of your head, caressing your shoulders, chest, arms, and
legs, and slowly drifting all the way down to your feet. Again,

feel the tingling of relaxation on the soles of your feet and know that you are going deeper in relaxation.

- Next picture yourself on a mist of soft yellow, with the coloured mist surrounding your body, starting at the very top of your head and drifting down across your cheeks, jaws, and mouth. Now the same quality of relaxation slips down across your shoulders, upper arms, elbows, and hands and wanders down through your abdomen, legs, and to the very bottom of the soles of your feet.

- Continue the visualisation until all the remaining colours of the rainbow have been envisioned—green, blue, and indigo, then white for clarity.

- Now slowly bring yourself back to the room, feeling alert and energised.

The Birth Companion's Reading

The Birth Companion reading can be alternative to the Rainbow. This reading is adapted from one originally composed by Henry Leo Bolduc for his wife Joan when they were preparing for the birth of their baby. The script appears in Henry's book *Self-Hypnosis: Creating Your Own Destiny*.

His reading was an outpouring of the awe with which a father views this wonderful miracle. Henry expresses sensitivity to perinatal bonding when he points out that the attitude and philosophy of the mother and the birth companion are as much a gentle suggestion for the child during birthing as it is reassurance for the mother.

Thanks to Henry for allowing me to incorporate a few HypnoBirthing images into his script.

New life is forming, growing and moving within you. You are part of the promise and the destiny of life itself. A very important event is taking place in your life . . . a wonderfully normal, natural, biological, and spiritual event. You're going to have a baby. What is happening now is the process of birthing and freeing the kicking, moving little being who's been a part of your body for so long.

Soon it will be time for the baby to become its own separate person. One cycle is ending and, immediately, another is beginning. What has been called "labour" is that in-between experience . . . the fulcrum . . . that small, short period of time and space between the baby's two worlds.

Change from one stage to another brings pressure, and then release. You will soon experience this as the change is completed and fulfilled. You can feel this and embrace it and welcome it as refreshing and totally natural.

With mind, you build a healthy attitude and happy expectation. Happy childbirth has much to do with a healthy, joyous, loving antici-pation. It is something remarkably beautiful. Being a channel of new life is said to be a spiritual experience. With this understanding, total relaxation, and serene breathing, all discomfort is lessened and often entirely absent.

As you begin labour, meditate on the tremendous universal force . . . the life force of nature with which you are in complete harmony during this experience.

Whenever you feel your body begin to surge, actively think "release" and "let go" of tension. There is a time for experiencing that uterine wave, flowing with it, and ultimately releasing and letting go.

You are learning to relax, to flow and melt with the very rhythm of life itself. With relaxation and positive expectation, you have come to know that all things are possible.

In your mind's eye, picture the shore of a lake or an ocean. Watch the endless waves softly brushing to the shore . . . the ebb and flow of the water. Observe it advancing and withdrawing over the sand. Become a part of it, flowing into it. Become a part of the rhythm of the waves within your own body . . . the surge and release.

Breathe in the natural relaxants of your own body . . . endorphins, many times more effective than the strongest drugs known to man . . . create your own serenity and release it throughout your body . . . breathing in and breathing through . . . giving birth to your baby.

With proper physical, spiritual, and mental exercise, you are preparing yourself for this wonderful celebration of life. As you get into the rhythm and work with your mind and body, the easier and smoother it becomes. Each time you hear your birth companion's voice and feel the gentle touch: the more easily your relaxation deepens.

Breathe . . . slowly, confidently, gently. Each time you breathe in, breathe in relaxation and peace. Each time you breathe out, breathe out stress, as the body's natural endorphins willfully breathe out tension and stress.

Feel only the sway of the wave that is bringing your baby closer and closer to birth. Relax and flow with your body's natural rhythm, confident in the fact that your body knows what to do. Give your birthing over to your body. Trust it. Relax and let it do its job.

With your mind's eye and your inner senses, mentally and emotionally feel yourself joyfully, totally aware and participating. See it as already accomplished. Listen with your mind's ear to that first sound of new life.

Create a vivid visualisation of the exhilaration you feel as you see your baby at the moment of birth. See the three of you bonding for the first time in this life. Now mentally see yourself stepping into this joyful scene. Become a part of this birthing . . . fulfilled. Feel it . . . sense it. This is your body, here, now. In your mind's eye, see and feel yourself totally enveloping that body . . . holding the baby on your breast. These are your arms enfolding your baby; these are your hands embracing this new little being.

You knew you could do it, and you did. You did well, and the feeling of ecstasy is one that will never be surpassed.

Join in with joy and amazement and watch the continuing mystery of creation unfold. The life force of nature is working in harmony with you. Now more than at any moment in your life, it is within you and with you. You are an integral part of nature, and nature is an integral part of your being. You are a part of the greatest celebration of life. You are a part of the promise and the destiny of life itself.

The Opening Blossom

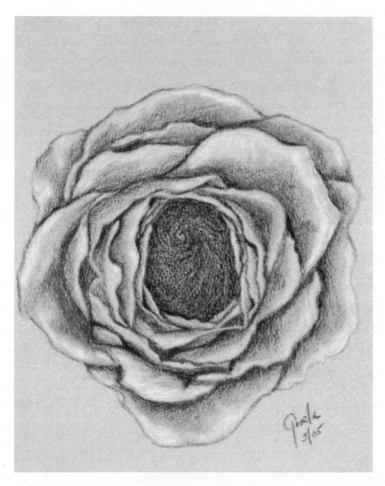

One of the most simple and effective visualisations is that of an opening rose. Use your breathing techniques to bring yourself into relaxation, then close your eyes and envision your baby moving gently down to the vaginal outlet. Imagine the gradual opening of the perineum to be like the gentle unfolding of the petals of the rose. This visualisation is recommended during the final days of your pregnancy to achieve the onset of labour, and also during the opening and birthing phases of labour.

Blue Satin Ribbons

Remember the lower circular muscle fibres that are drawn up and back to effect the thinning and opening of your cervix? Close your eyes and imagine the muscles not as fibres, but as soft, blue satin ribbons that gently and easily yield to the rhythmic draw of the vertical muscles, swirling up and back. You can practise this visualisation toward the end of your pregnancy so that it will be there for you during the surges of the thinning and opening phase of your labour.

The Arm-Wrist Relaxation Test

Because you don't really experience a particular sensation when you are in self-hypnosis, you will be amused and amazed at the Arm-Wrist Relaxation Test. It is very simple and, at the same time, very convincing. The technique is meant to assure both the birth companion and the mum that all the practice that you've been doing is working.

The Arm-Wrist Relaxation Technique

Lie on your back, with your arms at your side, your fingers gently cupped on the surface of the bed or sofa. Do not lie flat on your back for long periods of time or when you are in the late stages of pregnancy or in labour.

Once you are in a state of relaxation, picture that your birth companion has tied a giant, helium-filled red balloon to your right wrist. Almost immediately you will feel a tug on your wrist as the balloon

pulls upward. Now another helium-filled balloon—this one orange—
is added. The two balloons are tugging even harder on your wrist.
Your arm is beginning to rise upward. You sense that your elbow is
making a dent in the cushion or surface of your bed. The deeper the
dent, the more your wrist moves upward. With each tug, your arm is
being pulled higher. Still another balloon—a yellow one—is being
added. Each time a balloon is added, your arm begins to feel lighter
and lighter. The more you try to hold your wrist down, the more the
helium is pulling your arm upward. Your arm cannot resist the pull
of the balloons. Try as you may to hold it down, your wrist is being
yanked upward. Continue to picture more balloons being added with
all of the colours of the rainbow.

When your arm rises approximately six to ten inches off the bed,
place it back at your side. Each time you practise this exercise, fewer
balloons will be required to make your arm and wrist tilt upward.
At the end of each relaxation period, tell yourself that each time you
practise, relaxation will take over your body sooner than ever before.
Your goal should be to assume a deep level of relaxation within a very
short period of time.

Ultra-Deepening Techniques

These techniques have been found to be extremely effective in deepening relaxation to a point where the mother's body is totally limp, and she is in an almost amnesiac state. The expanded sessions of these exercises that you will practise in class with your practitioner will help you achieve the deep level of relaxation that you will use when you are nearing completion and beginning to use gentle Birth Breathing. This total relaxation allows the mum to go within to her birthing body and her baby. Often a mother will remain in this deep state while she breathes her baby down the birth path to the time for the baby to emerge.

To practise this combination of techniques, just breathe yourself into a state of relaxation. Once your body feels comfortably limp, you are ready to proceed.

Glove Relaxation

Glove Relaxation is the first of a combination of deepening techniques, and it is one of the best ways for you and your birth companion to plant an anchor for deep, soothing relaxation. It is also quite effective as a directive during labour and birthing. For this reason, I recommend that it be one of the primary elements of your practice sessions.

Glove Relaxation Technique

Imagine that you are putting a soft, silver glove onto your right hand—a special glove of natural endorphins. Immediately the fingers of your hand begin to feel larger and to tingle, as though there were springs at the ends of your fingers. The silver glove, with its endorphins flowing around your fingers, your palm, and the back of your hand, will cause your hand to feel numb, the way it would if you were to place it into a large container of icy slush.

As your birth companion strokes the back of your hand and arm, feel a tingling and then a numbness surrounding your hand and moving up your arm. Once your hand and arm lose all sensation, they begin to seem as lifeless and senseless as a piece of wood or a piece of leather. The silver mist of endorphins gradually drifts throughout your hand so that it can be transferred wherever you wish to bring about relaxation and comfort. To transfer the numbing effect, just visualise placing your hand on various parts of your body—each part now feels light, numb, and senseless. Even mothers who claim to feel uncomfortable when being touched fall into relaxation when the birth companion uses this technique and recites birthing prompts.

Practice will condition your body to react with calm when you feel your hand and arm being stroked. Go only with your breathing and your visualisations, not your body. Let your body continue to lie totally limp and senseless.

The Depthometer

The purpose of this exercise is to have you experience bringing yourself into an ultradeep state of relaxation—the kind you will use during the latter part of the opening phase of labour.

The Depthometer Technique

In your mind's eye, see or imagine within your body a large, soft, flexible, inverted thermometer. The bulb of the thermometer is just above your forehead. The flexible tube extends all the way down to your toes. Inside the bulb is a clear fluid of natural relaxation.

There are forty gradations on the thermometer. As you count down from 40 to 39 to 38, and so on, picture the fluid of relaxation gently flowing down from one number to the next, flowing out into your circulatory system and bringing your body into relaxation. To reinforce the concept of relaxation filling every cell, nerve, and muscle of your body, visualise more fluid flowing down into the tube of the thermometer. You will feel a deep relaxation gradually saturating your body as the fluid fills the space in the tube.

As you reach each descending decade number on the thermometer —30, 20, 10, and 0—you will experience the feeling of doubling your current relaxation as you go deeper. By the time you reach the lower teens, you will find yourself in a very deep relaxation. The final ten digits will bring you to the ultra-deep relaxation you will use during the latter part of the thinning and opening phase of labour.

When you reach this new ultradeep level you will find yourself in the control centre of your inner mind.

When your body is thoroughly relaxed, the feeling of calm flowing from the silver glove will drift around your wrist, your lower arm, and now all the way to your elbow. Your arm begins to feel almost as though it were not there. Once you experience this sensation, the relaxation can be transferred to other parts of your body, particularly the lower pelvic area. You can use this visualisation alone or with your birthing companion in practice or during labour.

The Sensory Gate Control Valve

While still in your inner control room, look around you, and you'll see in your mind's eye a large control panel with many lights and switches. In the middle of that panel is a large round valve, and above the valve are the words "HypnoBirthing Valve."

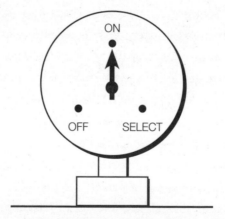

The Sensory Gate Control Valve

The Sensory Gate Valve Technique

This valve controls the messages that are sent from the brain past the sensory gate in the brain stem to all of the nerves in your body. You can use the indicator switch on this valve to shut off feeling throughout your body. Simply see yourself turning the switch on the valve to the "off" position at eight o'clock.

This imagery, combined with the Glove relaxation, helps to bring about a loss of sensation in selected parts of your body. The imagery of the control valve can be used for any number of things, such as keeping your blood pressure at a safe and healthy level, maintaining a safe amount of amniotic fluid and controlling your stress level. You might want to give it a test by suggesting to yourself that your right foot is just too numb and heavy. No matter how hard you try, it does not want to lift; it is stuck to the floor.

Be sure to return the switch to the off position and release all self-hypnosis and restore all normal functions to your body before attempting to move about.

You will experience practise with an additional ultra-depth for birthing script in your HypnoBirthing class session.

Time Distortion

We know that people who experience hypnosis rarely have a good sense of the length of time that they are in a session. This is a blessing to the birthing mother.

Once you have mastered the art of bringing yourself into relaxation, you may want to begin practising time distortion. When you are in a relaxed state, give yourself the suggestion that every five minutes will seem as one minute. During labour, when you are nearing the end of your thinning and opening phase, the birth companion will give you the suggestion that every twenty minutes will seem as five. Time distortion is an important part of birthing and is included among the prompts used by the birth companion.

This loss of a sense of time, and the accompanying state of amnesia, comes at a time in labour when you are so deeply relaxed that it is difficult for you to talk, and you lose a sense of the people around you. At this time, you will go more deeply into your birthing body and to your baby, and you will begin your journey together. This is a gift of nature that can occur with all birthings if the mother is willing to let go, bring herself deep enough, and turn her birthing over to her birthing instinct and her baby.

The partner's encouragement and practical help increase the effectiveness of labour-coping techniques, such as creative imagery and breathing patterns. The presence also increases the woman's chance of an emotionally fulfilling birth.

Carl Jones, *The Birth Partner's Handbook*

Nutrition

Contributions by Dr. Charles Swencionis

---

e've talked about the emotional, mental, and psychological aspects of birthing. These are all important to help you achieve a calm and relaxed birthing. But what you put into your body in the way of nutrition and how you prepare your body physically for birthing can make all the difference in the world in how your birthing plays out. Good nutrition is essential if you hope to have a healthy pregnancy and healthy birth and intend to sidestep many of the special circumstances of late pregnancy that can turn your birthing around.

Water: The Miracle Liquid

Consuming a sufficient amount of water is one of the most important elements in your daily health routine during pregnancy, and it's one of the easiest tasks that you can fit into your schedule. You need to consume water and other liquids, such as juices, to keep your body hydrated for better all-around bodily function. Hydration is paramount.

Approximately 60 percent of the human body is composed of water. It is one of the chief means of transportation within the body, carrying essential nutrients to the tissues and muscles that need them. Water aids in your digestion by moving food through the digestive system and then moving toxic waste products out of your body in elimination—two very important considerations when you are pregnant. Water acts as a lubricant, as well as a cushion for joints and muscles, and plays a major role in the spinal cord. It also helps to maintain a healthy body temperature. Because pregnancy changes the way your body stores and uses fluids, the kidneys are far more active in filtering toxins. Increasing your consumption of water can aid in this process and help avoid problems with toxemia later in pregnancy.

Water is one of the least expensive ways to maintain good physical health during your pregnancy, and it will help to ensure that you don't experience some of the inconveniences that some pregnant women may encounter, such as joint pain, constipation, muscle cramps, digestive problems, and a host of other common annoyances. It is far better to avoid these nuisances than to require steps to treat them.

Water is continually lost through exertion and body heat, as well as through the skin, kidneys, lungs, colon, and urination and perspiration. When you lose water through these means, it needs to be replaced because of the body's need for water. Amniotic fluid is replenished at least three times a day.

You will read and hear many recommendations concerning the amount of water that a pregnant woman should consume. Generally, it is recommended that a pregnant woman drink eight medium (200ml)glasses of water daily. You will need to consume more water if your activity level is high; if you live in a higher elevation; if the air where you live is less humid; if air temperatures are high; or if you consume a high-fibre diet; which you may be doing to ward off constipation.

The current thinking in determining how much water you should drink is simple. Allow your body to tell you what it needs, as it so nicely does in many other circumstances. You can easily tell if you are consuming a sufficient amount of water by checking the colour of your urine. A body that is properly hydrated releases urine that is the colour of light lemonade. If your urine is a deeper yellow, you need to reach for water more regularly and increase your consumption of protein. Pregnancy vitamins can affect the colour of your urine, so you will want to take that into consideration when assessing your colour. It's that simple.

You will also want to be aware of the quality of water—clean spring water or filtered water is optimal. Being faithful to this regimen can help prevent numerous pregnancy problems, as well as dry skin and other complexion problems.

Eating for Two

No single issue is more important as you carry your baby than the nutrition you provide for him as he develops and grows. You are building another little person made of bones, organs, tissues, muscles, blood, and cells. It doesn't matter how conscientiously you approach any building task and how carefully you think you're building, if the materials that go into the construction are less than the best, your project could prove to be less successful than you would like to see. Building a human being is even more exacting. There needs to be more attention paid to nutrition during the birthing year, and next to

nothing is focused on nutrition prior to conception, so now is the time
to take responsibility for good nutrition for your baby.

Since the HypnoBirthing philosophy is also one of avoiding late-
term consequences of a poor diet, we have set down a few general
suggestions that will help you and your baby to maintain good health.
It takes a healthy mother to have a healthy baby. Healthy mothers
have fewer low-birthweight infants, fewer incidences of premature
birth, fewer cases of PIH (pregnancy-induced hypertension) or simply
high blood pressure, and fewer incidences of toxemia. (The last two
are generally lumped together, though not accurately, and known as
preeclampsia.) In general, the pregnancies and births of healthy mothers are more apt to be "normal." The way to start on the road to good
pregnancy health, no matter where you are in your pregnancy, is to
realise that you are the single source of nutrition for your baby. If he
is going to be well nourished, it's going to have to be through you.

Of course, pregnancy vitamin supplements are fine, but they are just
that—supplements—which means that you should consume them in
addition to a wholly nutritious diet, not as a substitute for a good food
programme. It also means that, like most of the population, when you
do your grocery shopping, you have to do it defensively. Buy fresh
and organic foods as often as possible, rather than processed foods,
and become educated as to which fruits and vegetables may have been
sprayed with pesticides or treated with preservatives. As with everything in your pregnancy, ask questions. You need to protect your baby.

Note: Though these suggestions have been reviewed by a dietician
and have been suggested by nutritionists, if you are experiencing
a pregnancy that has special circumstances attached or if you have
special food considerations, you will want to consult a nutritionist or
dietician rather than follow the course of our suggestions. With no

intent to offend those who follow a vegetarian and vegan diet, I will leave those matters to the people who subscribe to that diet and who are far more knowledgeable than I in this matter.

Basic Formula for Good Nutrition

- Drink water

- Eat veggies!

- Eat at least 75–100 grams of protein a day.

- Be sure the fats you eat are mostly natural. Avoid processed industrial oils such as vegetable oil.

- Eat whole foods. Avoid processed foods that come in boxes and bags, and "wipe out whites": Eat no white food unless it's protein. This includes breads, rice, sugar, flour, white baked goods, and starches.

A Note on Food Quality

Let's focus on the nourishing foods we should eat. And while it's important to eat the right food groups, it's also essential to pay attention to food quality. Under each of the five main points below, we've included notes for selecting quality foods that will best nourish your baby while you are pregnant.

Pursuing perfection can be stressful, and therefore counterproductive for a healthy pregnancy. So do the best you can. Even if you incorporate one or two things from this chapter into your diet, you will be doing a service to your baby and yourself.

If you are interested in looking further, here are some resources for exploring this topic:

Deep Nutrition by Catherine Sahanahan, M.D.
Real Food and Real Food for Mum and Baby by Nina Planck
The Better Baby Book by Dave and Lana Asprey
Beautiful Babies by Kristen Michaelis
Food Rules, The Omnivore's Dilemma, and *Cooked* by Michael Pollan
It Starts With Food by Dallas and Melissa Hartwig
Nourishing Traditions by Sally Fallon and Mary Enig

Organic produce is preferable to conventionally farmed food if it is available and affordable. If not, keep in mind the "Clean 15" and the "Dirty Dozen."

The "Clean 15" foods have skins that chemicals can't penetrate easily; once washed and peeled, they can be safely eaten. These include: onions, avocados, sweet corn, pineapples, asparagus, cabbage, aubergine, grapefruit, sweet peas, kiwi, cantaloupe, watermelon, sweet potatoes, mango, and papayas.

The "Dirty Dozen" have skins that chemicals can penetrate easily; washing and peeling them won't necessarily remove the chemicals. These include: peaches; celery; strawberries; apples; spinach, kale and lettuce; potatoes, blueberries, nectarines, sweet bell peppers, cherries, cucumbers, and grapes.

High-quality proteins have proportions of amino acids that make building human tissue easy. Complete protein is possible by combining vegetables and grains. When we think of protein, we usually think of muscle meats and eggs, and that's true; those are excellent sources of high-quality, complete proteins.

But the ingredients for growing happy, healthy babies are found in a variety of healthy foods from each of the food groups. You should plan to increase your daily calorie intake by about 300 calories. Here are a few suggestions:

Eat:

Lots of protein—75 to 100 grams a day, taken in several snacks or light meals. Protein is the cornerstone of your nutrition programme. Protein includes such food items as cottage cheese, milk, ice cream, frozen yogurt, cheeses (except soft cheeses like Camembert, brie, and Roquefort), safe fish (see information to follow), peanut butter, lean red meat, poultry, pork, ham, bacon, lamb, veal tofu, eggs, butter, rabbit, vegetables, nuts and seeds (high sources), and fruits.

Celtic, Mediterranean, Pink Himalayan sea salt—with no minerals removed (salt your food to taste).

Safe fish—Increase your intake of safe fish or fish oils, which contain omega-3. Check before buying for possible mercury risks. (Don't eat raw fish.)

Green foods—dark, leafy raw foods, celery, green peppers, apples, broccoli, peas, avocado, string beans, Brussels sprouts, asparagus, broccoli, lima beans, collard greens, Swiss chard, grapes, limes, beet greens, courgettes, dandelion greens, lettuce, spinach (only occasionally as it can limit the absorption of calcium), watercress, snow peas.

It is believed that the darker and brighter the fruits and vegetables, the more nutrition they deliver.

Vegetables—Evidence suggests that children whose mothers ate more vegetables while pregnant found vegetables more palatable and had fewer aversions to eating vegetables later in childhood, setting up healthy habits for the years to come.

Orange foods—squash, yams and sweet potatoes, cantaloupe, oranges, peaches, apricots, nectarines, pumpkin, tangerines, carrots, peppers (raw and cooked).

Red foods—watermelon, strawberries (if not sprayed with pesticides), peppers (raw or cooked), tomatoes, apples, raspberries (drink red raspberry leaf tea), cherries, rhubarb, red potatoes, pimiento, radishes.

Coloured fruits—pineapple, pears, bananas, honeydew melons, kiwi, grapes.

Avoid:

- **Alcohol**

- **Caffeine**

- **Nicotine**

- **Processed meats**—hot dogs, luncheon meats, bologna, liverwurst.

- **Raw fish**—oysters, sushi, and others.

- **Unnecessary fats**—fried foods, French fries, fast foods.

- **White foods**—refined sugar, white flour products, white rice, white potatoes.

- **Sweets**—candies with empty calories that have no nutritional value.

Exercising and Toning

It is particularly important that you exercise during pregnancy. It is also crucial, however, that you don't build exercising into a routine that becomes an ordeal or a time-consuming chore. You will want to find ways to tone your body that are as natural as the birthing you are preparing for. Vary the exercises that you do and create a habit of doing them as often as you can as you go about your day-to-day activities.

You'll discover that many exercises can be practised incidentally. Some can even be done right on your bed as you awaken in the morning or just before you settle in for the night. If you are accustomed to brisk exercise, consult with your care provider to be sure that this kind of exercise will not compromise your baby's well-being.

One of the best ways to ensure that you are exercising regularly is to join a prenatal fitness and exercise group. Most of the time, the mothers in these classes are pretty upbeat about their pregnancies and upcoming birthings. Avoid any group that is given to commiserating over bad birth stories.

Walking

Walking is one of the best exercises you can do. It helps to strengthen your breathing, as well as your legs. You don't have to follow a strict regimen of walking, but you can look for ways to get in a little extra walking time, for example, by parking a distance from the entrance to your work or from the supermarket. Use an entrance that is not immediately adjacent to your destination. Rather than telephoning or taking an elevator to another area, find occasions to walk within the building at work. Walk as often as you can. Be sure that the surfaces you walk on are smooth and safe, and wear sensible shoes. Brisk walking is good from the beginning to the middle of your pregnancy. After that you may want to slow down a bit so that your baby is not jostled too much. When you engage in brisk exercise, your blood is directed to your arms and legs and away from the uterus, meaning that your baby is perhaps not receiving the amount of oxygenated blood that he should. Temper your time and pace.

Avoid Back Strain: Practise Good Posture

As your pregnancy advances, you will want to alleviate back strain by being aware of correct posture. Pregnant or not, a good assist to proper posture is to envision a string passing from a point at the front of the earlobe down through the shoulders and the hipbone to a spot just behind the ankle bone. Keeping your head in line with this imaginary string will prevent you from "leading with your head," and keep your pelvis tilted back and help you to avoid stooping as you gain in weight and size.

Don't lean back with your head behind the imaginary line; it will cause you to project your abdomen forward and will lead to the "pregnancy waddle." Many women assume this posture, with toes turned outward, as depicted in comedy skits and sitcoms, long before final "dropping" has occurred. Even then, awareness of how you carry yourself and your baby can make a difference in how you feel at the end of a day.

One of the best devices for maintaining good posture and for helping to ensure that your baby will assume a favourable position for birthing is to avoid slouching down into your pelvic area. This is not too easy to do with so many cars being equipped with bucket seats today, but it can be remedied by placing a pillow on the seat so that it is more level. Absolutely avoiding recliners is also good advice for the pregnant woman who is interested in achieving an optimal position for her baby at birth.

One of the best ways to practise good posture when sitting is to regularly sit on a birth ball (also known as an exercise ball). These handy balls can be bought at any number of locations, including most sporting goods stores, at very reasonable prices. The birth ball allows you to sit erect and, at the same time, tones your inner thighs and pelvic region. Use it at your desk or as a place to relax at home, instead of a chair. The birth ball comes in handy later in pregnancy, and it is a great place to rock during labour. It is one of the best and simplest tools you can buy. To ensure good balance while using the birth ball, fill the bottom of the ball with approximately 2 inches of sand. This will prevent your tilting one way or another and help you maintain that erect posture that is so important.

Another exercise that is helpful in relieving back strain is the "pelvic rock." This exercise helps to avoid back strain, strengthens abdominal muscles, increases the flexibility of your lower back, and promotes good alignment in your spine. There are several ways to do the pelvic rock. Instructions for two methods follow.

First Method: Using the back of a sturdy chair or other piece of furniture for arm support and balance, stand approximately two feet from the object. Bend your knees very slightly.

Lean forward from your hips and thrust your buttocks backward. Keep your back straight. Allow your abdominal muscles to relax for a few seconds while you create sway.

Bend your knees a little more and pull your hips forward, tucking your buttocks under as though you were being shooed from behind with a broom. Repeat the procedure several times.

Second Method: You can also practise the pelvic rock or tilt in a lying position during the early months of your pregnancy. Once your baby begins to take on some weight, you will want to avoid lying flat on your back.

On your back with your knees bent and your feet flat on the floor, tighten your lower abdominal muscles and the muscles of your buttocks. Your tailbone will rise, pressing the small of your back to the floor. Hold this position for a few seconds and then release the muscles. As you do this exercise, arch your back as much as you can. Repeat the procedure several times.

You will also find this an excellent technique for flattening the abdomen following birthing.

Toning the Inner Thigh and Leg Muscles

Toning your inner thigh muscles and legs is vitally important for a successful labour. At the end of your birthing when you are breathing your baby down and out of the birth path, you may find yourself in many positions that will call for you to use your legs in ways that are a bit unusual. The muscles in your inner thigh will need to be ready.

Position One: The best effect in toning can be derived from sitting on the floor or in the middle of a bed with soles of your feet together. Lean slightly forward and place your hands on your ankles. With your elbows resting on the inside of your knees, gently press your elbows onto your knees. Do not apply force as you stretch these important groin muscles. As you do these exercises over time, gradually and gently pull your heels toward your crotch until your heels and your crotch meet and your knees almost rest on the floor. Do not rush to make this happen. Take it slowly. Once you have achieved this muscle tone, you should straighten your back during subsequent practise sessions.

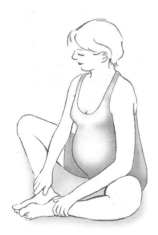

Toning the Inner Thigh Muscles

You can do this exercise alone, but it's more fun to get your birthing companion involved. Using the same technique as described previously, have the birth companion assist from behind you by placing his or her hands under your knees, pressing upward to create resistance. While this is happening, you gently press down on your knees. Then have your birth companion press downward on your knees while you bring your legs upward and push against the pressure.

Position Two: Resting on your tailbone with your knees bent and raised upward toward your shoulders, place the palms of your hands against the inner part of your knees and push your knees outward. Bring your knees together again and then push them apart. Do this about ten times in each practice session.

When you reach for low objects or lift an object or a small child, bend with your knees, rather than from the waist. Do not attempt to lift heavy objects.

The Leaping Frog

The Leaping Frog position comes to us from midwives in the Virgin Islands. This easy, forward squat is used in many places in the world. Not only does this position help to tone your muscles, but it also provides you with one of the best positions in which to labour during the birthing phase.

While women in other cultures regularly use a squatting position for birthing, you must remember that these women use this posture for much of what they do on a daily basis. Western women are not naturally inclined to squatting, so this posture needs practice. There are two ways of assuming the Leaping Frog stance—with your arms thrust forward inside your spread knees or with your arms behind you at the side of your hips. The second position is an ideal position to assume for birthing as it relieves all pressure from the buttocks and provides open and clear access for both baby and attendant. The time that you spend in practising this modified form of squatting will be well spent.

Assuming the Leaping Frog position during labour offers benefits for both you and your baby when you are Birth Breathing. Just a few of the benefits of the Leaping Frog include the following:

- Widens the pelvic opening

- Relaxes and opens the perineal tissues

- Helps to avoid tearing and lessens the need for an episiotomy

- Relieves strain in the lower back

- Increases the supply of oxygen to your baby

- Shortens the birth path

- Allows you a clear view of your baby's birth

- Makes good use of the effect of gravity

Though I recommend the Leaping Frog position, attempting to adopt it for any length of time when your muscles are not adequately toned could result in pain or injury to your leg muscles. If you choose to birth with your arms behind you, you will want considerable practice so that your arms will be able to support you. A variation of this is to lean with your arms on your companion's knees so that you can slowly lower yourself into the squatting position. The companion can also stand in front of you, holding your hands to assist as you slowly lower your body into position.

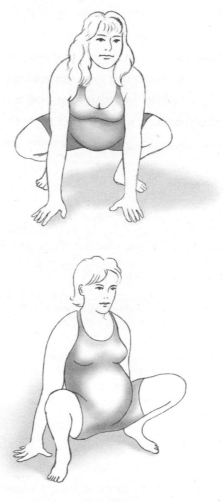

Leaping Frog Positions

From a standing position with your feet spread about a foot and a half apart, assume a squatting position on your toes with your knees spread outward. Place your hands on the floor on either the inside or the outside of your legs.

During birthing, you may wish to place pillows beneath your hands and your knees.

This same position nicely converts into a Polar Bear position if there is need to assist baby to shift position during birthing. This is easily accomplished by leaning your chin and your forearms on the pillows in front of you, while your buttocks extend into the air.

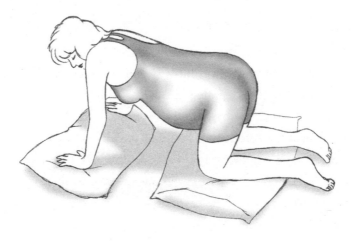

Hands and knees position

Pelvic Floor Exercises

Not enough attention is paid to pelvic floor exercises, sometimes called Kegels. They are among the most important of all the prenatal muscle toning. Designed to tone and strengthen the muscles used during the birthing phase of labour, these exercises involve the network of muscles that form a figure eight around the entire vaginal and anal region.

Toning the pelvic floor muscles also serves the very important function of quick return to their normal size after labour and can be helpful in preventing some of the urinary problems connected with aging.

Control of this area can actually enhance lovemaking after having a child. You will enjoy the confidence derived from a well-toned anal and vaginal region as your pregnancy advances and there is more pressure on the bladder and bowel. These sphincters are the same sphincters that you will use while practising Birth Breathing on the toilet. As you breathe down, you will want to open both the vaginal and anal outlets, keeping them open during the intake of the next soft breath.

Technique

In a sitting position, start by constricting the lowest muscles of the anal and vaginal tracts as tightly as you can. Keep tightening the vaginal muscles until you can feel the constricting muscles all the way up into the top of the vagina. When working with anal muscles, draw in until you get the sensation of pulling the anus into the rectum. It is helpful, though not necessary, to count from one to ten as you do these exercises, tightening a little more with each number. When you have tightened the muscles in the area, hold the contraction for a few seconds and then release slowly.

These muscles are the same ones used to stop the flow of urine. To see if you are doing this exercise correctly, attempt to stop the flow of urine while you are urinating. Do not continue to do this once you have established that you are doing the exercise correctly. To do this more than is necessary could result in a urinary tract infection. Be sure to practise this exercise several times a day, doing the exercise five to ten times at each practise. Frequent practice is all to your benefit. These exercises can be done easily at anytime, anywhere, whether at work or at home, while driving or while walking. The important thing is to DO IT.

Perineal Massage

erineal massage is one of the oldest and surest ways of improving the health, blood flow, elasticity, and relaxation of the pelvic floor muscles. Practised in the latter part of your pregnancy, approximately six to eight weeks prior to term, this technique will also help you to identify and become acquainted with the tissues you will relax and the region through which you will birth your baby. Perineal massage is vitally important to the success of your HypnoBirthing. Do not take this exercise for granted.

Massaging with oil helps the perineal tissues to soften and thereby gently unfold with no resistance as they open during birthing to allow the passage of the baby. As you or your partner do the massage, you can teach these muscles to relax and open outward in response to pressure.

This massage increases your chances of birthing your baby over an intact perineum. When your perineal rim is soft and relaxed, the perennial folds easily open, and your baby slips past the rim and out of the vagina. The perenial tissues gently unfold. Attention to this massage will pay off. It is simple, yet so effective. You will want to take it seriously. The massage should be done every day for at least five minutes.

Because of your increased size and the awkwardness of bending around your abdomen, it may be easier to have someone else do the massage for you. If the massage is done gently, there is no need for discomfort. I suggest that couples make it part of their lovemaking.

If you are doing the massage by yourself, you'll find it easier if you use your thumb. Place one foot on the seat of a chair, with the other approximately two feet away from the chair. This allows you to work around and under your abdomen from the back.

Be sure that fingernails are smooth and short when doing the massage. A rubber glove will ensure that there are no rough surfaces to irritate the vaginal tissue. You may use virgin olive oil, sweet oil, almond oil, apricot oil, or a lubricating gel. Avoid perfumed oils.

Technique

Pour a little of the oil into a custard cup or shallow bowl. (Be sure to discard oil that is left after massaging—do not reuse.)

Sit with your back resting against pillows and get comfortable. It's a good idea to use a mirror during the first few times that you do this exercise. It will assist you in identifying the muscles involved and allow you to observe the easing of the edge of the perineum.

Dip your thumb into the oil and thoroughly moisten it. If a partner is doing the massage, the first two fingers will be used. The thumb or fingers should be dipped into the oil to the second knuckle and inserted into the vagina approximately two to three inches, pressing downward on the area between the vagina and the rectum. Rub the oil into the inner edge of the perineum and the lower vaginal wall.

Maintaining a steady pressure, slide the fingers upward along the sides of the vagina in a U, sling-type motion. This pressure will stretch the vaginal tissue, the muscles surrounding the vagina, and the outer rim of the perineum. Be sure to reach the inner portions as well as the outer rim of the perineum. In the beginning you will feel the tightness of the muscles, but with time and practice, the tissue will relax.

Practise relaxing the extended muscles by picturing the perineum opening outward as pressure is applied. The opening rosebud is a good visualisation to use during this exercise.

Selecting Your Care Providers

*Birth is the last frontier in a woman's
quest for freedom. A woman needs to be free to
birth her babies as she chooses.*

LORNE CAMPBELL, SR., M.D.

You Can't Grow Orchids in the Arctic

You probably have never given much thought to growing orchids; but for the sake of conversation, let's assume that you have decided to devote your life to growing orchids. Without any in-depth thought as to the people you will work with or the surroundings in which you will be working, you choose to take your project to the Arctic Circle.

It will not be long after your plane touches down that you discover that the Arctic is little more than large, barren fields of ice. The people who brought you there confirm that the Arctic is no place to grow orchids. The freezing temperatures offer a bitter cold welcome. You know that you've made a huge mistake. The Arctic is definitely not conducive to your fulfilling of your dream to grow orchids. So you leave, saddened and disappointed but not defeated.

When you get home, a little bit of inquiry and research clearly indicates that Singapore would have been the better choice. The people there are entirely supportive, and the surroundings and environment are conducive to growing orchids. So you confidently take your seedlings and head for Singapore convinced that Singapore is all you are looking for.

Approaching your upcoming birthing day without exploring these same factors—the attitudes of the people who will attend you, the physical surroundings and the general environment of your birth facility—is not unlike attempting to grow orchids in the Arctic.

This is your baby's first birthday, and as a parent, it is your responsibility to do all you can to ensure that the right people attend the birth and that the birthing facility is a perfect match for the birth you are envisioning. All other decisions that you will be making will pale in comparison to the importance of these factors. The most important question you must ask yourself is "How certain am I that my primary birth attendant will listen to my requests and honour me and my baby as a birthing family?" The philosophy and management style of this person and the policies and procedures in effect at the facility are the most essential.

Parents often will ask "But how can I find that really caring birth professional?" We say listen and pay attention to your gut sense. If it feels right, you have found the right person. If when you leave the provider's office, you feel anything less than enthusiastic about this person, your inner knowing is sending you a message.

A member of the HypnoBirthing faculty, Lori Nicholson, of Bethesda, Maryland, offers the following thought-provoking scenario to her parent classes. She suggests this approach:

Imagine yourself employed in an important position in a fairly large organisation. The Chief Administrative Officer of the organisation has called you into his office to explain that he is interested in becoming involved in an important project that will require hiring a key person to oversee this project. He is appointing you to act as the hiring manager.

The first candidate whom you interview starts the interview by telling you that he is very familiar with the project but feels that its objectives are flawed. He feels that the project has very little likelihood of success and suggests that his approach should be adopted. He states that he is very well educated, and he has good experience and a good work history. He has a good personality and feels that he is the person for this job of Project Overseer. Based on your conversation with this person, would you hire him for this job? Would he be the person that you feel you could trust to bring about a successful and happy conclusion?

As a parent of your unborn baby, you are the hiring manager whose job it is to select the very best person for the position of the overseer of your birthing. The person you select can either make or break the success of the birthing day.

As birthing parents, you can achieve that freedom only when you take responsibility for seeing that the people you surround yourselves with are people who hold the same view of birth as you do and who are willing to respect and support your dreams. You do have choices, and you need to identify them.

Even in an ideal situation, you may need to keep reminding the caregiver that you are planning for a HypnoBirthing. Mention your birth preferences early and often, without being irksome. Health-care providers are busy people who see many families. They sometimes need that gentle reminder.

If you've had a surgical birth previously and truly want to birth vaginally this time, seriously look into having a VBAC (vaginal birth after caesarean) and actively seek a doctor or midwife who will encourage you. The HypnoBirthing method is especially favourable to VBACs because the breathing techniques are gentle all through the opening phase, and you will not strain with forced pushing during the baby's descent—another plus for the VBAC mother.

Many providers who have never seen HypnoBirthing are more than happy to keep an open mind and support your wishes if the benefits are presented to them in an inviting, rather than demanding, way.

YOUR OPTIONS - AND YOU DO HAVE CHOICES

There is no one system of care that covers the entire UK. Several systems are in place; but it is true to say that midwife-led care is the norm for most healthy, low-risk women in the National Health Service (NHS). Midwives are considered the guardians of normal birth and will do their utmost to see that normal birth is achieved. Their philosophy is sometimes shared with the general practitioner; but, for the most part, it is the midwife who is seen as the birthing expert.

The clientele of the midwife is mostly healthy women in a low-risk category. However, midwives are trained to detect possible abnormalities and make an appropriate referral to a doctor.

There are choices for midwifery services. When making your decision, look into your heart, consider your birthing wishes, and be sure that you feel comfortable with your choice. The following options are legitimate from both a safety and comfort perspective:

Community Midwives: Community midwives are organised into groups of six to eight midwives. Their services include antenatal appointments at clinics in the community, as well as home visits for anywhere from 10 to 29 days following the birth of the baby. Women working with community midwives may choose to give birth at home, and will have an opportunity, in most cases, to meet the group of midwives prior to their birthings.

A small percentage of women who choose to birth in the local hospital will be cared for by a team member, the others will be cared for by a staff midwife at the hospital.

The idea of team midwifery is popular with women preparing to give birth since they are able to get to know the person who will attend their birth and they are able to discuss their preferences beforehand. Midwives are guided by the women's choices for birthing and are equally comfortable giving support to a woman wishing a fully natural birth, as with a woman who feels that she may need some degree of medication.

Midwife-led Birth Centres: Another option in some areas is an NHS midwife-led birth centre. These units are made as homelike as possible. They have pools for labour and/or birthing and are staffed solely by midwives and health-care assistants or maternity-care assistants.

Independent Midwives: The concept of working with an independent midwife is also another option. Independent midwives are trained by the NHS and must practice by their standards. Most support natural birth and encourage the use of a birthing pool and homeopathy to enhance the experience.

You may hire an independent midwife by contacting the midwife and arranging a private agreement for her services. The agreement may be dependent upon whether all or only part of the care is to be covered by the midwife, and fees are charged accordingly. (For more information visit www.imuk.org.uk.)

If your pregnancy is categorised as high risk, you will probably need to have a caregiver who attends births in the hospital.

Midwives work in close conjunction with physicians in the event that a birthing does require a medical referral. Midwives usually are quite receptive to listening and supporting the wishes of birthing parents, but this, too, can differ with individuals.

My three recent trips to England to teach HypnoBirthing certification classes have allowed me to observe an entirely different approach to birth than what we experience in the United States. It is interesting to note the attitude toward midwifery and birthing in the United Kingdom and contrast it with ours in the United States. In the United Kingdom, midwives are the principal attendants at births and have a legal obligation to attend a birthing mother wherever she wishes to birth. In the early 1990s, the House of Commons in the UK officially mandated that the needs of birthing mothers be the central focus of maternal health-care providers and that maternity services be fashioned around them, not the other way around. Refreshing!

In the United Kingdom and other countries that operate under a National Health System (NHS), your birthing attendant could be one of any number of midwives. A midwife in the United Kingdom works with the NHS, serving women with normal pregnancies and labour. In addition to doing all of the antenatal clinics and attending births, he/she will also cover the postnatal period up to twenty-eight days. While their clientele is mostly healthy women in a low-risk category, midwives are trained to detect possible abnormalities and make an appropriate referral to a doctor. Under this system, healthy women with healthy pregnancies can be attended by midwives, and most women never need to see a doctor. Almost three quarters of women birthing in the Netherlands are attended by midwives.

One of my mums had her first baby last Sunday at home. She completed the course with me only two weeks earlier ... She went into labour spontaneously and called the homebirth midwife to come and check her because she was "getting some strange sensations"! The midwife stayed for an hour and concluded that there was no way the mum was in active labour. The midwife could not tell when the mum was having surges and had to ask her to indicate them by squeezing her husband's hand so that the baby could be monitored.

Baby and mother were so calm that the midwife said that she would leave them for a few hours and to call if things progressed. The mum then said, "Before you go, can you just tell me — is it normal to want to push at this stage?" The midwife was compelled to do an exam and found that the mum was fully open and the head was visible!! A beautiful baby boy was breathed into the world twenty minutes later.

Later, as the midwife was leaving, she said to a very ecstatic, proud and alert mum, "Well, I have never seen anything like that before. You are obviously made to have babies." To which the mum replied: "Yes, I'm a woman!"

Vanessa, Wales, U.K.

In some areas, you may have the option of a midwifery system called the Domino scheme, whereby community midwives are attached to a hospital. The Domino scheme provides the same continuity of care as for a home birth, but provides the opportunity for a woman to give birth in hospital, if she feels that is where she will be most comfortable. This option can mean that all antenatal services will be conducted by midwives, with the possibility of seeing a different midwife at each visit. If your labour is prolonged or spills from one shift to another, you could have more than one midwife attend your birthing.

I was in my fortieth week of pregnancy and had looked forward to a planned homebirth, but a late test result indicated that it couldn't be. I needed to change plans fast for birthing with a midwife and seek a physician. I felt this would not be an easy task at this late date.

I called my family physician, Dr. Barrett, and made an appointment to see him on Friday morning. The man earned high honours in my book for being willing to take me on as a patient at exactly forty weeks. I knew him to be a wonderful doctor and a very compassionate man.

Friday afternoon, I began to have surges. This was nothing new to me, as I had had surges off and on for many weeks, but these were two to three minutes apart and felt different. We got packed, got into the car and headed for the hospital.

We arrived a little after 3:30 and were admitted. Much to my delight, the surges continued to get longer and stronger.

→

Our doula, Missy, showed up soon after. Our nurse was puzzled that I could walk, talk and smile through surges, and seemed flustered to think that I was going to birth without an epidural. She said that unless the cervix is changing, it isn't real labour. I'm sure that she didn't believe that I was in true labour — too quiet and too relaxed. She called Dr. Barrett when I declined to answer the questions on the pain scale and told him that I had a very bossy doula who was telling me that I could refuse things. He supported my position.

When my membranes released at 6:40, I began to feel pressure. Missy recognised the signs and felt that this was going to be a really short labour. Reluctantly the nurse called Dr. Barrett. As soon as he came into the room, I released and began to nudge the baby down. Two surges later, our baby was born. I held him in my arms and cried with happiness for love of him and relief that he was here, alive and healthy.

Dr. Barrett spent the next two hours with us, as did Missy. He personally secured warm blankets for me, made sure I had food, gave me his pager number and did all the sweet things you would expect from a good friend. He was supportive of all the things I wanted. I gave birth without an IV or medication, ate throughout labour and had no anaesthesia.

This birth was different from what I had envisioned and hoped for a few weeks earlier, but it was the birth that our baby needed, and a beautiful birth at that.

Melanie, Salt Lake City

Obstetrician: Obstetricians are medical doctors who have graduated from an accredited school of medicine and have completed two to three years of advanced study in the field of gynaecology and obstetrics. They are highly trained surgeons and are proficient at detecting, diagnosing and treating gynaecological and obstetrical problems that require specialised procedures. They are skilled specialists who are called upon when special circumstances arise in birthing that require specific medical or surgical procedures. Because they are prepared and trained for surgical births, they would be most likely to see a large number of mothers who are in the category of high risk.

Obstetricians see pregnant women for examinations, testing and other antenatal care, as well as postnatal checkups. If a surgical birth is deemed necessary, an obstetrician will perform the caesarean section. Obstetricians do not need backup from another surgeon, except in rare or unusual circumstances.

I was concerned that I might not find a doctor who would understand our wanting to birth naturally, but Dr. Adams was wonderful. He had never heard of HypnoBirthing, but asked if he could take our book home with him to share with his wife who is preparing to become a doula. He was very accepting of our birth preferences.

My "Guess Date" was May 6, and on May 11, with my blood pressure rising, our doctor suggested induction. I was already at 4 centimetres open, and he knew that labour was near.

$\longrightarrow$

We arrived at the hospital at 7:00 the following morning. Dr. Adams said that he would rupture the membranes rather than give me something stronger.

We spent the day walking when I wasn't being monitored. My husband said that I looked like I was drugged because I was so relaxed. When a surge came, I simply stopped walking and talking and closed my eyes. I visualised waves rolling in and out on a beach. I was 6 centimetres opened at 6:00 P.M., but I wasn't told what stage I was in. I didn't want to know.

At 7:00 P.M., I felt I needed to be checked. I asked the nurse not to tell me how open I was because I didn't want to be disappointed or to ruin my frame of mind. She checked and said, "Well, I'll say this. I need to call the doctor and tell him to come quickly." Our baby was on his way down. When I crowned, I pushed two or three times, and my baby was born. I had an eight-pound baby boy at 8:36 P.M.

Throughout the whole birthing, I felt about one second of pain. I was scared by the sensation of tearing. I had two tiny tears that healed in a couple of days.

I did not need to practise time distortion because the whole day was a blur. I couldn't believe that twelve hours had passed. Our doctor and the nurses were truly amazed.

Our baby is easygoing, a good sleeper and nurses well, which I attribute to his calm, drug-free birth.

Thanks to a supportive doctor and to our HypnoBirthing practitioner for a miracle to be treasured always.

Teresa, Vermont

Here are a few questions you might ask the person(s) you are considering selecting to get a feel for their openness to normal birthing:

- We are planning to do HypnoBirthing — a natural birth; will you support us in that?

- How often do you perform caesarean births? What is the most common reason?

- Considering ten of your patients, how many do you feel will need to be induced? Need augmentation? Have a caesarean section?

- If our baby is strong, and I am fine, will you postpone discussion of induction until forty-two weeks?

- If release of membranes is the first sign of labour, how long are you willing to wait for spontaneous onset of labour? Why do you choose that number?

- During the birthing phase, I will be breathing the baby down to birth rather than forcefully pushing. Are you comfortable with that?

- I would like to eat light snacks for energy while in labour. What is your feeling about that?

Doula: A doula is a person who knows birthing and, from behind the scenes, helps parents achieve the uninterrupted birth they are seeking. A doula frees the birth companion to focus his or her attention upon the mum, while the doula tends to details of seeing that the mum has a cool facecloth that is refreshed regularly and reminds her to change positions or to empty her bladder. One of the most important roles that a doula plays is that of liaison with hospital staff when parents have a request or need help interpreting the situation. Just the presence of a doula helps to avoid the suggestion of intervention and allows parents to relax in the confidence that they are in good hands. (For more information on hiring a doula, visit www.doula.org.uk.)

Preparing Birth Preferences

Birth in a Sanctuary? Why not!

Imagine...
  A place where everyone
  Honours you and the work you will
    do in labour,
  Speaks quietly and moves slowly
    and gently,
  Respects your need to be spontaneous—
    to eat, drink, make sounds, move around, cry, shout, laugh,
  Treats you and your baby as fully conscious and sensitive beings.
  Giving birth is as intimate as lovemaking
    You will need privacy and support and tenderness
  Labour is not a spectator sport
    Your partner is not your "coach"
  It's the journey of a lifetime for your baby and you
    Don't settle for a typical birth
  Find out more... home birth... birth centres
    Safe alternatives to epidurals... Seek out a midwife
    Arrange for a labour companion/doula to stay with you...
Protect your baby and empower yourself!

SUZANNE ARMS

CHOOSING YOUR BIRTHING ENVIRONMENT

In-Hospital Birth Centres: Some hospitals have an entire unit devoted to birthing and the care of newborn babies — these are midwifery-led units. They have discarded the old "Labour and Delivery" signs and replaced them with names that indicate a softer, less medicalised atmosphere. A great deal of money and effort have been put into making these units appear attractive, comfortable and homelike. This is very appealing, but you must evaluate more than the decor. Matching curtains and bedspreads give an air of charm and a homelike appearance, but unless the people who come into this setting to attend the birthing families have a matching attitude of kindness, are family-oriented and view birth as normal, the decor becomes only window dressing, disguising the equipment, instruments and machinery that may be in full force during your birthing.

Supporting the belief that healthy women with healthy babies can safely birth outside the "geared-for-emergency" protocol, there are hospitals that are truly committed to natural birthing and family-friendly care and attention. Some of them have even allocated a sizeable segment of the birthing unit, and in some cases an entire floor, to families who want to birth naturally. These rooms are free of monitors and other medical equipment and apparatus. Mums are not immediately stripped of their clothing, put to bed, strapped to a machine and outfitted with an IV. Staff members are carefully selected to support the families who choose to birth there.

A hospital in Rochester, New Hampshire, is so commit-
ted to gentle birth that nearly half of all of their births are
HypnoBirthings. Thanks to the efforts of caring nurses and
administrators, as well as the goodwill of a few HypnoBirth-
ing practitioners, a hospital in San Diego, California, has
an entire floor devoted to families who want to birth in an
atmosphere that is as close to normal as possible. A large hos-
pital in Chicago has an ABC unit (Alternative Birth Center),
as do many others across the country. The trend is growing.
You will want to be sure that the hospital you select is truly
HypnoBirthing-friendly, lending an atmosphere that says birth
is normal and not an emergency waiting to happen.

William and Martha Sears, authors of The Birth Book, suggest
that "parent power" is the answer to making care providers and hospital administrators more sensitive to this need. When millions of
expectant families call the hospital of their choice and ask for such
accommodations, including a staff that supports normal birth, it will
happen. Parents need to be aware, however, that, on occasion, the
same hospital that teaches gentle birthing in their childbirth classes
may meet the couple with "routine" procedures when they arrive at
the hospital to birth their baby. Parents need to address this inconsist-
ency, and it is a good idea to set the stage early. Ask the caregivers
and the hospital staff, as well as parents who have birthed in that
facility, if the facility is family-friendly and endorses the belief of
normal birth.

If possible, tour more than one birthing facility and talk with the staff, just as you did when you selected your medical care provider. The answers to these questions will tell you about the hospital's philosophy. It's a good idea to do this early: You may want to change your plans based on your findings. Don't wait until just before your birthing time to inquire about these things.

Here are some questions for you to consider:

- Is there flexibility in policies and willingness to accommodate HypnoBirthing preferences in the absence of special circumstances?

- Are there midwives on staff who are partial to natural birth?

- Do they have a pool?

- Do they have birthing balls or can you bring one?

- Will you be fed if your labour lingers? Are snacks available?

- Are you free to walk outside or within the hospital?

- May you remain in your own clothes during labour?

- Is immediate, skin-to-skin bonding time allowed with the baby?

- Are doulas welcome?

- Is there a provision for the partner and baby to stay in the same room as the mum?

- Are statistics on inductions, augmentations, epidurals and caesarean births available?

Free-standing Birth Centres: The birth centre is more likely to afford you the opportunity to birth without intervention. You will want to ask the same questions of a birth centre staff member as you do of hospital staff. Because the birth centre focus is on healthy women with healthy pregnancies, they don't have to be equipped with all of the high-tech apparatus that is needed for women with pregnancy complications. Birthing in a birth centre, however, is as safe as hospital birthing.

Homebirth: There is much misunderstanding and misinformation about homebirths. Among them are the myths that homebirthing is dangerous while hospital births are safe.

A study done by Dr. Lewis Mehl-Madronna in 1976, in conjunction with researchers at Stanford University, compared the safety of homebirth with hospital births. The results showed that morbidity outcomes of the 2,092 births studied were identical. The study also showed that only 5 percent of the mothers birthing at home received medication, whereas 75 percent of the in-hospital births received medication. Even more revealing, three times as many caesarean sections were performed on the mother in hospital births as there were in the planned homebirths that required transfer to a hospital. Babies born in hospitals suffered more foetal distress, newborn infection and birth injuries than did those born in homes. Interestingly, 66 percent of the homebirths were attended by doctors, which would suggest that when women are relaxed in the comfort of their own homes and are allowed to birth normally, what is looked upon as a medical incident can evolve into something quite natural and safe.

Also, not commonly known is that the community midwife who attends homebirths is required to carry the same equipment and drugs that are used to meet the most common special circumstances that occur in hospitals, although their need for it is very rare.

Baby's Choice: Occasionally, while their parents have plans that are quite different, HypnoBirthing babies may decide that it is all right to be born en route to the hospital or even in the comfort of their own homes.

It is important to know that there is nothing about this situation that creates an emergency or that is necessarily cause for panic. As many taxi drivers and policemen will attest, babies can be born safely wherever they choose. Should your baby decide that your bedroom or the backseat of your car, away from the hustle and bustle of other people, is perfectly fine with him, you can remain calm and offer the same gentle birth you had planned earlier.

We suggest that when you set out for the hospital, drape the backseat of your car with plastic bags underneath a sheet, and be sure to bring pillows. It is better to pull over to the side of the road than to risk rushing through traffic. If you are at home, it is better to just get off your feet with something underneath you and relax where you are in your home than to risk having the baby emerge while you're running to get to the car. Baby will be much happier, and you will be better able to maintain the calm and joy of his birthing.

Since much of the apprehension over an unplanned out-of-hospital birth lies in questions about how to handle the umbilical cord, it is important for you to know that leaving the cord attached, even for hours, as is done in some cultures, is safe and quite beneficial to the baby. Your practitioner can offer more details.

A pregnant woman is like a
beautiful flowering tree, but take care
when it comes time for the harvest that you
do not shake or bruise the tree, for in doing so,
you may harm both the tree and its fruit.

Peter Jackson, R.N.

Australia

The Management Styles
of Labour—Compared

This chapter has been included at the request of parents who expressed a feeling of being well prepared for natural, instinctive birthing, but who felt totally unprepared to meet the protocols that could be imposed in a less-than-natural setting or with a provider who subscribes to Active Management of Labour (AML), and to a lesser degree, even in a standard birth setting.

You can avoid encountering a confrontational situation and/or disappointment if you have prepared thoroughly and discussed these issues with your care provider to determine if the provider is, in fact, on the same page as you are on in regard to gentle birthing. As parents, you need to take responsibility for making choices based on knowledge and questioning. You need to know if the birthing environment and the provider that you are presently with is, in fact, a true fit with your wishes and for how you want the birth of your baby to pay out for mum, baby, and dad.

Management Models

—Active Management of Labour
—Management for Standard or Conventional Birth
—Management for Instinctive-Physiological Birth
—Parental Self-Management for Unassisted Birth

We will explore the various management styles of those care providers who attend births.

Active Management of Labour

• This method of labour involves a concerted effort to forcefully cause the birthing body to do what it already has the innate ability to do with ease, comfort, and dignity if left undisturbed.

• Developed in the late 1960s and 70s in Ireland in an attempt to reduce the number of caesarean sections. It was assumed that mothers who had long labours were traumatised.

• A normal birth, according to AML standards, was about 24 hours. Over the years, that timeline was considerably shortened to 12 hours.

• AML has not decreased the caesarean rate, but instead has had the opposite effect.

• Today, only a few providers in Ireland are becoming more aware of the natural rhythm of birthing and respect that birthing belongs to the family, not to the provider.

Birthing in a hospital does not necessarily mean that your birth will be a managed birth. Some hospitals have gone to great lengths to provide an environment that fits with the goals and wishes of the parents and, not all hospitals, doctors, or midwives engage in Active Management Labour procedures. Many providers refrain from this approach unless circumstances of the birthing deem it necessary in cases of high risk. However, it is sadly true that a very large percentage of hospital facilities and care providers today are needlessly using some, or all, features of AML rather than exercising patience and allowing labour to play out naturally.

If you have chosen a birth attendant who subscribes to AML you are more likely to experience the protocols and interventions that are listed on the management chart that follows this discussion.

Standard or Conventional

The management style that most couples will meet if they choose to birth in a hospital will follow protocols which can be a blend of the regimen of Active Management of Labour and a less strict instinctive physiological labour. Which one of these they encounter depends wholly on the philosophy of the birth attendants. These, too, are listed on the management chart.

Management for Instinctive Birthing

Instinctive births are managed when the need arises. Most care providers who subscribe are happy to honour parents' requests for unmedicated and unintervened births. Parents and medical professionals work together as a team and there is an understanding that should there be a medical indication for intervention, they will have the full cooperation of the parents.

These births are calm, joyful, and peace filled. Babies born in this manner a mellow, content and happy. Parents report that they are easily cared for.

Providers' Management Styles

Active Management of Labour	Standardised Labour
Hospital Setting	**Hospital or Birth Centre**
Physician Managed	Physician/Midwife
Little/No Parent Input	Possible Parent Input
Induction is Scheduled	May/May Not Induce
Early Rupture of Membranes	Release of Membranes
Mandatory IV/Heplock	May Possibly Decline IV
Continuous EF Monitor	Mandatory/Intermittent EFM
Fragmented Labour	Fragmented Labour
Total Food Restriction	Possible Food Restriction
Early Augmentation	Augmentation
Frequent Augmentation	Possible Frequent Augmentation
Chronological Insistence	Some Chronological Expectation
Routine Epidural	Epidural Available
Coached, Forced Pushing	Coached, Forced Pushing
Frequent Infant Heart Decels	Frequent Infant Heart Decels
Use of Oxytocics Post-Birth	Probable Oxytocics Post-Birth
Suctioning of Infant	Probable Suctioning of Infant
Episiotomy is Routine	Infrequent Episiotomy
Immediate Cord Clamping	Probable Immediate Cord Clamping
Land Births Only	Probably Land Births

—A Comparison

Natural, Instinctive Labour	Pure Birth
Free-Standing Centre or Home	**Home Setting**
Midwife/Parent Team	Unassisted
Parents/Provider Team Input	Parents Manage
Spontaneous Onset	Spontaneous Onset
Spontaneous ROM	Spontaneous ROM
No Needle Insertions	No Needle Insertions
Manually Monitored	Self-Monitored
Labour is a Continuum	Labour is a Continuum
Food Allowed	Food Allowed
Natural Augmentation	Natural Augmentation
Augmentation Only as Needed	Augmentation Only as Needed
Clock is Irrelevant	Clock is Irrelevant
No Epidural Use	Natural Relaxation
Body's Natural Expulsive Reflex	Body's Natural Expulsive Reflex
Less Frequent or No Heart Decels	Less Frequent or No Heart Decels
No Oxytocics Used	No Oxytocics Used
Necessary Infant Suctioning Only	Necessary Infant Suctioning Only
Infrequent Episiotomy	No Episiotomy
Delayed Cord Clamping	Delayed Cord Clamping
Water Births and Land Births	Mother's Choice

When Baby Is Breech

In preparation for birthing, sometime between the thirty-second and thirty-seventh weeks of pregnancy, the baby turns from its upright position into what is called a vertex position in preparation for birthing. With this turn, the baby's head is properly positioned down at the mouth of the cervix. Because the head contains the brain and the skull, it is the heaviest part of the baby's body. Once the baby is almost fully developed, the natural pull of gravity is usually sufficient to draw the head down.

Most of the time this turning goes without note, especially if it occurs while the mother is sleeping. The turn can be delayed, however, if the mother is experiencing fear or tension, or if there are circumstances in her life that are upsetting.

Some mothers, for any number of reasons, are reluctant to "let go," and so their uterus remains taut and the baby is not able to complete the turn. When this happens, the baby, deprived of adequate space in which to turn, is unable to complete the rotation and remains in the original, upright position. The baby's buttocks remain at the neck of the uterus in what is called "breech presentation." Sometimes the baby completes only a partial rotation, leaving a shoulder, an arm, or one or both feet positioned at the lower part of the cervix.

A breech position, if not reversed, calls for important decisions. The options are limited to making every effort to help the baby turn, to birth the baby in the breech position, or to resort to a surgical birth. Since few medical providers are trained in the birthing of breech-presented babies, most resort to caesarean births, but this doesn't need to be the first avenue to explore. Many women birth their breech-presented babies vaginally with homebirth midwives.

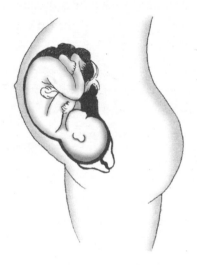

Proper Vertex Position

Helping the Breech-Positioned Baby to Turn

Many babies have been coached to turn with the help of Hypno-Birthing techniques. A special session has proven to be very effective in helping the breech-presented baby to spontaneously reposition into vertex position on its own. This concept is buttressed in a study, presented by Dr. Lewis Mehl-Madronna, formerly of the psychiatric department of the University of Vermont Medical School and Arizona University School of Medicine. The study included 100 women who were referred from practising obstetricians and an additional 100 who responded to an advertisement. Only women who were found to be carrying their babies in breech position at thirty-six weeks gestation or more were included. Mehl-Madronna approached this study looking at reports on serial ultrasound examinations and abdominal palpation that suggested that the likelihood of a breech-positioned baby turning after the thirty-seventh week was no more than 12 percent.

One hundred women in the study group used hypnotherapy. The comparison group consisted of 100 women had no hypnotherapy, though some did have ECV (external cephalic version), a procedure whereby the baby's head is manually manipulated from outside the abdomen to bring about the downward turn.

In the study group, the mothers, while in hypnosis, were led through guided imagery to bring about deep relaxation. Suggestions were then given that they visualise their babies easily turning and see the turn accomplished, with the baby in proper vertex position for birthing. The mothers were helped to visualise the uterus becoming pliable and relaxed in order to allow the baby sufficient room to make the move. The mother was asked to talk to her baby, and the therapists encouraged the baby to release itself from the position it had settled into and to turn downward for an easy birth.

The study ended with 81 of the 100 breech babies in the study group having turned spontaneously from breech position to vertex position. It was originally thought that each mother would require approximately ten hours of hypnotherapy in order to accomplish the desired result.

As the study unfolded, the average number of hours spent with each woman was only four, and half of the successful 81 turns required only one session.

In the comparison group of 100 women who did not participate in hypnotherapy, only 26 babies turned spontaneously. An additional 20 were turned with ECV. It should be noted that it is not uncommon for the baby who is turned through ECV to turn back into breech position. The figures arrived at through this study are considered medically quite significant.

From these findings we see that, in addition to working with visualisation conducive to relaxing the uterus, mothers with babies in breech position can be helped through release therapy. Release therapy is an integral part of the HypnoBirthing programme, where mothers are helped to identify and release negative emotions. If your baby is in breech presentation and there is talk of a possible surgical birth, seek the assistance of your HypnoBirthing practitioner, who will help you with a special hypnosis session that has been found to be especially successful in achieving the desired turn. When the turning of the breech baby is achieved through relaxation and tension release, the baby usually remains in vertex position.

Your practitioner can also help you with finding community resources, acupuncturists, acupressurists, and chiropractors who perform the Webster technique and reflexologists and others who can help with turning techniques. Inquire about "tilting" techniques and other methods for helping the baby to turn. Then, and only then, consider ECV, which is a last resort to avoid a caesarean section. It is not usually a procedure of choice for most women, but it is preferable to surrendering to a surgical birth.

Before Labour:
When Baby Is Ready

From working with HypnoBirthing mothers over many years, I find that our mothers welcome the early signs that labour is near. Sometime prior to term, the mother begins to sense various signals that nature is playing its part in tuning up for the main concert.

Early Signals

Practice Labour: Much talked about but little understood, these surges are nature's way of preparing the uterus for your baby's birthing. They are much like the tightening sensations that are felt during labour, and for that reason we call them practise labour. For first babies, these tightening surges will probably show up sometime during the end of the seventh month. For subsequent pregnancies, they may appear as early as the sixth month.

From day to day you'll experience more of the practise labour surges. As you move and walk, you may even feel a sharp jolt as the pelvic area begins to make room for the baby's journey. This is the pubis bone moving forward and pulling at a ligament here or there. Your body is telling you that it, too, is "getting ready."

Until the final month of pregnancy, these surges are usually erratic and infrequent. As you come near to term, however, you may find that the intervals between them become shorter, and then finally become as frequent as ten- to twenty-minute intervals. Interestingly enough, these surges will sometimes give you a jolt with their pressure like waves, but they are not accompanied by pain. This makes one wonder if the painless pre-labour sensations are further proof of the mind-body connection—the mind knows the body is not ready for labour, so no pain impulse is emitted.

While most people don't consider these surges to be labour, there are many who would disagree and support the belief that the body is already involved in a labour practice that does, in fact, result in the cervix beginning to open. Some mothers will welcome the opportunity to remain relaxed and greet the surges with ease. As you reach term, you will want to take more notice of these sensations so that you don't dismiss what could actually be labour. Many mothers at this time get tuned in to their bodies, and they depend upon this and their instincts to let them know when the real thing has arrived.

Lightening: Several weeks before actual labour begins, the baby "drops" into the lower pelvic area. This is called "lightening." This is usually accompanied by mixed reactions on the part of the mother. It does, indeed, relieve that cramped feeling under the rib cage, and breathing is much easier. However, it also brings about much more pressure on the lower pelvis, and walking becomes a whole new experience. In spite of adjustments that you will have to make for this new position of your baby, you will find, like most other mothers, that your excitement begins to build.

Vaginal Discharge: Occasionally, you may experience more than a slight vaginal discharge that can be clear or whitish. This is another signal that your body is preparing for birth, and it is due to a higher volume of blood flow to that region of your body—another signal that your body is preparing for birth.

Looking at Your "Due Date"

What if your Estimated Due Date (EDD) arrives and labour doesn't start? A whole new set of feelings can spring up. Emotionally and physically, you feel ready "to go"—to birth your baby—but it isn't happening. If you take your due date as gospel and you're not prepared for a possible delay, these days of anticipation can take a toll on you. You may find that anxious, well-meaning family members begin to call regularly to check; your midwife and doctor will begin to take a more watchful eye; fears concerning the baby's well-being can creep in; and each day can start and end with a feeling of disappointment.

Perhaps you'll hear many stories from your friends who chose to be induced when the baby was "overdue." You may even be tempted to accept the subtle suggestions that you don't really need to wait any longer or that "you can be home for the holiday or the weekend." The important thing for you to do is to continue to relax and wait. Your baby knows when it's time to be born. Trust him or her.

Before overreacting to outside pressures, remember that the estimated due date is just that—an estimation. One of our doctors calls it "The Guess Date." Some suggest that it would be more realistic to refer to a birth month or to a segment of the month— "toward the end of September. . ." or "Sometime during the first part of October. . . ."

There are several reasons why your due date is only an estimation. To begin with, the selected date is usually calculated by recalling the date of the first day of your last menstrual period (which may not be accurate), counting back three months from that date and then adding seven days. However, recent studies suggest that for first-time mums, fifteen days should be added, and ten days should be added for mums who have birthed previously.

There are several factors that can skew this estimate: a) Actual calendar months differ in length; b) Menstrual cycles differ in the number of days between periods and in the duration of a period; c) The length of gestation can vary; d) Detection of a heartbeat or foetal movement may seem to support the timely development of the baby at a given point, but it must be remembered that just as children differ in their development, so, too, do babies in utero.

It's interesting to note that the number of babies who arrive on their due date is only around 5 percent, so if your birthing is not "on time," relax. You will be among the 95 percent of parents whose babies are born in advance of the EDD or sometime after the appointed date. The gestation period for 95 percent of normal babies lies within a very broad range of 265 to 300 days from the first day of the mother's last period. The average, taken from those figures, is the 282 days usually used to estimate the due date.

Also interesting is the fact that so many women today are being given as many as three different "due dates" as they proceed through pregnancy. That is certainly an indication that estimates are not solid. How many times did your conception date change?

You need to be able to focus on the fact that the range is between thirty-seven and forty-two weeks. You are not actually "Post Date" until you reach forty-two weeks. Remember, too, that if you are a first-time mother it's not unreasonable to expect that you may go a bit beyond the routine forty-two weeks. Many physicians will not even consider artificial initiation of labour in the absence of any special circumstances until you are at forty-two weeks. Your EDD has no magical significance, and as long as your baby is strong and healthy and you are strong and healthy, don't allow yourself to be pressured into thinking that every day beyond the EDD is a precarious time.

For your baby's sake, resist the temptation to bring medical intervention to your pregnancy when you pass your Guess Date, and certainly don't even consider induction prior to the EDD without a valid medical indication. Induction should occur only when a medical necessity exists for you or your baby. The artificial induction of labour for a baby whose term has been mistakenly calculated could result in birthing a premature baby. It can also mean further medical procedures if your cervix is not "ripe" and ready for birthing.

If it is suggested that you be induced, you owe it to yourself and your baby to have a valid explanation of the reason. You will want to ask about the risks of induction at the time it is recommended, as well as the benefits. Ask to know what your rating is on the "Bishop's Score," which is used to determine the degree to which your body is ready for labour and the probable success of your being induced. Inductions with low Bishop's Scores could mean that the induction could be difficult, leading to lengthy, painful labour and an increased possibility of surgical birth. A score of 8 or 9 would indicate that the induction probably would be successful, but it could also indicate that

your baby's birth is near. An induction should be considered only if
there is some true medical indication for it.

If you've done a good job initially at securing the support of your
caregiver, this should not become a problem for you.

This chart of the Bishop's Score shows the categories that are
considered.

Cervix	Score			
	0	1	2	3
Position	Posterior	Midposition	Anterior	Anterior
Consistency	Firm	Medium	Soft	Soft
Effacement	0–30%	40–50%	60–70%	80+
Dilation	Closed	1–2 cms	3–4 cms	5 cms+
Station	–3	–2	–1	+1, +2

Bishop's Score Chart

Neither your body nor your baby understands arbitrary timetables or
charts, so take the due date in stride and let Mother Nature and your
baby play out their intended roles in their own time. It is the safest
and most natural way. Once intervention is introduced in the way of
artificial induction, you have already moved away from normal birth.
Even the casual suggestion of "just popping that bag" or "doing a
little sweep," or helping your labour to start with a "little jump-start,"

can change the whole ball game for your birthing. These seemingly benign procedures can also result in a labour that is prolonged and sometimes painful if your body is really not "ready to go." When labour is delayed because the cervix is not opening, you may find yourself hearing further suggestions because "Your cervix just doesn't seem to want to open," or your cervix is taking an "inordinate amount of time to get started."

The best advice in looking at your due date is "don't."

Letting Your Baby
and Your Body Set the Pace

Mothers, hold on to your bag of waters.
It is there for a reason.

WILLIAM AND MARTHA SEARS, *THE BIRTH BOOK*

The actual trigger for the beginning of labour is not entirely known, but it is believed that a hormone secreted from within the baby's body triggers oxytocin, the natural labour-initiating hormone within the mother's body, and the miracle unfolds. That is all part of the master plan—a plan that has a designated flow, but not a designated schedule.

A labour that is slow to start or, later, a resting labour, does not automatically call for the introduction of a chemical stimulant to start or speed up your labour. Nor do these indications necessarily mean a complicated labour. If you experience a latent period when your surges are not starting, or if later the distance between the surges is lengthening, it doesn't mean that your birthing has gone askew. It simply means that the uterus and your baby are not so sure that this is the time yet.

Discussion of rushing in to "jump-start labour" or "move things along" or "augment sluggish surges" can actually bring about the opposite effect and cause a total interruption of the kind of labour that you are planning. If you allow yourself to succumb to these suggestions, you can easily find yourself in the middle of a chemically and chronologically managed labour. If such a comment is made, you or your birthing companion can nicely explain that unless there is a medical urgency, you would like to stay with your birth preferences and that you are in no hurry. One father, when told that if they didn't agree to inducing labour, they could be there all day, commented, "Oh, that's okay. We're not going anywhere." Nature will have its way, and calm is what you need.

Occasionally a mother will find that even when she accepts the suggestion of rupturing her membranes or of using a vaginal gel or Syntocinon drip, her labour still does not move along. Perhaps her body is being prompted into a labour for which it is not quite ready. Since the development of your baby's brain cells is accelerated during the last eight weeks of pregnancy, it seems prudent to let the baby complete this development in utero and not rush birth.

Once artificial induction or augmentation has been introduced in any form, you may find that you have surrendered your choices. Before agreeing to the introduction of procedures or drugs into your body and, therefore, your baby's body, weigh the possibility that you may be placing yourself and your baby on a very slippery slope. Hopefully these issues have weighed heavily upon your decision when you selected your care provider. The birthing room is no place to find that you should have questioned earlier or more often during your pre-natal office visits.

Some women find that by accepting even the smallest doses of synthetic oxytocin, they are able to continue to call on their HypnoBirthing relaxation techniques; others tell us that they tried, but, eventually, Syntocinon won out and they were into even larger doses. They had to request an epidural. This is one of the best reasons for not agreeing to it in the first place unless there is a true medical indication to consider. And, again, we turn to the argument for employing the right caregiver. When the family and caregiver are working together, this discussion will be moot. You will trust that such recommendations will be given only in the event of a situation that genuinely requires a change in the course of your labour.

Few expectant parents really take the time beforehand to explore the risks of deciding to use drugs for faster birth. Parents rarely seek an opportunity to talk with their caregivers about the effects of narcotics upon their pre-born and, subsequently, newborn. No parent would ever choose to give drugs to his or her newborn baby needlessly, but fear of labour can be strong enough to make it simpler for the pregnant family to avoid questions concerning the risks of inductions or epidurals. Similarly, few doctors take the opportunity to explain the adverse side effects of labour drugs with their patients. The matter becomes the medical version of "Don't ask; don't tell."

The well-respected Physicians' Desk Reference (PDR) clearly states that at this time there are no adequate and well-controlled studies for the use of these drugs with pregnant women. The PDR also points out that it is still not known whether these drugs can cause foetal harm when administered to labouring women. There is no hard evidence to support most of these procedures.

Even pills, or any of the injected drugs used to "take the edge off," can suppress a labouring mum's efforts to work with her body's surges, as HypnoBirthing mums are trained to do. An epidural, used to quell the effects of Pitocin/Syntocinon, may offer relief, but it also has a downside. These narcotics can cause reduced muscle tone and prolong labour. Because of the numbing effects of drugs, the labouring woman is less aware of her surges and may not be able to efficiently assist in working with them to facilitate opening. This can prolong labour and often results in increased administration of Pitocin/Syntocinon, leading to continued pain relievers, and so on. A very vicious cycle is established. If she is unable to feel surges and assist in the birthing phase, she could end up with a surgical birth.

Foetology experts are now saying that the disorientation that a baby experiences when his mother has accepted drugs can result in disconnection between mother and baby and cause a long-term feeling of abandonment on the part of the baby. Epidurals, in addition to causing dysfunction in the birthing process, can also cause a woman to run a fever. If this occurs, there is very little remedy except to get the baby born quickly.

If there is talk of induction, turn to the suggested natural means of bringing on labour in the next chapter. Don't dismiss these natural means of initiation, especially professional acupuncture, chiropractic, and acupressure. If you are already in labour, but are being offered augmentation, ask for time to be able to use some of the same natural methods used to initiate labour. Ask for privacy so you can use natural methods—hugs before drugs. As long as indications point to a healthy, strong baby and you are in no danger, be willing to protect your baby from the assault of drugs.

It is important for parents to meet all diagnoses and recommendations with curiosity. They should pause and consider the effects upon the mother and the baby, as well as the overall impact of the birthing experience. It is sometimes difficult for those medical care providers who subscribe to active management of labour to adjust to waiting and "standing by" in the event that they are needed. But if this is how you see your labour advancing and it differs from what you envisioned, you will want to rethink the path that you are on. If you are already beginning to sense that your birthing may go this way, you may want to make some changes now.

When Nature Needs Assistance

While simply going beyond your due date is not by itself cause to bring about medical intervention, on rare occasions a medically risky situation could occur in late pregnancy that should not be brushed aside or ignored as being "nothing." If you experience any of the signals listed below, call your care provider at the earliest possible time. Let your caregiver decide if, indeed, it is nothing or whether your condition requires medical attention.

Such instances include:

- Premature labour (three or more weeks early)
- Diminished foetal motion for more than six hours
- A prolonged period of time from release of the membrane without the natural start of labour
- Persistent and severe headaches—possibly elevated blood pressure
- A strong odour, colour, or significant amount of meconium (greenish-brown, tarlike substance) in the amniotic fluid

- Excessive vaginal bleeding
- Evidence of a prolapsed cord (Get off your feet, raise your buttocks, and call 999.)
- Indication of infection or fever
- Persistent or excessive vomiting or diarrhoea
- Dizziness or blurred vision
- Severe swelling of hands, face, ankles or feet
- Considerably darkened urine
- Unrelenting anxiety over mother's or baby's well-being
- Suicidal thoughts (call 999)

Initiating Labour Naturally

Without these factors, your relaxed attitude can work wonders in bringing about a natural start to your labour along with safe, labour-inducing techniques that you can use naturally and easily:

Hot and spicy foods. Mexican, Indian or Italian foods with "lots of hots" have had more than occasional success in starting labour. By stirring up the digestive processes in your body, you also stir your birthing muscles and your body into action. (Ask your HypnoBirthing practitioner for the special Italian recipe.) This is a good method to combine with any of the other techniques.

Lovemaking (hugs before drugs). If your membrane hasn't released, make love. Semen contains the hormone prostaglandin, which helps to soften the cervix. Here we see nature going full circle—what entered the uterus to help make the baby can help get it out. Kissing, hugging, fondling, and gentle finger or oral nipple or clitoral stimulation triggers the hormonal connection between the breast and vagina, producing the natural oxytocin that can start uterine surges. It is helpful to bring the mother to orgasm. If the stimulation of one nipple is not sufficient to start surges, try stimulation of both nipples simultaneously. However, prolonged or vigorous nipple stimulation of both nipples is not advised as it can have an adverse effect on your baby by creating hyperstimulation.

Visualisation. While your nipple or clitoris is being stimulated, use the rosebud visualisation, focusing on the rosebud's slowly unfolding and opening. Gently direct your breath down into the vaginal region while visualising.

Walk. Walk, walk, and then walk some more.

Bath. A medium-hot bath often provides the relaxation you need. You or your partner can scoop the water over your nipples and your abdomen. Take a shower, directing the hot water over your abdomen.

Fear release. Have your birth companion take you through a fear-release session similar to the one practised in class so that you can search your thoughts to see if there are any lingering fears, emotions, or unresolved issues that you need to release. Locked-up emotions can make you feel uptight and cause your body to produce inhibiting catecholamine. Your tension can translate into a tense cervix, preventing the flow of your natural relaxants. If you feel you need professional help, call your HypnoBirthing instructor for an individual fear-release session or ask for a referral to a hypnotherapist. It works wonders. Use this time for talking to the baby.

Acupressure. An acupressurist can facilitate the natural onset of labour almost immediately and yet afford you the time to make whatever preparations you need. Using the services of a professional will improve your chances of having the most effective points used and of obtaining faster results. It can also be helpful for use during labour. Do not apply pressure to these points other than at a time when you are ready to initiate labour.

Acupuncture/auricular therapy. Like acupressure, there are points that an acupuncturist or an auricular therapist can activate for the easy and effective induction of labour. These are relatively easy procedures and offer a much smoother entry into labour. Like the acupressure points, it is important that these points not be stimulated during pregnancy except for the purpose of induction when labour is slow to start or during a labour that has slowed.

Seeking the services of homeopathic and naturopathic doctors can be beneficial in collaboration with the recommendation above when these other recommendations have not been sufficient.

When you have exhausted all these means of natural initiations of labour, and it is determined that artificial induction by Pitocin/Syntocinon drip is an absolute necessity, you may request that only a minimal dose be administered and that it not be increased without your consent. You will also want to ask that the Pitocin/Syntocinon be withdrawn once your body has taken over. Many of our mothers report that the HypnoBirthing relaxation techniques that they mastered saw them through even with an induced labour, but it should be a last resort.

The Onset of Labour

L abour is usually defined as that period from the time that your cervix actually begins to thin and open until the moment that the baby is born.

HypnoBirthing recognises only two phases of labour: the Thinning and Opening Phase, and then the actual Birthing Phase, where the baby descends as his mother assists with Birth Breathing.

For the purpose of this study, I am covering in this chapter the more familiar aspects of labour as experienced by most couples. Much of the material applies to most birthing women whether they are birthing in a hospital setting, free-standing birth centre, or in their homes.

Labour will start with the first phase anytime between 37 and 42 weeks of pregnancy. The 40-week estimation of term is called EDD (Estimated Due Date). From 40 weeks, gestation period is expressed as 40.1; 40.2; 40.3; and so on. First-time mums average a gestation period of 41.3. A woman is not post date, or late, until she has reached 42.0.

The most common signs of the onset of labour are:

The release of the membranes (can be leaking or a sizeable gush).

Release of the uterine seal and birth show.

Uterine surges often up to 30 minutes apart.

A feeling of constipation or loose stooling.

Surges that form a pattern.

None of the above (some women report only tightness around the abdominal area).

Sometimes the release of membrane is an early sign of labour; for others, it may not occur until just before the baby is born. Babies can even be born "en caul," with the membrane surrounding them like a veil.

If the release of your membranes is the first signal that your labour is beginning, you will want to check the fluid to be sure that it:

1. is clear with no particles, except for an occasional show of white vernix, the cheeselike covering that surrounds the baby in the sac;

2. has no colour;

3. has no putrid odour.

When the membranes release, call your care provider to report that you have examined the fluid, and it meets all of the conditions mentioned above. Assure the caregiver that you wish to remain at home until your labour is under way and that you will call before leaving for the hospital. If you have hired the right caregiver, this should be the end of the conversation.

You may begin to hear of the danger of infection. This often is followed by the suggestion that you come into the hospital "to be checked" so that antibiotics can be administered to prevent infection or so that you can be monitored. While infection is a possibility, it is a very rare one, and it is not imminent. Bacteria have to be introduced into the body in order for infection to take place. As one doctor says, "The vagina is not a straw." Another advises, "The vagina is not a sponge." When you step out of the bathtub, there is no flow of water that has gathered in the vagina. One of our doctors reminds his mothers that bacteria are not sperm, and they don't swim. Don't be intimidated by talk of early infection if there is no indication of infection.

Accepting a vaginal exam can be the first step toward artificial induction. Often being checked translates to "check-in," followed by pressure to jump-start your labour. If you remain at home until your labour really starts, you will avoid both of these interventions.

Sometimes there is a considerable delay between the time that your membrane releases and active labour starts. This doesn't mean that something is wrong. In the event that the onset of labour is delayed, refer back to the suggestions for initiating labour naturally. Don't buy into the notion that labour must be started immediately. Chances are, labour will start on its own within twenty-four hours. Buy time and request that you wait for another couple of hours or so. Your temperature can be monitored. If your labour is delayed for a long period of time, and you are being pressured to have your labour induced, request that antibiotics be administered. Politely decline any vaginal exams. It's that simple. It is not necessary that an induction procedure be initiated, barring any other indications of a need to do so. Agreeing to that first intervention or to an artificial induction in the absence of medical indication could turn your plans for a calm birth upside down.

You will know that the onset of true labour has arrived when you experience uterine surges that are rhythmic—tightening and releasing in a distinct pattern. You may or may not feel your uterine surges starting. Some mothers report feeling only a tightening sensation in and around the abdomen at the onset of their labour. For many HypnoBirthing mothers, these sensations are not accompanied by discomfort. They are not convinced that their labour has actually begun. Some report only that they feel constipated and need to relieve their bowels.

Before or after you experience your first uterine surge, you may discover that the uterine seal that prevents bacteria from entering the uterus has dislodged. "This birth show" is a stringy discharge that can be clear, tinged, slightly pink, or bright red.

From the time you were admitted at the hospital or birthing centre, your assessment will be judged by how long you have been in labour. Don't allow yourself or your birth companion to become overly caught up in the mechanics of timing and charting. You will sense when the intervals between surges are becoming shorter if you listen to your body frequently.

The months of conditioning and practice are now paying off. Your positive attitude and confidence will allow you to remain calm and relaxed.

When your surges begin, use relaxation and Slow Breathing to increase the efficiency of each surge, visualising the opening rosebud and breathing gently down toward your vagina. This will encourage the uterus to start surging.

The calm HypnoBirthing approach to birth inhibits secretion of catecholamines, so it is likely that your digestive functioning will not be arrested. You need energy and you need to snack; drink lots of fluids to avoid dehydration and keep your bladder empty.

At your signal—usually closing your eyes—your birth companion will know that you are in surge and will stroke your arm while reciting the cues that are on the Birth Companion's Prompt Card (available from your HypnoBirthing instructor). It's not necessary to follow the prompts line by line. These are suggestions for the kinds of phrases that will assist you in remaining relaxed.

The most important factor to consider during labour may be what you sense and feel, not what you see or hear. As your birth companion gives prompts, trust your body and go deeper within each surge that you breathe up, maximising each surge to the fullest. Trust your body, as it knows and will tell you when it is the best time to move to a birthing facility. If you are birthing at home, continue to relax and stay at home.

The illustration that follows shows a comfortable birthing mother lying in a lateral position during labour.

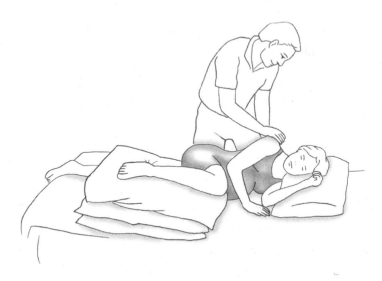

Lateral Position During Labour

As Labour Advances:
Thinning and Opening

Prepare for a no-fault birth. . . .
If you confidently participate in all the
decisions made during your labour and delivery—
even those that were not in your birth plan—
you are likely to look upon your birth
with no blame and no regrets.

WILLIAM SEARS AND MARTHA SEARS, *THE BIRTH BOOK*

A s you move through the Thinning and Opening Phase of your labour, you will find that your many weeks of preparation are now stepping in to assist you as you turn your birthing over to your baby and your body. You call upon your natural birthing instinct and literally "do nothing" but allow your body to remain loose and limp. Creating a nest, as you did when you practised, can greatly assist you in reaching a wonderful feeling of lightness and buoyancy. Nesting is illustrated earlier in this book.

Instead of looking upon your labour in fragments, as is the case in most other programmes, you will see your labour as a continuum. You may hear mention of centimeters and discussion of how "open" your cervix is. Pay no attention to those numbers. HypnoBirthing mothers blow those figures right out of the water. One can be at only four centimeters at one vaginal exam and, surprisingly, at seven or eight at the next exam. The number tells you little or nothing, and certainly they are not a valid gauge of how long your labour will last. They tell you only where you are at that given moment. Relax and just visualise the cervix opening in a continuing manner, as shown in the illustration.

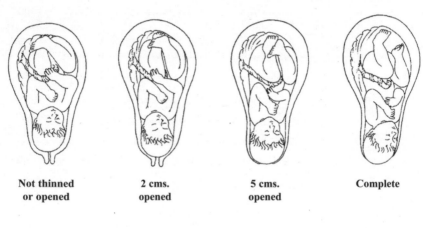

| Not thinned or opened | 2 cms. opened | 5 cms. opened | Complete |

Hallmarks of Labour

During this period, you will probably experience at least one or more of the hallmarks of labour—those milestones that tell you that your labour is moving along. They are all very natural and good messages from your body. Your birth companion will remind you of the hallmarks as you pass each one. It's exciting.

- Your body heat will rise and/or drop alternately. One minute you will be kicking off bedding; in another you'll be requesting a warmed blanket.

- When you get up to empty your bladder, there may be a spot of blood on your sanitary pad. The body is directing its efforts downward.

- You may begin to hiccup, burp, feel nauseated, or even vomit as your diaphragm has an initial reaction to the lower pulsations in your body that will soon move your baby down to birth. The good news is that it doesn't last long. (It happens rarely with HypnoBirthing mums because their bodies are calm and not in tumult.)

- Regardless of how calmly and well you have approached your birthing, you may all of a sudden feel the need "to escape." Even a mum who is having a fantastic birthing has been known to express the thought, "I don't think I want to do this any longer" or "I can't do this anymore." This last hallmark is one of the most exciting. It means that the birth of your baby is right around the corner. Your birth companion will remind you of this hallmark, and the mood changes for everyone in the room. Your baby is almost here.

What Is Happening?

The cervix is thinning. The longitudinal fibres of the uterus continue to draw back the circular fibres so that the cervix increasingly thins and opens.

You will continue to experience the wave of each surge. Your abdomen will feel as though it is surging upward, tightening, and then receding back down again. These surges usually last no more than thirty-five to forty-five seconds at this point. Keeping your body limp and relaxed allows this stage to pass with little or no discomfort. Intervals between surges can vary considerably.

Clutching, clenching, or curling up in a foetal position all create tension in your body that is counterproductive. You will also want to avoid getting caught up in activities and options that hospital staff will offer with kind intentions (unless those activities or options appeal to you). Mothers frequently say that suggestions that they take walks, spend time in a rocker, or "get things moving" distracted them and broke their deep level of relaxation.

You will hear that your muscles will work more efficiently if you walk and remain active. In 1997 a study in Texas, conducted through the University of Texas Southwestern Medical Centre, found that there were no significant differences between the length of labour of women who walked and those who remained sitting, relaxing, or resting. I have never observed animal mothers walking halls. Instead, they seem to go deeper into relaxation.

HypnoBirthing mothers find that their cervixes seem to open more easily and quickly as a result of giving those muscles the necessary relaxation and oxygenated blood flow needed to open.

If you feel that you would like to walk, then do so, but not because you are being pressured to get on your feet and get those muscles moving.

Attempting to overcome or manipulate labour can cause fatigue and discouragement. If you have spent a sufficient amount of time conditioning your mind and body, the art will be there for you. Follow the techniques that you learned, and trust in yourself and your body's ability to birth. You'll be fresh, alert, and fully energised when that wonderful moment of birth arrives.

"Tubbers"

I spoke to a labour and birthing nurse recently who couldn't rave enough about how successful her "tubbers" were at combining HypnoBirthing and water birthing. We are seeing many women choose the comfort and ease of water birthing. It is an extraordinarily good complement to HypnoBirthing, enhancing your relaxation and allowing the baby to be born into an environment that makes for an easy transition from life within the womb to air breathing. There is no doubt about the merit of the weightlessness and buoyancy that water provides. When women use this combination, their minds are free and relaxed, and their bodies are better able to benefit from the softening effect that water has on the birthing muscles and on the folds of the perineum. One therapy contributes to the efficacy of the other.

The association between water and sensuality is also not wasted on couples who are birthing. That's because it is understood that water gives us a feeling of pleasure, contentment, and well-being. Water will help this phase of labour pass in a way that is beyond comparison.

Slow or Resting Labour

I t is not uncommon for a labour to slow, then to accelerate, slow again, and then reach completion. The best way to manage a slowed or resting labour is to meet it with patience. The one thing you don't want to see happening is that you succumb to the notion that this is a trouble sign and the labour must be augmented. Most HypnoBirthing families are better able to get through this without intervention because they do not have continual Electronic Foetal Monitor (EFM).

Introduced onto the birthing scene in the 1980s, these machines were devised to help monitor the labours of women who were high-risk; but now with one in every room, the devices have become a huge drawback for the family who is not at risk. The biggest drawback of having an EFM in the birthing environment is that some medical care-givers tend to get overly caught up with tracings and patterns. There is the mistaken belief that a woman's cervix must open according to some regulated pattern or time frame, or it needs to be "fixed." The baby often ends up on the short end of the fixing.

A resting labour later does not mean that immediate steps need to be taken to restart the labour. Nature will have its way, and calm is what you need. After experiencing the calm of a nap, many mothers resume an active and even accelerated labour.

If you should experience a slow or resting labour, ask for time to be able to use some of the same natural methods used to initiate or restart a resting labour. Ask for privacy so you can use natural methods—hugs before drugs. As long as you and your baby are healthy and strong, and you are in no danger, be willing to protect your baby from the assault of drugs.

Occasionally, when a mother accepts the suggestion of rupturing her membranes or of using a Syntocinon drip, her labour does not move along more rapidly.

Unless it's a true medical urgency, the family should pause and consider the effects of any intervention upon the mother and the baby, as well as the overall impact of the birthing experience.

In addition to employing some of the suggestions in the section on inducing labour naturally, there are several ways in which you can pass time during a slow or resting labour that actually enhance your comfort and contribute to the opening and spreading of the pelvic area. For example:

The Birth Ball: The birth ball serves many purposes: It can offer you an alternative to remaining in bed during a prolonged labour; it is an excellent prop for you to support yourself by the side of your bed while your birthing companion applies Light Touch Massage; and it relaxes the pelvic muscles. Many hospitals provide birth balls for labouring mothers. Feel free to request one or bring your own. They're fun and so beneficial.

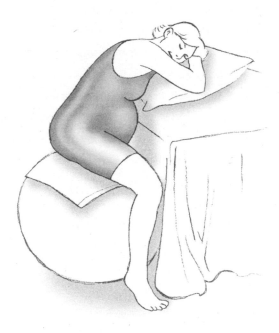

Labouring Mother Resting on a Birth Ball

Bath or Birth Pool: The benefits of the bath or birth pool have already been explained. Many mothers delight in spending a good deal of time in them if their labours are taking time. In order to derive the most benefit from your stint in the bath, place a towel from the tips of your nipples down to your thighs to keep the protruding parts of your body warm. While gently scooping water over your body, your birthing companion can recite the usual prompts during your surges.

Shower: A warm shower, with the water directed to your abdomen, is also a good way to pass time and gives the effect of effleurage.

Humour: The breathing produced by laughter is one of the best means of relaxing. Pack several pieces of humourous reading. Humour increases the production of endorphins, which, in turn, block the intro-duction of catecholamine.

Nipple Stimulation: The stimulation of one or both nipples triggers the hormonal connection between the breast and the vagina, producing your body's natural oxytocin that can enhance your uterine surges. Ask for the privacy to be able to use nipple stimulation. Your medical caregivers will be neither surprised nor embarrassed at your request.

If Labour Weakens

There may come a time when all accommodation to your wishes has been extended, but, for some reason, an obvious pattern of decreased or severely weakened uterine activity forms; and your baby is not weathering it well. In such an instance, it may be determined that your birthing needs medical assistance.

In this kind of situation, you will find that being a part of the decision-making team will help you accede to whatever preparations need to be made. You will remain calm and in control of your circum-stances. This is HypnoBirthing.

Nearing Completion

You are reaching the end of the Thinning and Opening Phase. Your surges are closer, stronger, and more beneficial. The wall of your cervix has completely thinned, and the cervix is continuing to open sufficiently to allow the baby to begin to move down. When this happens, your body sends a message that it's time to change from Slow Breathing to Birth Breathing—the gentle, but firm, breathing down that will help you to bypass lengthy, difficult, and fatiguing "pushing" techniques used by other methods.

Time distortion usually sets in, and you lose track of time. You will be more aware of the working of your uterus, with waves rising almost as though your birthing body is separate from the rest of your body; you may or may not be aware that the surges are becoming longer and higher. As you breathe each one up to the fullest, they become more efficient. The touch and voice of your birth companion will guide you through each surge. Your journey becomes more encouraging, as labour from this point can move along very quickly, especially as you deepen your relaxation.

You drift into an almost amnesiac state, focusing on your birthing experience. You will find that conversations in the room become fuzzy; and even if you are spoken to, it just seems like almost too much effort to respond. You go deeper and deeper, and your mind relaxes and rests. At this point you are fully birthing instinctively. You just get out of the way and let your body do the work. At the end of this phase, as your cervix becomes fully opened, you will feel the fullness within your body and, unless you experience a resting time, you will instinctively feel the need to change your breathing pattern to the downward Birth Breathing to assist the baby in his descent. It is essential that you understand that from this point on there is no pathological reason for discomfort, unless you allow yourself to slip out of this amnesiac state and assume the tension within your body.

During this time your body assists you with its natural expulsive reflex (NER). It is important more than ever that you do nothing and allow your body to do its job of taking charge of your baby's descent. To help you further, the vaginal wall becomes lubricated and expands. The rhythmic pulsations move the baby down.

What Feelings You May Experience

Your mood will remain calm and nearly euphoric. You may go through this final phase of opening in an almost dreamlike state. Nature's amnesia will lull you so that you seem to drift in and out of alertness. It becomes even easier to place your awareness only on your baby and your birthing body.

As time distortion clicks in, the length of the surge will be distorted, and your time consciousness will fade. Twenty minutes will, indeed, seem like five. This is nature's way of helping you remain placid and serene. At the end of this phase, your shift to Birth Breathing will give you a feeling of well-being, as you and your baby work together.

How You May Participate

At this time, you really settle into birthing. Your conversant stage has passed, and you are easing into the business of having a baby. Deep relaxation and a thoroughly limp body help you to block out your surroundings and go even further within to your baby.

By this time, many women have already adopted a lateral position. If you choose to stay on your back, your birthing companion needs to be sure that the head of the bed is elevated so that you are not lying flat. Lying flat can limit the supply of oxygen to your baby. Your birthing companion will help you to adjust your position if you slip down in the bed.

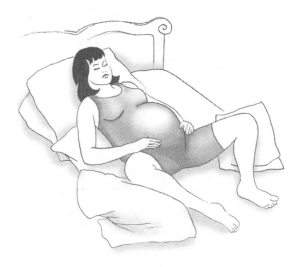

Semi-Reclining Position Modified

With deepened relaxation, you let go and let your baby and your body do what each can do best during this time. You will continue to breathe up with your uterine surges until your cervix opens, but it will seem almost effortless. With the signal of downward lower fullness, you will know instinctively that it is time to change your breathing to Birth Breathing. Your birth companion will assure staff that you are not going to push at this point; and it is safe for you to change to a Birth Breath.

With no effort, you move closer to a place of utter comfort, moving in harmony with your body.

When your body sends the message that it is time to begin to nudge your baby down, you will follow the lead of your body and work with the shift of your pulsations that now direct your breathing downward in contrast to the upward breathing that you have been doing up until now. Often this is all accomplished with little notice; you continue to work with your surges quietly and serenely without changing position.

You should not be alone, even though you may appear to be perfectly relaxed and simply resting. That look can be deceiving, as few others are aware that you are breathing your baby down to the vaginal outlet.

The Pelvic Station

The location of the baby's head within the pelvic region is measured by what is known as the Pelvic Station. You will hear reference to the Pelvic Station both before and during your birthing. As the baby journeys downward, his progress may be explained to you as being at -1 or +1 or +2. Positive numbers are below the midsection of the pelvis; negative numbers are above the midsection. The measure is determined by where the "presenting part" or top of the baby's head is. If you are told that the head is high, it means that the position is still in the minus level. The head is said to be engaged when the head is at 0.

The Pelvic Station

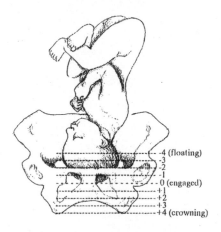

-4 (floating)
-3
-2
-1
0 (engaged)
+1
+2
+3
+4 (crowning)

Every child is unique. Every child must pass through the same stages, leading from an enclosed world to the open one, from being folded in on itself to reaching outward.

Frederick Leboyer, M.D., *Birth Without Violence*

Practice Positions
Also Used in Birthing

What Is Happening?

W hat is happening is **birth**! Your baby gradually descends to the rim of the perineum, and the baby's head becomes visible (crowning). With the head nearly or fully crowned, you are ready now to give those final few breaths that will bring the baby past the perineal rim and into the world. After birth, your baby is placed immediately on the skin of your abdomen or lower chest for embrace and bonding with you and your birth companion. When the umbilical cord stops pulsating, the cord will be cut, and you, your baby, and your birthing companion continue to bond.

The more nature is able to take its course, the less likely you are to need an episiotomy. In the same way that the neck of the cervix needed to be gradually thinned and opened, the thick rim of the perineum needs to gradually thin and unfold through each surge by natural pressure of the baby's head until, at last, the folds open fully to allow the baby's head to pass through. It appears to be a slow unraveling, but, to the contrary, it is more swiftly accomplished with Birth Breathing than by any other means. HypnoBirthing mums talk of three or four Birth Breaths to bring the baby past the perineum and out.

Birth Breathing is the opposite of Slow Breathing, where you drew the surge up and worked with the upward wave. Now, instead of breathing up, you will take in a short, deep breath and breathe down. Your birthing companion will prompt you to direct your breath and love downward to help your baby move smoothly down to crowning. As you exhale, breathe down and visualise the opening of your vagina like the petals of a rose, folding outward as your baby moves to the perineal rim.

If the move is going smoothly, you may choose to remain in a lateral position (see illustration to follow) and simply breathe down until the baby's head is visible, or you may wish to adopt the Slanted "J" position, being sure to rest just above your tailbone to allow the baby plenty of room to move out. If your baby needs some help in moving down smoothly, you may want to adopt some of the positions that are described and illustrated in the following pages. Some of the recommended positions are designed to help the muscles and pelvic structure to spread and open more freely. Many of the positions call for your birth companion to assist you so that the two of you can take part in your baby's birth together.

Toilet Sitting Position

This position that you have been using throughout your pregnancy on a daily basis will also prove to be a very comfortable one to alternate with other positions during your birthing

Many women find a great deal of comfort in Toilet Sitting while they are still in the opening phase and while breathing their baby down.

The body naturally responds to this position as it is conditioned to release and let go when toileting. The two sets of muscles are closely related, and the Natural Expulsive Reflex (NER) present in birthing is supported by Birth Breathing. This position can offer the kind of spread that helps your pelvic area, opens your vagina, utilises gravity, and relieves you from having to support yourself on your legs. Just place a pillow or two behind your back and relax. As you near the crowning period, you will have to assume another of the birthing positions in order to safely birth your baby.

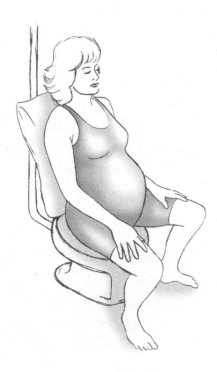

Toilet Sitting

Additional Relaxation and Birthing Positions

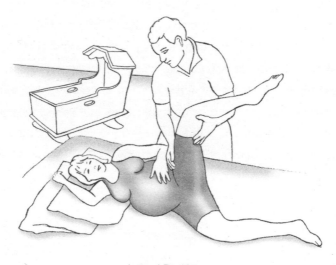

Lateral Position

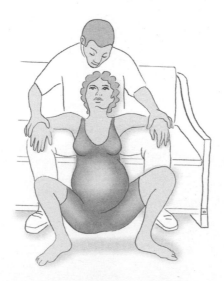

Companion Supported Squat Position

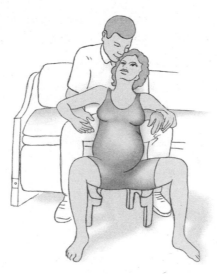

Supported Position on Birthing Stool

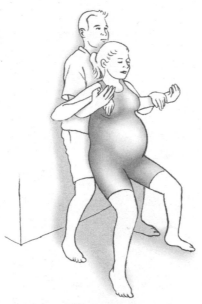

Companion Supported Upright Position

These are additional positions to use during the birthing stage that can be adopted by the birthing mother without the assistance of her companion. They are as follows:

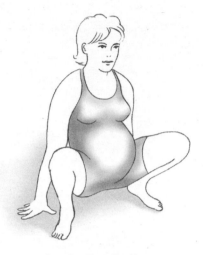

Leaping Frog Positions

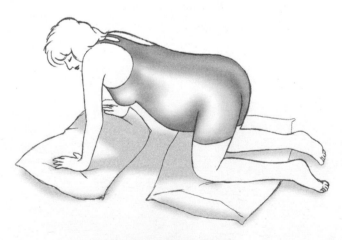

Hands-and-Knees Position

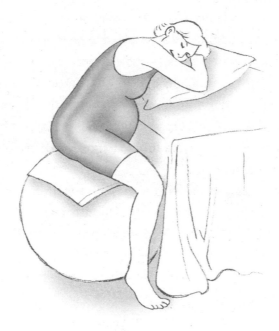

The Birth Ball

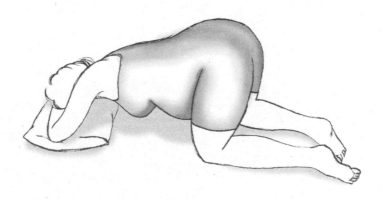

Polar Bear Position

Polar Bear: While the Polar Bear position is not a birthing position, it can be helpful if the baby is found to be in a less than optimal position for emergence. This favourable position can be assumed from a Hands-and-Knees position by placing your forearms on the floor in front of you and resting your forehead on your hands. Both the Polar Bear and the Hands-and-Knees position allow your baby to move back from the lower pelvic area and turn to a more beneficial position for birthing if this is needed.

If the baby does need an assist to move to a more optimal position, the Rebozo technique can be nicely utilised while mother is in the Polar Bear position. The technique, developed by midwife Guadalupe Trueba, is well known in Mexico and is fast making its way into birthing rooms in the United States. It is simply done by placing a long scarf under the mother's abdomen at the area of the pelvic region and lifting upward. This manoeuvre lifts the baby out of the present position and provides her with an opportunity to, in effect, back up and return to the birth path in a more favourable position for easy birthing.

Your Baby Crowns and Births

This is the first time that you "see" the results of your labour as the tip of the baby's head becomes visible. You will feel encouraged when you reach this point. The natural pulsations of your body will slowly urge your baby forward as you continue to direct the breathing that assists your baby to crowning.

When the top of the head is fully visible, one or two more surges are usually all that are needed to gently birth the baby's head. It is amazing how easily a head can pass through the elastic-like perineum if you remain relaxed. Tears in the skin can be avoided if the mother has practised perineal massage and there are no rushed, violent pushes.

The birth companion will continue to help you return to a relaxed state between surges. Birthing prompts are repeated here also. The entire pelvic area should be kept as relaxed as possible. Directing your breath toward the vagina and helping the baby to move forward will help the perineum to unfold.

If everything is fine, the baby should be birthed fully before suctioning or other routines are performed, and one of the parents should receive the baby if that is their wish. The handling of the baby by someone other than a parent should be minimal and utilised only if necessary. This will help make the baby's transition into her new surroundings less traumatic. Many caregivers now are happy to assist a parent in this.

Bonding

If you don't already know if your baby is a boy or a girl, you'll not have to wait long, for as soon as the baby is born, your birthing companion will announce the sex of the baby to you. You'll share this happy time together while caregivers visibly observe the baby's condition and assess mum's needs.

The baby is placed immediately on your bare chest or abdomen for bonding. Remarkably, studies called Kangaroo Mother Care, out of Australia, have found that the mother's body heat adjusts to the needs of her newborn.

At this point the birthing companion places his hand on the baby's back to offer the security of skin-to-skin bonding that is so important during these first few moments. Handling by others should be minimal, if not absent entirely. The baby needs to feel safe among the people whose scents and energies she is most familiar with.

There is no need to rush to "clean" the baby, nor to cut the cord. It is more important for the newborn to experience skin contact with both of its parents, if possible. The vernix caseosa, that cheesy covering that makes your baby look like a channel swimmer, will simply be absorbed into the baby's skin—it is a gift from nature. Any excesses will be removed later when baby has her first bath.

You will experience exhilaration beyond compare in these first few incredible moments as you and your birth companion touch and hold the baby, watching her begin to stretch and move and unfold, gaining a tactile sense of her new environment, one arm and one leg at a time.

Bonding during those first few precious moments of your baby's life will provide a natural high that defies description, and the feeling that you and your companion experience will remain with you for the rest of your lives. This is when the relationship that began before your baby was born is reaffirmed with actual skin-to-skin bonding—mother and father and baby (or other birthing companion) embracing in loving union.

It is during this time that a loving relationship is affirmed, and this wonderful happening should not be rushed. Through your caresses, gaze, and soft conversation, you validate your infant's acceptance and approval. The baby feels this love, and her feelings of security and self-worth are validated.

HypnoBirthing practitioners who have witnessed that first gaze when the infant's eyes meet with his parents' cite this as one of the most spiritual times in their lives as birthing educators.

Like all mammals, babies are genetically and instinctively programmed to take to the breast. You may wish to bond with your baby in this way, while the birth companion continues to support the baby's body with his hand or becomes involved with the cutting of the cord. Allowing your baby to complete the crawl to the breast has physical, as well as psychological, benefits. This contact and stimulation at the breast causes your uterus to begin to contract, helps to expel the placenta, and appropriately closes blood vessels to avoid any possible excessive bleeding. Your midwife will offer suggestions and assistance to help you and your baby as you experience your first feeding.

More is written on the importance of secluding yourselves with your baby to help her adjust to this new earthly environment in the chapter "Birth Afterglow."

Baby Is Born

You should be informed of the first appearances of your baby's head in a calm manner. There is a tendency for those in attendance to begin to direct this phase with loud, animated cheers. I stress that birthing is not an athletic event. Voices should not be raised. This is as much for your baby as for you. Your baby hears every sound; the sounds that he hears should not frighten him.

What You Will Feel

There is no need for discomfort during the birthing phase of labour. The cervix has already thinned and opened, and now the gradual descent of the baby is conducted in such a way that there is no strain on the tissues and sphincters of the birth path. Movies and television notwithstanding, if this descent is completed as you have practised, there is no reason for pain or any other sensation. Most women experience this birthing phase calmly as they breathe down and ultimately help the baby to emerge. There is no doubt that this is the most beautiful time of birthing. This is the culmination of everything you've planned and waited for during the last nine months.

Birth Breathing

For a good portion of the birthing phase, your body and baby will be working in harmony, as the natural expulsive reflex (NER) takes over and moves your baby down the birth path. You will assist by using the breathing technique that you have been practising for some time. Once your baby's head becomes visible, you will continue to use this downward nudge breath until the baby is gently breathed past the opening folds of the perineum and emerges in birth.

This phase cannot be taken lightly if you wish to birth easily and efficiently. Just as you needed to practise Surge Breathing to bring yourself past the thinning and opening phase, you will need to practise Birth Breathing. While in labour, you will follow your body's lead and work with it when you feel the onset of a surge. Here are some helpful hints:

- The best place to practise this breathing style is on the toilet as you are moving your bowels. Become aware of the pulsations that move the stool down and out. Your breaths are short intakes with gentle nudging breaths downward—nothing forceful. Practising in this way will show you that it actually accomplishes the task more easily and quickly.

- Your eyes may remain closed if you choose to stay in deep relaxation through this period. Since you will not be forcefully pushing, there is no need for you to keep your eyes open to avoid tearing the tiny blood vessels in your eyes.

- Placing the tip of your tongue at the place where your front teeth and palate meet will help your lower jaw to recede so that you remain free of tension in your mouth and jaw area. This will also help to relax the vaginal outlet.

- When you feel the onset of a surge, follow it. Take in a short, but deep, breath through your nose and direct the energy of that breath to the lower back of your throat and down through your body behind your baby in the form of a "J"—down and forward. Allow all the muscles in your vaginal area to open as though you were letting the breath out through them or moving your bowels. Don't ride out or hang on to a breath beyond its effectiveness; and don't allow those lower muscles to tighten.

- Repeat this process by taking in another short, deep breath and breathe down in the same pattern as above—and then another.

- Repeat this motion several times with each surge as your body leads you through this part of birthing your baby down to crowning. Continue to work with your body as long as it is still surging. Breathing down only once during a surge can cause you to lose the effectiveness of the surge, prolong the birthing time, and waste your energy.

- Firmly direct your breathing down through your body. Don't let the thrust of your breath escape through your mouth. These are not shallow breaths, but they are also not strenuous. These are deep breaths, with the energy of the breath going right down to your vagina.

- You may experience the sensation of needing to move your bowels, and that is exactly the region to which you need to direct the thrust of your breath. That is the reason we ask you to practise on the toilet.

- With the exhalation of each breath, your birthing companion will prompt you to breathe love and energy down to your baby, to open the path and to nudge your baby down to birth.

Your baby is now ready to come out and must be allowed to come easily. The head births first; the vulva gradually distends without discomfort; the baby's body emerges, often requiring only more gentle bearing down.

Many HypnoBirthing mothers who have thoroughly mastered relaxation and deepening techniques are surprised to learn that none of the steps described above are necessary. A relaxed body can actually propel the baby through the path to emergence on its own.

Post-Birth Activities

Still at work for you, your body reacts to the euphoria you are feeling by stimulating the uterus into the final stage. The umbilical cord is cut after it stops pulsating. With one or two more surges, the placenta is born. You and your birth companion bond with your new baby.

From this point on, all who share this wonderful miracle experience a very enjoyable high. Often doctors and midwives who witness HypnoBirthing express awe at participating in the experience. An indefinable feeling of joy and pleasure sweeps in and takes over. You and your birthing companion may be oblivious to the activities of medical caregivers at this point as you experience getting acquainted with your new baby.

It is important that the clamping and cutting of the cord be delayed until after it stops pulsating. When the cord is prematurely cut, it abruptly cuts off the flow of blood to the baby, depriving him of that source of oxygen and of the many nutrients that will affect his health for a lifetime. Allowing the baby to take his first breaths with the continued benefit of oxygen from the placenta eases the task of taking air into his lungs once he is outside the womb. It is an easier and more comfortable introduction to breathing.

Your baby is put to the breast. HypnoBirthing babies, alert and comfortable, usually take to the breast within minutes of their birth.

Dr. Lennart Righard's Delivery Self-Attachment video, resulting from a study in Denmark published in 1990, shows the ability of newborns who were not medicated during labour to crawl to the mother's breast, just as other mammals do, and suckle. On the other hand, even with help, the babies whose mothers were medicated lacked the ability to crawl to the breast and were unable to suckle even with assistance.

When the cord has stopped pulsating, it is clamped. Your companion, if he or she chooses, may take part in cutting the cord, separating the baby from the cord and placenta.

The expulsion of the placenta should be allowed to occur naturally with just one or two pushes as your uterus continues to surge. You may or may not be aware of these continued surges as your placenta is birthed. These final surges help your placenta to loosen from the wall of the uterus and assist the uterus to begin to assume its normal size. Allowing your placenta to break away in this normal manner can take anywhere from five to thirty minutes. In the event that the placenta is not birthed within a reasonable amount of time, your medical caregiver may suggest a medical assist. The cord should not be pulled in order to effect an extraction.

Your midwife or doctor will examine your placenta and then the abdomen to determine the "status" of your uterus.

An indescribable feeling of joy, excitement, and even giddiness sweeps in and takes over. Congratulations! Your miracle is complete.

Breastfeeding Is Best Feeding

Contributed by Robin Frees,
Lactation Consultant, HypnoBirthing practitioner

I t is your baby's "birth" day. If you could ask your baby about the best gift he could get from you, what would that be? Your baby would want to breastfeed. So before making a decision about infant feeding, consider the following thoughts and information. Give breastfeeding a try; and make an informed decision about your long-term goals for nurturing your child.

Breastfeeding is the perfect gift of love, security, and health all in one simple act. Just as your womb nourished your child for nine months, now your breasts are ready to continue that connection of food and nurturing for your baby. Just as your amniotic fluid acquired tastes and smells from your diet and your infant swallowed this while in the womb, breast milk also has flavours from your diet; and after birth, your baby continues to experience many new tastes. This is a gift that money can't buy. Whether you decide to breastfeed for a few weeks, months, or years, this is your first opportunity to give your baby a gift with benefits that will last a lifetime. Earlier we discussed your baby's need for connection; what better way to meet his many needs than to be held and breastfed?

In recent years, research has confirmed that breast milk is truly a unique food that cannot be duplicated. Formula is not equal to breast milk. The evidence of this fact became so overwhelming that in 1997 the American Academy of Pediatrics adopted a policy statement recommending that children receive breast milk for twelve months or more. The World Health Organisation recommendations on the priority of infant nutrition are in the following order:

1. mother's own milk directly from the breast

2. expressed mother's milk fed to infant another way

3. other human milk (from a milk bank)

4. infant formula

One of the outstanding benefits of human milk is that it is custom-made for each infant. Mothers with premature infants make milk that is specifically composed for their infant with extra antibodies and proteins. Breast milk contains not only carbohydrates, fats, and proteins but also has growth hormones and special substances that enhance visual and brain development, as well as antibodies to fight infection. Scientists are unable to put these valuable substances into formula. Studies have shown children who breastfeed have fewer instances of ear infections, diarrhoea, and upper respiratory infections. The advantages carry over into later periods in life. Adults who were breastfed have lower cholesterol and fewer occasions of heart disease. Studies have also shown that women who breastfeed have lower rates of breast cancer and cervical cancer. In addition to experiencing fewer common illnesses and diseases, breastfed children have higher IQs.

You may not have considered the financial value of this resource that your body makes at no cost to you. If you were to bottle-feed formula to your infant for a year, it may cost between $1,200 to $2,700, whereas human milk obtained by a doctor's prescription from a milk bank would cost about $36,000 for the same period! No wonder mothers call breast milk "liquid gold." Your body provides your baby this perfect diet absolutely free.

Normally, breastfeeding is a skill that is easy for you and your baby to learn. Mothers and babies have been doing this for thousands of years. As with any skill, like dancing or driving a car, the more you do it, the better you get at it. Getting through the first couple of weeks may seem natural or, at first, seem awkward, but given time, you and your baby will enjoy this special experience more and more.

During the first couple of days, your body has a small amount of early milk called colostrum. This is the time when your infant can practise latching on and sucking before the milk begins to increase in volume from teaspoons to ounces. Colostrum is an effective laxative that can help clear the meconium (baby's first stools) from your baby's system. It is also full of antibodies to protect your baby from illness. If your baby is sleepy and uninterested in eating, you can always express your colostrum onto a spoon and feed it to your baby to entice him to want to feed. Holding your baby skin-to-skin is another way for your baby to become interested in feeding. Studies show that the breast secretes a smell similar to amniotic fluid to attract the baby.

Learning a new skill is easier when someone is helping you. You didn't learn to drive a car by yourself. Remember to ask for help. Watching other mother's breastfeed before your baby is born will help you learn faster, too.

You may experience some breastfeeding challenges during the first week, but as you did during your pregnancy, keep a positive attitude toward breastfeeding. It soon becomes a gift to both mother and baby alike. If you experience discomfort, know that it is not a normal part of breastfeeding and indicates that you need attention. The earlier a problem is identified, the easier it is to solve. Lactation consultants and breastfeeding support volunteers are available in most communities. A supportive health-care provider or hospital staff will have information and can refer you to a breastfeeding expert in your area. Setting up your support system before your baby is born and learning about breastfeeding from knowledgeable sources like the La Leche League can minimise problems.

If problems do occur, there are two things that you can do while you are looking for help. First, maintain your milk supply. As long as you remove milk from the breast five to eight times a day, you will make more milk. If your baby cannot feed from the breast, remove milk with hand expression or use a breast pump. The second thing you need to do is feed your baby. You can use the milk you have expressed, or you may find that you need to supplement with formula until your supply increases. A baby who is gaining weight will be eager to learn to breastfeed. Support and timely "hands-on" help will create a positive learning environment for him.

It is important for people close to the mother to be emotionally supportive of her decision to breastfeed. Many fathers and grandparents today want to play an active role in caring for the new baby and wonder how they can be more involved if the baby is motherfed. There are many ways they can participate in other daily activities besides feeding. Walking, holding, rocking, and burping the baby after feeds can support the mother in these activities and allow the baby to get to know others in the family. While changing nappies may not be as appealing, it is another way for others to show they care! Baby's bath at the end of the day is a wonderful way for fathers to connect with their children.

Remember your reasons for learning about HypnoBirthing? You were looking for a birth experience that is calmer and safer for you and your baby—one that will give you more confidence than other experiences that your friends and relatives may have had in their birthings. The same is true with breastfeeding. Well-meaning acquaintances may have had difficulty breastfeeding because they could not find help or information when they needed it, but don't let that stop you from making this important decision for your baby. After the birth of your baby, Mother Nature assumes you will breastfeed and provides you with an abundance of milk. This is the time to go with breastfeeding and see how much you and your baby enjoy this special bond. It is a most special gift that you and your baby will surely appreciate, and it will build a bond that will last for a lifetime.

The Birth Afterglow

Together you bond in love
Each one defined as three;
All three connected as one . . .

A Celebration of Life

M uch is said of the adjustments that parents of newly born infants must make in meeting the changes in schedules and the life tasks that are all of a sudden just there.

However, one doesn't often hear of the significant adjustments that your new little infant will be making as he emerges from the life of ease and security that he knew in his womb life and enters into the earthly environment.

During those months in which your baby has been developing within your womb, he's been comforted by the closeness and warmth of the wall of the membrane that softly caressed, soothed, and nestled him. Your baby has felt the gentle stimulation of the swirling waters, and he's been lulled by the subtle movement of your body. He has heard and felt the love that you offered as you talked and played together.

Birth has brought an abrupt ending to that safe, secure period of life within the womb. At the moment of birth, your baby emerged from his unencumbered world into a whole new series of experiences.

What your baby felt as he made his way into the world was a profusion of sensory encounters that can help make his transition easy or cause him to tremble, jerk, and cringe in fear. This experience can leave your baby with a birth memory that will affect his entire life, his personality, and his spirit.

The baby startled as he took that first breath on his own, felt air brushing across his skin, and bristled to the roughness of fabric used to rub the protective vernix from his body.

The manner in which you laboured and birthed, and the atmosphere into which your baby was born, should have offered the same love and care that you provided as you carried him. Only you can ensure that your baby's initial adjustment into his new surroundings is made as gentle as possible by planning and directing how his welcome will proceed.

Today's movies and television shows portray birth as comedic or traumatic; but no one realises the effect upon the emerging baby. The birthing environment following his emergence should have the same respect and calm as a place of worship. Great or humble, the decorum and protocol surrounding the birth of each and every baby should be conducted in a manner of reverence.

From the moment of birth, those first few seconds, minutes, hours, and weeks can be enormously important in shaping your baby's perception of what life is. This is his first lesson, and there should be a conscious effort on the part of all who are involved to ensure that it is a lesson that says his world is one of love, respect, and gentility.

Your baby's entrance is not always as genteel as we would like to see. As a result, the adjustments that he needs to make are enormous, but not all participants are cognizant of his worldly or his spiritual experience at this time. As parents you need to see that he is protected from the hustle and bustle that can exist in a birthing room after a baby is born. Voices should be subdued, and the room immediately returned to the soft lights and calm environment that existed prior to his birth.

At this time, assuming all is well, the only arms and hands that should hold your baby are yours and those of your partner. For some time, the baby needs to be sheltered from what could be a frightening experience of being introduced to the scent and the energy of others. Most hospitals today assure parents of at least an hour to become acquainted with their new baby before the onslaught of well-intentioned friends and family. All participants must keep in mind that these situations are frightening and disturbing to a newborn who is just getting accustomed to breathing and absorbing his new life outside of the womb. One hour is not nearly enough, one week is not enough. In some cultures parents and babies seclude themselves for as much as two to three weeks where their baby is kept in dimness and calmness, knowing only the soothing voices and gentle touches of his parents.

When parents kindly educate others in the family and close friends of what a traumatic time this is for a newborn baby, most will readily understand and honour the parents' explanation. Grandparents and friends can visit and observe and extend their well-wishes, but the baby should not be handed from one to the other until he is well on his way to accepting and adjusting to his new environment.

Responding to your baby's needs and learning that his cries are his way of communicating that he needs comforting and support are important. It is essential that he learns that he is accepted and that he is a loved and loving human being.

Some childbirth educators more affectionately call this special time a "babymoon." Much like a honeymoon, this is a time to get to know each other.

Because there is a considerable development continuing within your baby's brain and in her body even after birth is completed, it is important that you keep in mind the transitions that she is facing.

Some babies seem content in their new world, while others seem to experience the transition with difficulty. Allow your baby some time to adjust to her new life by making it as simple as her life in the womb as possible.

Your entire focus in these first few weeks should be on your baby's adjustment and not on hosting well-wishers. The privacy and the moments of exploring and getting acquainted are just as important now. You all need calm and peace and bonding as much as you did before your baby's arrival.

To begin with, minimise contact with the outside world. Simplify your daily life to meet your basic needs. Wear your pyjamas all day and order in food. This is not the time to have a constant stream of coworkers, friends, and relatives drop in. Guests, especially female, tend to want to hold new babies, but it needs to be remembered that babies are making a tremendous adjustment. They need to get accustomed to the scent and the touch of their parents and to become acclimated to their new surroundings.

Allow friends and relatives to visit only if they are bringing you a meal, want to do laundry, go shopping for you, or clean your house! Having these needs met makes the next leg of your journey into parenthood enjoyable and rewarding, and helps to create a transition into your new roles as parents and your infant's new role of going from pre-born to newborn.

Birth Preference Sheets

The following pages are copies of the worksheets that your HypnoBirthing practitioner will provide for your use in designing your birth preferences. It is a good idea to complete the Birth Preference Sheets prior to touring the facility you will use for your birthing. You may wish to discuss some of the items with the person conducting your tour.

This plan has been developed for use throughout the United States and in several foreign countries. For that reason, you will find items on the plan that may not apply to you or the facility at which you will birth. Several of the items that are listed have been adopted by most hospitals and staff long ago. However, many of the requests that are routinely honoured in some geographic areas are as yet unheard-of in other areas of this country and outside of the United States. You may skip these items, mark them N/A, or extract only those that apply to your own preferences.

Dear Health Care Provider:

My birthing companion and I have chosen you, our health care provider, and you, our birthing facility staff, as the people we want to attend us when our baby is born. We have chosen the HypnoBirthing® method of quiet, relaxed, natural birth. From everything we have heard from others, we truly believe that you will do your utmost to help us attain our wish for a joyous, memorable, and most satisfying natural birth.

The information that follows is a copy of our Birth Preferences. We have given careful consideration to each specific request in our plan, and we feel that it represents our wishes at this time. We realise that as labour ensues, we may choose to change our thinking and wish to feel free to do so.

We're looking forward to a normal pregnancy and birth and understand that these choices presume that this will be the case. Should a special circumstance arise that could cause us to deviate from our planned natural birth, we trust that you will provide us with a clear explanation of the special circumstance, the medical need for any procedure you may anticipate, and what options might be available. In such an event, please know that after we have had an explanation of the medical need and have had the opportunity to discuss the decision between ourselves, you will have our complete cooperation. In the absence of any special circumstance, we ask that the following requests be honoured.

Please attach these requests to my prenatal record. I will provide other copies for:

❏ Hospital admissions
❏ My midwife
❏ Birthing clinic staff

Please make this information known to any other physicians, nursing staff, or midwives who may be attending the birth should you not be attending us.

Signed: _____
                    Parent(s)

Signed: _____
                    Care Provider

Birth Preference Sheets

Mother's and Birth Companion's Names:

We have chosen you to be our care providers, and we thank you in advance for honouring our birthing preferences and assisting us in achieving a gentle and natural birth.

Welcoming our baby:

We are preparing for our baby's arrival with HypnoBirthing®, and we anticipate a calm, natural birth. We will be using special breathing techniques and relaxation, including self-hypnosis. My birth companion will be actively involved in our birthing. He/she has been fully prepared to support me in decisions and techniques regarding our baby's birth. Please include him/her in all discussions as labour advances. We ask for your understanding and accommodation to the requests outlined below, allowing our labour and birth to unfold as naturally as possible. These preferences are forwarded with the understanding that should an unexpected special circumstance arise, you will have our full cooperation after discussion and explanation. With this goal in mind, we list the following preferences:

Onset of labour:

❑ To allow labour to begin naturally unless induction by medical means is truly needed for the safety of my baby or me.

❑ To remain at home until labour is well established

Admission to hospital:

❏ To return home if labour is not well established at 4 cm to 6 cm

❏ To have birth companion ensure that mother maintains fluid intake and output

❏ To enjoy only intermittent foetal monitoring, unless medical indication requires otherwise

❏ To discuss my "comfort level," rather than a "level of pain" or being shown a pain scale

❏ To feel free to dim the room and have soft music playing

❏ To have bed rails lowered to encourage perinatal bonding

During Opening and Thinning:

❏ To feel free to walk, move about, and to find the most comfortable and effective positions

❏ To allow for an undisturbed rhythm and flow of natural labour with few or no vaginal exams

❏ To labour in tub if one is available—if not, to choose the shower

❏ To be relieved of blood pressure cuff and foetal monitor belts between readings

❏ To snack and drink as desired if labour is prolonged

❏ To forego medical interventions, including rupturing of membranes and augmentation, without clear medical need. Membranes to remain intact until baby is fully born.

❑ To use natural means before moving to intervention if baby requires more optimal repositioning

❑ To exercise patience if labour slows or rests, and use only natural means to stimulate labour if needed

❑ To have full explanation and discussion of medical need and alternatives before moving to intervention

During Descent:

❑ To assume a position of my choice, change position, or remain in a relaxed pose

❑ To breathe my baby down to crowning with prompts from only my birth companion

❑ To bear down only when my body is in surge, using the natural expulsive reflex

During Birth:

❑ To allow baby to emerge physiologically, free of assist unless needed

❑ To suction airway only if medically necessary

❑ To have father or mother receive baby once head and shoulders are born

❑ To allow time for the placenta to be released physiologically

❑ To use artificial oxytocin injection to prevent hemorrhage only if there is clear indication of need

For Baby:

❑ To dry or wipe baby gently with a soft fabric if necessary

❑ To have baby placed directly on mother's abdomen. Dad will join in.

❑ To allow cord pulsation to cease before cutting cord

❑ To allow baby to crawl to breast and self-attach for first feeding

❑ To apply prophylactic eye medication after family bonding time

❑ To use oral Vitamin K in multiple doses or delay Vitamin K injection

❑ To have baby remain with mother and birth companion at all times

We thank you in advance for your kind support and assistance in helping us meet our goal of a beautiful, natural birth.

About the Author

M arie Mongan was a clinical hypnotherapist and recipient of the 1995 National Guild of Hypnotists President's Award. She founded the HypnoBirthing Institute in the US in 1989 and it now operates globally. She was the mother of four children, all born using the techniques upon which HypnoBirthing is based. Marie Mongan passed away in June 2019.

Bibliography

Books

Barber, Joseph, Ph.D., and Cheri Adrian, Ph.D., Eds. *Psychological Approaches to the Management of Pain*. Levittown, Pa.: Brunner/Mazel, 1982.

Barstow, Anne Llewellyn. *Witchcraze*. San Francisco: Pandora, 1994.

Bieler, Henry G., M.D. *Food Is Your Best Medicine*. New York: Random House, 1965.

Birch, William G., M.D. *A Doctor Discusses Pregnancy*. Chicago: Budlong Press, 1988.

Blaustone, Jan. *The Joy of Parenthood*. Deephaven, Minn.: Meadowbrook Press, 1993.

Bolduc, Henry Leo. *Self Hypnosis: Creating Your Own Destiny*. Independence, Va.: Adventures into Time Publishers, 1992.

Bradley, Robert A., M.D. *Husband-Coached Childbirth.* New York: Bantam Books, 1996.

Capacchione, Lucia, and Sandra Bardsley. *Creating a Joyful Birth Experience.* New York: Fireside, 1994.

Carmack, Adrienne, MD. *Reclaiming My Birth Rights.* Adrienne Carmack/USA, 2014.

Carola, Robert, et al. *Human Anatomy and Physiology.* New York: McGraw-Hill Education, 1990.

Carpenter, Carl. *Hypno Kinesiology: A Holistic Approach to Healing.* New Delhi, India: Sterling Publishers, 2003.

Contey, Carrie, PhD., and Takikawa, Debby, DC. *CALMS-A Guide to Soothing Your Baby.* Hana Peace Works, 2007.

Chamberlain, David. *The Mind of Your Newborn Baby.* Berkeley, Calif.: North Atlantic Books, 1998.

Charpak, Nathalie. *Kangaroo Babies: A Different Way of Mothering.* Great Britain: Souvenir Press, 2006.

Curtis, Glade B., and Judith Schuler. *Your Pregnancy Week by Week.* Cambridge, Mass.: DeCapo Press, 2004.

Davis, Elizabeth, et al. Heart & Hands: *A Midwife's Guide to Pregnancy and Birth.* Berkeley, Calif.: Celestial Arts, 2004.

Dick-Read, Grantly, M.D. *Childbirth Without Fear.* London: Pinter & Martin Ltd., 2004.

Dunham, Carroll, et al. *Mamatoto: A Celebration of Birth.* New York: Viking-Penguin, 1992.

Dunstan, Priscilla. *Dunstan Baby Language*, 2006.

Dye, John H., M.D. *Easy Childbirth: Healthy Mother and Healthy Children*. Buffalo, N.Y.: J. H. Dye Medical Institute, 1891.

Ehrenreich, Barbara, and Deirdre English. *Witches, Midwives and Nurses*. New York: The Feminist Press, 2010.

Ellerbe, Helen. *The Dark Side of Christian History*. Berkeley, Calif.: Morningstar Books, 1995.

Gaskin, Ina May. *Spiritual Midwifery*. Summertown, Tenn.: Book Publishing Co., 2002.

Goer, Henci. *The Thinking Woman's Guide to a Better Birth*. New York: Perigree Books, 1999.

Goulding, Joane. *SleepTalk*. Pennon Publishing, 2004.

Hawk, Breck, R.N., midwife. *Hey! Who's Having This Baby, Anyway?* Phoenix, Ariz.: End Table Books, 2005.

Harper, Barbara, R.N. *Gentle Birth Choices*. Rochester, Vt.: Healing Arts Press, 1994.

Hoke, James H. *I Would If I Could and I Can*. Glendale, Calif.: Westwood Publishing Co., 1980.

Idarius, Betty, L.M., C. Hom. *The Homeopathic Children Manual*. Idarius Press, 2nd Edition, 1999.

Jones, Carl. *The Birth Partner's Handbook*. Deephaven, Minn.: Meadowbrook Press, 1989.

———. *Mind over Labor*. New York: Penguin Books, 1987.

Jordon, Brigitte. *Birth in Four Cultures*. Waveland Press, Inc., 1993.

Kerr, Mary Brandt. *The Joy of Pregnancy*. New York: Golden Apple Publishers, 1987.

Krasner, A.M., Ph.D. *The Wizard Within*. Irvine, Calif.: American Board of Hypnotherapy Press, 1990.

Kroger, William, M.D. *Childbirth with Hypnosis.* North Hollywood, Calif.: Wilshire Book Co., 1970.

Lazarev, Michael, M.D. *Sonatal*. Bloomsbury, N.J.: Infinite Potential, Inc., 1991.

Leboyer, Frederick. *Birth Without Violence*. Rochester, Vt.: Healing Arts Press, 2002.

Lennart, Righard. *Delivery Self-Attachment*. Sunland, Calif.: Geddes Productions, 1992.

Lesko, Wendy, and Matthew Lesko. *The Maternity Sourcebook*. New York: Warner Books, 1985.

Longacre, R.D., Ph.D., F.B.H.A. *Client-Centreed Hypnotherapy*. Dubuque, Iowa: Kendall/Hunt Publishing Co., 1995.

Losier, Michael J. *Law of Attraction*. Victoria, B.C., Canada: Michael Losier, 2003.

McCubbin, Jack H., M.D. *The Unborn Baby Book*. E.P. Dutton, 1987.

McCutcheon, Susan. *Natural Childbirth the Bradley Way*. New York: Plume, 1996.

Mitford, Jessica. *The American Way of Birth*. New York: E. P. Dutton, 1992.

Nathanielsz, Peter, M.D. *The Prenatal Prescription*. New York: HarperCollins Publishers, 2001.

Northrup, Christiane, M.D., Ph.D. *Women's Bodies, Women's Wisdom*. New York: Bantam Books, 2002.

Odent, Michel, M.D. *Birth Reborn*. Medford, N.J.: Birth Works Press, 1994.

O'Toole, Marie T., Ed. *Miller-Keane Encyclopedia and Dictionary of Medicine, Nursing and Allied Health*. Philadelphia, Pa.: W. B. Saunders Co., 2003.

Peterson, Gayle, Ph.D. *An Easier Childbirth*. Berkeley, Calif.: Shadow and Light Publications, 1993.

Schwartz, Leni. *Bonding Before Birth—A Guide to Becoming a Family*. Sigo Press, 1991.

Sears, William, M.D., and Martha Sears, R.N. *The Birth Book*. Boston, Mass.: Little, Brown, 1994.

Shanley, Laura Kaplan. *Unassisted Childbirth*. New York: Bergin & Garvey Paperback, 1994.

Simkin, Penny. *The Birth Partner*. Boston, Mass.: Harvard Common Press, 2001.

————, et al. *Pregnancy, Childbirth and the Newborn*. Deephaven, Minn.: Meadowbrook Press, 2001.

Stone, Merlin. *When God Was a Woman*. Orlando, Fla.: Harcourt Brace & Co., 1976.

Straus, Roger A., Ph.D., *Strategic Self-Hypnosis*. New York: Simon & Schuster, 2000.

Strong, Thomas H., Jr., M.D. *Expecting Trouble*. New York University Press, 2002.

Sutton, Jean, and Scott, Pauline. *Optimal Foetal Positioning*. Birth Concepts: New Zealand, 2nd Edition.

Thomas, Clayton L., Ed. *Taber's Cyclopedic Medical Dictionary*. Philadelphia, Pa.: F. A. Davis Co., 1997.

Vander, Arthur, et al. *Human Physiology*. New York: McGraw-Hill Publishing Co., 1997

Vaughn, Kathleen. *Safe Childbirth*. London: Bailliere, Tindall & Cox, 1937.

Verny, Thomas, M.D. *The Secret Life of the Unborn Child*. New York: Dell Publishing, 1981.

Weil, Andrew, M.D. *Spontaneous Healing*. New York: Ballantine Publishing Group. 1995.

Wessel, Helen. *The Joy of Natural Childbirth*. Bookmates International, Inc., 1994.

Wildner, Kim. *Mother's Intention: How Belief Shapes Birth*. Ludington, Mich.: Harbor & Hill Publishing, 2003.

Wirth, Frederick, M.D. *Prenatal Parenting*. New York: HarperCollins
Publishers, 2001.

Worth, Jennifer. *Call the Midwife*. Phoenix, 2008.

THE
SHANGANI
PATROL

JOHN WILCOX

headline

First published in 2010 by
HEADLINE PUBLISHING GROUP

First published in paperback in 2010 by
HEADLINE PUBLISHING GROUP

1

Cataloguing in Publication Data is available from the British Library

ISBN 978 0 7553 4562 5

Typeset in Sabon by Avon DataSet Ltd,
Bidford on Avon, Warwickshire

Printed and bound in the UK by CPI Mackays, Chatham, ME5 8TD

Headline's policy is to use papers that are natural, renewable and
recyclable products and made from wood grown in sustainable forests.
The logging and manufacturing processes are expected to conform to the
environmental regulations of the country of origin.

HEADLINE PUBLISHING GROUP
An Hachette UK Company
338 Euston Road
London NW1 3BH

www.headline.co.uk
www.hachette.co.uk

In memory of my friend Liam Hunter

Acknowledgements

I owe a debt to my editor at Headline, Sherise Hobbs, for her infinite attention to detail and, in particular, her intuitive sense of pace, of knowing where passages need more action and less of my regrettable tendency to let my characters talk too much. I must also thank my copyeditor, Jane Selley, for her care in tidying up my prose. I wouldn't be a writer without my agent, Jane Conway-Gordon, and I appreciate her constant support. As I do that of my wife, Betty, my devoted research assistant, proofreader and first critic of all my work.

These four have been a constant in most of my writings so far, but in the case of this particular book, my biggest vote of thanks must go to Dave Sutcliffe, an ex-Rhodesian now living in Newcastle, KwaZulu Natal, South Africa. For various reasons, I was unable to get into Zimbabwe to carry out basic research, and Dave, ex-surveyor, naturalist, guide and historian in his own right, did not hesitate to fill the gap by supplying detailed maps and local knowledge. Any mistakes that may have crept into the narrative concerning historical events and flora and fauna, however, are mine, not his.

As always, the London Library proved invaluable in supplying books about the period. However, I could find few definitive accounts of Rhodes's invasion of Matabeleland and Mashonaland either in the UK or during an all too brief visit to South Africa. Nevertheless, contemporary copies of *The Times*, kept in a pristine state at the London Library, proved useful, as did the following books:

A Flag for the Matabele by Peter Gibbs, Frederick Muller Ltd., London, 1955

To the Victoria Falls via Matabeleland, the diary of Major Henry Stabb, 1875, edited by Edward C. Tabler, C. Struik (Pty) Ltd, Cape Town, 1967

Rhodes by J. G. Lockhart and the Hon. C. M. Woodhouse, Hodder and Stoughton, London, 1963

Cecil Rhodes by John Flint, Hutchinson, London, 1976

And that great old stand-by, *The Colonial Wars Source Book* by Philip J. Haythornthwaite, Arms and Armour Press, London, 1995

Alas, many of these books will be out of print, but the London Library and the British Library should be able to help.

Chapter 1

They stood in silence in a rough half-circle on the beaten earth in the centre of the kraal, all eyes on the tall, thin figure of the black man with a long stick on the edge of the circle. It was not yet quite light and the stars were still pricking the indigo blue of the darkness above them. Simon Fonthill, ex-soldier, army scout and leader of the group, shivered – and not just because it was bitterly cold in these few minutes before dawn.

'Lion,' said Mzingeli, their guide. 'We go to kill him but he very dangerous animal. He also very shy . . .'

'Ah well,' murmured 352 Jenkins, 'then p'raps it would be rude to bother 'im, eh?' Jenkins, Fonthill's long-standing comrade, was the inevitable jester of the group. But this time no one smiled.

'. . . and he run from us in daylight. But at night he can see in dark and we cannot. So he attack us then without fear. That is why we go now, in light, just as sun comes up.' The tall man looked at them in turn. 'We hear him and his ladies roaring in bush last night and we know he make kill. So we follow his spoor now until we find where he lie down to sleep his meal

1

away, and then you, Nkosi,' he nodded to Fonthill, 'or you, Nkosi,' he inclined his head towards Jenkins, a touch less deferentially, 'will kill him.'

No one spoke. Mzingeli was their servant, but he spoke with an air of quiet authority that shrugged off questions of rank, class or race, and it would have seemed an act of lese-majesty to have interupted him at this point. His name meant the Hunter, and he looked the part. Some six feet tall, he was slim and probably older than his athletic frame suggested, for the tightly curled hair that lay close to his scalp was now quite grey and his eyes seemed to reflect the sadness of great years. His nose was long, with flared nostrils, and his lips were thin. He wore the dress of the Afrikaner – dirty corduroy trousers and a loose flannel shirt – but his feet were bare, showing white patches between his toes as though from the touch of a paintbrush, and totemic beads hung around his neck. An old Snider rifle was slung across his shoulder, but now he was drawing in the dust with the end of his stick.

'This is animal,' he said, and suddenly the silhouette of a male lion appeared at their feet. He stabbed at a point just above the left front leg of the animal. 'Here you shoot. Here is heart and lungs.' His stick moved again quickly, and the impressive outline of a charging lion, head on, materialised. 'Lion can jump twenty feet,' he went on, 'so you do not want to see him like this. Only way to kill him like this is here.' He jabbed the stick between the eyes of the animal. 'No good down here,' he gestured at the chest beneath and behind the mane, 'because chest has about nine inches deep of muscle, and although your bullet may kill charging Zulu,' a smile appeared, showing perfect white teeth, 'it no go through lion chest.'

Fonthill shot a quick glance at Alice, his wife. She was

listening with rapt attention, a tiny pink sliver of tongue showing between her lips. But he noticed that despite the cold, small beads of perspiration had appeared on her forehead. Like him, she was apprehensive but exhilarated. Why the hell had she insisted on coming? She would have been safe enough staying here in the kraal. Then he gave a slight shrug of the shoulders. He knew well enough now that Alice Fonthill could never be dissuaded from a course of action on which her mind was set. But Mzingeli was continuing.

'We hunt lion and two lionesses. We find the kill then we track spoor. We do not make noise. Walk in straight line. I lead, then come Nkosi Fonthill, then,' he nodded at Alice, 'Nkosana, then Nkosi Jenkins, then my boys.' The two black bearers stood leaning on their spears, not understanding a word. 'When we find lions, I do not point with hand or move quickly. I point gently with head and eyes. Watch me. Then, Nkosi, you walk very quiet ahead and kill animal.'

Simon nodded. 'Yes . . . hum . . . yes. Yes, of course.'

'Very quietly,' added Jenkins.

'Mzingeli,' Alice interjected.

'Nkosana?'

'You said that there is one male lion and two lionesses who have been attacking the cattle compound.'

'Yes, Nkosana.'

'Are there no cubs? Do they not form a pride?'

Mzingeli nodded at the relevance of the question. 'It is usual, yes. But this is just one man and two ladies. Male must have fought with previous lion and killed him, or perhaps other lion was old and died. New one now comes in and kills all cubs and starts again with these lionesses, so no family yet.'

Alice wrinkled her nose. 'How disgusting. Does this

mean . . .' and her voice faltered for a second, 'that we must kill all three?'

The black man shook his head. 'No, unless they all attack us. We kill only lion. His ladies then go away and find another mate. I don't think they come back here.' Mzingeli looked around enquiringly, as though waiting for further questions. Then his eyes widened and he added slowly, 'This dangerous. Everybody go very, very careful.'

As though on cue, the tips of the mopane trees fringing the compound became suddenly alight as they caught the first rays of the rising sun. The little party turned to leave and began making for the opening at the edge of the thorn hedge that encircled the village. There, as if from nowhere, the village *inDuna*, or headman, materialised, spoke briefly to Mzingeli and then smiled and nodded to Fonthill.

'He thank you for what we do,' said the tracker.

Simon returned the smile and gave an acknowledging nod. But he felt not at all confident about their mission, and despite Mzingeli's competence, nor did he feel assured that they could bring it to a successful conclusion. When they had recruited Mzingeli in the Transvaal – on the warm recommendation of an old army acquaintance in the Cape – they had had no intention of hunting lion or other big game, or even of crossing the lazy Limpopo into the wilderness that was Matabeleland. They had merely wished to travel in a leisurely manner through the rolling grasslands of the veldt, shooting a few guineafowl and buck, camping under the stars and breathing the fresh, clear air of the country. A holiday, but also a way of forgetting the sadness they had left behind them at home in Norfolk. A brief change of direction for the three of them: Simon, Alice and, of course, Jenkins, Fonthill's former batman, now lifelong friend, and survivor, with

Simon, of a dozen or more dangerous encounters on campaign with the British Army. This was to have been a few weeks of indulgence, far from danger, and with a first-rate tracker to guide them through the country and help them find game when they needed it.

It had been Mzingeli who had suggested that, as they were so near to the Matabele border with the Transvaal, they should cross the river and spend a couple of nights at his home village, thus allowing him to see again his elderly father, who was the *inDuna* there. There would be no need to seek permission from the all-powerful Matabele king, Lobengula, to enter his country. They would slip in and move out again without detection. The tracker had explained that he himself was a member of the Malakala tribe, a minority clan who lived on either side of the Limpopo. A non-militant, reclusive people, they had been completely subjugated by the Matabele, who used them as a source of plunder and slaves. His fellow tribesmen, he said, would see that the party were completely hidden from the king's men during their short stay.

Fonthill gave a wry smile as he trod carefully behind the tall figure of Mzingeli. He was still unsure whether the tracker had known, as he neared his old home with his employers, that his village's slender stock of cattle – those few still left to them by the Matabele – was being ravaged by the lions, or whether it was a mere coincidence that they should arrive when the white man's legendary firepower and hunting skills were so sorely needed. Either way, Simon had felt quite unable to resist the request that they should rid the village of this terrible scourge. He smiled again. He felt a little like the young hero of a medieval tale, called upon to slaughter the terrible dragon that was terrorising the hamlet and taking away the young maidens. Except that he knew nothing about dragon-slaying and even less about lion-killing. Thank God for Mzingeli – except that, of course, they wouldn't be in this mess in the first place if it hadn't been for the crafty old tracker. He shrugged. Ah, well. He and Jenkins had been in more dangerous situations than this and survived. If only Alice hadn't insisted on coming too!

He turned and tried to smile reassuringly at his wife. They were walking in single file, as Mzingeli had instructed, except that for some reason, the two bearers, Ntini and Sando, carrying their spears and light shoulder packs, had overtaken Jenkins, leaving the latter at the back. Fonthill caught the Welshman's eye.

'I'd be grateful,' said Jenkins, in a hoarse whisper that seemed to boom back at them from the trees, 'if I could be relieved of this postin' at the back, see, before we come up with these bleedin' lions . . . oh, beggin' your pardon, Miss Alice.'

Alice sighed, stopped and turned. 'Three five two, if you're going to apologise every time you swear, it is going to make for a very long day. Let me remind you that I am a brigadier's daughter, I have served as a war correspondent on almost as many campaigns as you and Simon, and I have heard language that might make even your hair curl. So do feel free to swear as much as you bloody well like.'

Jenkins bit into his huge black moustache. 'Yes, miss. Sorry, miss. It's just that I'd rather be up front to face the bugg . . . beggars when they come than at the back 'ere, with me arse sort of exposed, look you.'

Mzingeli held up his hand. 'No talk now.' He spoke curtly in his own language to the two bearers, who sheepishly moved behind Jenkins. Then they all moved on.

Within what seemed like only moments, they had been

swallowed up by the bush. Mzingeli had called this terrain mopane woodland, named after the mopane itself, a deciduous tree with butterfly-shaped leaves that cattle loved to chew, and he had told them that it stretched in a broad belt for miles along the low veldt north of the Limpopo. Yet it bore little resemblance to any woodland that Fonthill remembered from England. The mopane jostled for space with the much larger baobab tree and the smaller thorn trees and bushes. Visibility was only about one hundred yards, and the terrain could not have been more different from the rolling grassland that they had left behind them in the Transvaal.

The night had brought them little sleep, for the bush had been alive with noise: the squeal of hyenas, the barking of baboons, the grunting of dozens of other, unknown animals, and above all, the roar of lions – that primeval sound that made them pull their blankets under their chins and ensure that their rifles were within reach. Lions feared no one; even elephants were likely to form a defensive circle when the king of beasts was on the hunt. Now, however, as they walked, the woodland had turned into a sleepy, seemingly quiet environment. But it was not a tranquil place. They trod carefully yet they continually disturbed guineafowl, which suddenly flew up ahead of them, squawking, flapping and sending their hearts into their mouths. Simon became aware of a distinctive smell of . . . what? Ah yes – cinnamon. He realised that it emanated from the miniature kopjes of dried clay constructed by ants that now began to appear among the trees. The rainy season had long since passed, and underneath their boots the soil was dry and powdery. Strange new country. Good country for lions. He licked his dry lips and gripped his rifle tightly.

None of them carried weapons ideal for big-game hunting. They had set out originally armed mainly with light rifles, like the small-calibre Westley Richards that Alice now cradled. Ideal for bringing down antelope and buck but capable only of wounding a charging lion. Mzingeli's Snider was an old rifle that had been replaced as British Army issue long before the Zulu War ten years ago, and although the man had already proved himself to be a good shot with it, it too seemed inadequate for today's purpose. The bearers had their assegais, razor sharp but best used for skinning and cutting up a carcass rather than killing. That left the Martini-Henry rifles carried by Fonthill and Jenkins. These had been used by the pair at the end of the abortive Sudan campaign four years ago, and thrown into the back of their wagon almost as an afterthought when they had set out from the Cape, merely a precaution in case danger should ensue from hostile natives. They packed a heavy .45 cartridge that, as Mzingeli had reminded them, could be effective against a charging Zulu. But a lion . . . ? Fonthill looked down and checked that he had inserted a round 'up the snout'.

Simon himself, at thirty-four, was no longer the apprehensive young subaltern who had first landed in South Africa exactly ten years ago. The decade spent as a highly irregular army scout in Zululand, Afghanistan, the Transvaal (twice) and Egypt had lined his face a little and brought a light dusting of grey to his temples. Some five feet nine inches tall, his figure had filled out a little but his waist was slim enough, his shoulders broad and he carried himself lightly. He certainly looked the part of a hunter, in his light khaki shirt and trousers. The brown eyes, narrowed now under his wide-brimmed Boer hat as they peered into the bush, still, however, carried a trace of uncertainty, although the Pathan musket that had broken his nose had left it hooked and given his face a predatory air.

He turned his head to look at his wife stepping behind him. Exactly the same age as Simon, Alice Fonthill had matured into a fine-looking woman: erect, slim, with long fair hair tied into a serviceable bun behind the brim of her bush hat, her grey eyes steady and meeting those of her husband with a ready smile, although they too displayed a hint of something – sadness? – that gave her face a haunting, perhaps melancholy element. Alice's chin was perhaps a little too strong and square to bestow conventional beauty, but she carried herself with an air of charismatic attractiveness that had served her well in the masculine world of journalism, especially during her time covering the campaigns of Queen Victoria's army over the last ten years.

Behind them both, Jenkins carried his rifle at the slope over his shoulder, as befitted an ex-soldier of Her Majesty's 24th Regiment of Foot. It was at the regiment's hospital on the Welsh borders that he had met Fonthill, becoming the young subaltern's servant-batman, mentor and friend. Always known as 352 – the last three figures of his army number, and used to distinguish him from the many other Jenkinses in this most Welsh of regiments – he was some four years older than Simon, although no flecks of grey had yet dared to fight their way through the thicket of black hair that stood out vertically on his head, or into the great moustache that swept across his face. Seemingly as broad as he was tall (he stood at about five feet four inches), Jenkins exuded strength. He was as muscled and broad-chested as a pit bull terrier – Welsh, of course.

Now the three walked in self-absorbed silence, slowing a little in pace with Mzingeli, who had changed direction to the right and begun pushing through the thorns into a little clearing. As he did so, two hyenas squealed and ran away in their hangdog way and, in an indignant beating of wings, a brace of vultures rose into the air. Underneath them, the bones of an impala were picked almost clean.

Mzingeli held up his hand to keep them away from the carcass. Then he bent his knees and began examining the sandy floor near the bones, squatting and peering carefully at the earth, occasionally poking at it with one long black finger.

He stood and beckoned Simon. 'The three killed here,' he said. 'Maybe three hours ago.'

'Are they nearby still?'

'No. They go to find somewhere in shade to sleep. Look.' He pointed to the ground. 'Big lion – probably more than four hundred thirty pounds. See here, where he lies down. Big mane.' Fonthill bent to examine the scuffed sand but could see nothing distinctive.

'Were the two lionesses with him?' he asked.

'Oh, yes. They kill impala. Old lion just come up and do eating when hunting is done. Good life for him.'

Ntini called from the edge of the clearing. Mzingeli nodded. 'Good, we have spoor. We follow.' He addressed them all now in a soft voice. 'I do not know how far away they are. I think not far, maybe half a mile. So we go very quietly. Very dangerous now.'

'Oh blimey,' murmured Jenkins. 'Let me come up front with you, bach sir.'

Fonthill shook his head. He was under no illusion that Jenkins was concerned about his own safety. The Welshman had the heart of a lion himself, and Simon knew of only three things that daunted him: water (he couldn't swim), heights and crocodiles. No, he would wish to be near Fonthill to protect him. A crack shot, he knew that Simon was still only a moderate marksman and that the opportunity of firing off a second round after a missed first shot was unlikely to present itself. By the time the second cartridge could be inserted into the breech of the single-shot Martini-Henry, the lion would have sprung. He wished to take up his post, familiar to him over the years, at Fonthill's shoulder.

Simon smiled. 'No thanks, old chap. Stay just there. Behind Alice.'

In single file again, they moved off. This time the two bearers, who previously had been conversing in very low voices so that Mzingeli could not hear up ahead, were silent, the whites of their eyes showing prominently and their assegais held firmly across their bodies. They had dropped back a little from the quartet ahead. They were undoubtedly apprehensive. Perhaps their fear had communicated itself to the others, for everyone was now stepping with great care and peering cautiously into the foliage that pressed in on them on either side – everyone, that is, but Mzingeli, whose eyes remained fixed on the sandy track ahead of him.

Eventually, after half an hour, he raised his right hand slightly in a signal to halt. The bush had thinned noticeably, and ahead of them the track had widened until it admitted a rocky outcrop. The tracker, his eyes still fixed to the front, motioned over his shoulder for Fonthill to join him.

He nodded to the ground ahead and then whispered, 'See mark in front of lion's paw, like brush mark.' Simon squinted but could see nothing of the kind. 'Lion tired,' continued Mzingeli. 'He drag front of his paw as he lift it up.' The tracker gently nodded his head. 'I think they found place to rest and digest meal, up there, behind rocks.'

'What about our scent?' asked Fonthill.

'We are upwind. They do not smell us.'

Fonthill felt a hand on his shoulder. Alice whispered in his ear, 'They're up there, aren't they? Up in those rocks?'

'Yes. Mzingeli believes so.'

'Don't go in alone. Take 352 with you.'

Simon fought back a flash of irritation. 'No. He must stay here with you. I can kill this damned lion. In any case, Mzingeli will probably come with me—'

He was interrupted by the tracker, who turned, his finger to his lips. 'We go together round to right,' he whispered. 'Stay very close. Be ready to shoot quickly if lion sees us. Very quiet now.'

Gesturing to Jenkins to stay close to Alice, Fonthill gave a twisted smile to his wife – somehow the muscles on his face seemed to be set rictus-like, not allowing him to give her the reassuring beam he intended – and followed Mzingeli at a crouch, his rifle clutched across his breast. The two men stole away to the right of the rocks, the tracker gently pulling away branches and holding them until Simon could take them in turn and pass through. They climbed a little through the bush and moved in a semicircle until they began to edge around the end of the highest rock, some ten feet away from it. Mzingeli was ahead, his bare feet making no sound as he placed each one carefully in front of the other on the now stony ground. Then he froze and, his eyes staring ahead of him, motioned for Simon to come alongside

Ahead of them was the lion, stretched resplendent in the shade of the overhanging rock. His great head lay away from them, the tangled mass of the dark brown mane contrasting with the tawny colour of the body, and he seemed huge in that confined space, the end of his tail almost, it seemed, within reach. His head rested on one side; the one eye that could be seen was closed, and his chest rose and fell in gentle rhythm. There seemed to be a look of beatific satisfaction on the giant beast's face in repose. It had been a good meal and he was sleeping it off. Of the lionesses there was no sign.

A smile creased Mzingeli's face. He gestured with both hands to Simon as if tracing a circle, and mouthed, 'Big.' Then he moved slightly to his right and nodded his head forward. The signal was clear: kill. Kill now.

Fonthill licked his dry lips and inched forward, raising his rifle to the shoulder. Where was the target spot? Ah yes, just above and behind the front leg. Not easy to define from the rear, with the mane spreading so far down the body. He squinted through the foresight. Damn! It was set at one hundred yards. At point-blank range he would overshoot by miles. Feeling Mzingeli's disapproval radiating towards him, he lowered the rifle and, with infinite care, pushed down the sight, then raised the rifle once more and focused on the sleeping animal. His finger tightened on the trigger . . . *squeeze, don't pull* . . . and there it stayed, until the end of the long barrel began to sway a little with the weight of it.

The lion was sleeping, *sleeping*. Fonthill had killed many men in the heat of battle or in one-to-one combat over the preceding years, but he had never killed anything that was not erect and facing him. This magnificent beast lay a few yards from him in perfect somnolence, completely unaware of the danger. It seemed somehow unfair, completely unfair, to kill him like this. It was not a killing, more an execution. He could not do it. Give the animal a fighting chance, at least.

So Fonthill shouted, 'Get up, you lazy bastard.'

Immediately the sleeping thing became alive, very much alive. The lion was on its feet within a second, turning its great head towards the danger, its mouth open showing yellow incisor fangs and emitting a roar that boomed back from the rocks around. At that moment, Fonthill fired.

The bullet tore through the muscles just behind the

animal's head, cutting a furrow through the mane and causing blood to spurt. Then, with one bound, the beast had gone, leaving behind the echo of the shot and a bloodstain on the rocky ground. From the other side of the rock came two responding roars and a scuffle as the lionesses, unseen, followed him.

Fonthill and Mzingeli were left staring at each other. Neither spoke for a second or two, then Simon cleared his throat. 'Sorry. I just couldn't kill him while he was asleep. It seemed so . . . so . . . unfair somehow. I am sorry, Mzingeli.'

Slowly, a smile spread across the tracker's face. 'I think I understand, Nkosi.' Then the smile disappeared. 'But now we have big problem. We cannot leave wounded animal. We must follow into bush and finish him. If he stay alive with wound, he cannot chase properly to hunt and he turn to eating men. Becomes man-killer. We must track him now into bush. Very dangerous.'

'What happened?' Alice and Jenkins had suddenly materialised, Alice's eyes wide. Behind them – at some distance – appeared Ntini and Sando. 'Oh, thank goodness you are all right.' Alice clutched Simon's arm. 'What happened?'

'Well, I . . . er . . . missed. That's it really. No, it isn't.' Fonthill's face was crestfallen. 'The fact is, I just couldn't kill the bloody thing at point-blank range when it was sleeping.'

Mzingeli's face was once again illuminated by his great grin. He interjected, 'Nkosi shouted, "Wake up, lion" to make it fair. It is the English way, I think. I don't see this before.'

'Well,' Jenkins's expression was lugubrious, 'it's not the bloody Welsh way, I can tell you, Jelly. I would 'ave shot 'im up the arse if necessary, see.'

Fonthill cleared his throat again. 'Yes, well. I couldn't do it and that's that. Then I missed, although I wounded the beast. Now I must follow him and finish him off. It should be quite easy. I will have a blood spoor that will lead me to him, and this time I promise I won't miss. You must all stay here because the lionesses are still about, but I would like Mzingeli to come with me, please.'

'Don't talk nonsense, Simon.' Alice's voice was quite determined. 'We will all come with you. This time it will be more dangerous because the animals will be alerted – and they will probably be in the bush, and not,' her voice took on a gentler tone and her eyes were soft, 'lying on a nice clean rock waiting for you to shoot. Don't worry, my love, the odds will be much more equal this time.'

'Oh bloody 'ell,' said Jenkins.

Mzingeli gestured to the two bearers and spoke to them in their own tongue. Then he turned to the others. 'I think we take cup of tea and something to eat before we follow. There will be time.'

They set off again within the half-hour, moving more quickly this time. The trail was easy to follow and it led in a straight line, deeper into the bush. Then, after a while, the drops of blood became more irregular until finally they disappeared and Mzingeli was forced to deploy his arcane tracking skills again. Not that this was too difficult, because the three animals seemed now to be moving abreast through the bush, flattening the long grasses that had become a feature of the terrain.

As they progressed, a new and deeper air of tension began to pervade the little group. The bush seemed very, very quiet now, as though all of its occupants were standing off, silently waiting for the denouement that was surely to come. Somewhere a jackal barked, and high above an eagle wheeled, but otherwise the eerie stillness seemed to grow as they trudged along, watching carefully to ensure that they did not tread on a puff adder that might lurk in the sandy hollows that were becoming more prevalent and whose bite could be fatal. On either side of them the grasses seemed to have become longer and more impenetrable.

They reached a little clearing and Mzingeli held up his hand. He nodded at the ground. 'He stop bleeding,' he said. 'Not hit bad, then, and maybe close. He very dangerous now. I think he very angry.' As he spoke, the others were aware of a strange, musky smell.

'Yes,' said Jenkins, 'well I would be if I'd 'ad a bullet through me—'

He was silenced by the most frightening sound Simon, Alice or Jenkins had heard since they had first landed in South Africa. From somewhere nearby, out in the bush but beyond their vision, came a low, rumbling growl. Its source was hard to place, but it was immediately followed by another from a different direction and then a third, again with a different origin. The sound was other-worldly – malicious and menacing, as though Satan himself was watching them from the surrounding bush and giving a warning of intent. The three Europeans all immediately felt a prickling at the nape of their necks.

'The buggers 'ave surrounded us,' breathed Jenkins.

Fonthill pulled Alice to his side and looked at Mzingeli. The tracker's eyes were wide and he was turning slowly, examining each section of the undergrowth in turn, his rifle at the ready. The six had instinctively moved together now, so that they stood in a tight circle, almost back to back, except for Sando, who for some reason had stayed slightly apart, his eyes fixed on some long grass underneath a thorn tree.

In a flash of tawny flesh, the lioness broke out of the grass, ran towards the bearer and then sprang on him. Sando just had time to sink on to his haunches and dig the butt of his long spear in to the earth, its blade pointing at an angle of about forty-five degrees straight at the lioness. It seemed that the animal hit Sando and the blade of the assegai at exactly the same time. The spear head penetrated its throat, snapping the shaft, but the lioness seemed to engulf the bearer, knocking him backwards, its jaws seeking his throat, despite the tip of the blade protruding from the back of its neck.

With speed matching that of the lioness, Ntini plunged his own assegai into the side of the beast, at the top of and just behind its foreleg. He withdrew it quickly and then thrust it into the stomach, this time twisting it as he pulled it out with that familiar sucking sound, *iklwa*, that Fonthill had first heard on the battlefield of Isandlwana a decade before. The lioness became suddenly still. From underneath its body, a bloodstained Sando began the struggle to free himself.

The others, however, had no time to help him, because the little clearing now erupted into a maelstrom of action. From the right, the lion broke cover with ferocious speed and sprang at Fonthill, as though recognising him as his earlier tormentor. Instinctively Simon leapt aside, firing as he did so. At such short range, the force of the bullet had the effect of making the beast twist in mid-air, although it had only entered that mass of muscle under the chin, not quite penetrating it. As the lion hit the ground, however, Alice's much lighter cartridge took him at the side of the head. The second shot had the effect of stunning the beast for a moment, and fumbling a second round into the breech of his Martini-Henry, Fonthill had time to leap forward and deliver the *coup de grâce* at point-blank range into the lion's heart. The beast's head sank forward with a sigh and he lay still.

From the left, the second lioness had timed its attack to coincide exactly with that of its mate and it bounded towards Jenkins. The latter's shot took her just above the right eye and that of Mzingeli directly in the open, snarling muzzle. She lay as still as the others.

'Well,' gasped Jenkins, 'we weren't very quiet but we seem to 'ave done the job, isn't it?' In moments of great anxiety, Jenkins's Welshness always seemed to increase.

Simon gathered Alice into his arms. 'Well done, my love,' he murmured into her ear. 'Good shooting. I doubt if I could have finished him myself. Are you all right?'

'Quite all right, thank you. Well done yourself.' But her voice carried a tremble. She gently disentangled herself. 'What about Sando?'

Mzingeli and Ntini, with gun and spear, were labouring to lever the dead lioness off the struggling bearer, who eventually emerged covered in blood, although whether his own or that of the lioness it was difficult to tell. Closer inspection, however, disclosed an ugly strip of flesh hanging from his shoulder, like an unbuttoned epaulette, although his teeth were flashing in a broad grin. He was clearly going to live to fight another lion on another day.

Mzingeli looked up and grinned. 'Very good shooting,' he said to Fonthill. 'Better this time. Not easy to move *and* fire. Nkosana very good too.'

'Thank you,' said Alice, then she frowned. 'But I am sorry we had to kill the females, too. Why did *they* attack us, Mzingeli?'

The black man shrugged. 'I think they knew we going to kill lion. They frightened too, you know.'

'Ah well.' Alice looked down at Sando and then bent and examined his shoulder.

'Mmm. Not good. This will need stitching. Where's my medical bag?'

Jenkins picked up the pack that Ntini had dropped and presented it to Alice. He looked at the wound and wrinkled his nose. 'Blimey, miss. There's not much you can do with that, is there?'

'Oh yes.' Alice rummaged through the pack and extracted a small but quite heavy leather bag. 'I took an instructional course in basic medicine at the London Missionary Society before we left,' she said. 'Just as well, I would say, the way this so-called holiday is going. Here, hold this.' She held out a small bottle. Jenkins wiped his hands on his trousers and took it, then received a small package wrapped in oiled waterproof paper.

Alice kneeled down beside the stricken bearer, whose face was now creased in pain. His eyes widened in anxiety when she produced another bottle from her bag, and then a small, tube-like instrument with a thin needle point at its end. She called to Mzingeli.

'Please come and interpret for me. Please explain to Sando that this is not witchcraft but white man's medicine to make him better. Tell him that I will use this needle.' She turned to Simon and Jenkins, now watching with as much anxiety as Sando, and held up the hypodermic syringe. 'It's still quite new, I think; it's called the Pravaz syringe back home.' She showed it to Mzingeli. 'I will use this to put some fluid into his veins that will stop the pain. Then I will very carefully clean the wound and sew the skin and flesh back on to the shoulder. He will feel no pain while I do this, although later on it will hurt a little. He must not touch it afterwards.'

Mzingeli nodded and translated. Sando, the whites of his eyes showing and his mouth open, said nothing, but watched Alice with awe as she went about her work: first pouring a little water on to her hands, washing them with a tiny bar of soap from her box and drying them, then slipping the needle end into the little bottle, pulling the morphine into the syringe and, with great care, injecting the fluid into the arm. The bearer winced but seemed as fascinated by the procedure as the four others, who were all looking on, quite engrossed. Alice poured a little liquid from the bottle on to a swab from the package that Jenkins held and then gently dabbed it on the open wound to disinfect it. This also had the effect of stopping the bleeding. Wiping the wound dry, she selected a needle from her box and then threaded it with a fine gut.

'Simon,' she called, 'wash your hands and put a little of this disinfectant on them. Then pull back the flesh that is hanging down and hold it in place while I sew. Three five two – if you're going to be sick, I would rather you did it away from my patient, thank you.'

'Thank you, miss. Oh bloody . . .'Ere, Jelly, 'old this bottle, quick.'

The operation continued until the flesh had been sewn into place, with Sando's head nodding now, his eyes half closed, as the morphine took effect. 'There,' said Alice, making a tight little overstitch to complete the sewing. 'Just as well that I was always a good seamstress.' She looked up at Fonthill. 'Don't you think, darling?'

Simon shook his head and blew out his cheeks. 'Not to put too fine a point on it, my love, I think you are bloody marvellous. Killing a lion one minute, then performing surgery on your knees the next. You continue to amaze me. I may have to marry you again if you go on like this.'

'Very good, very good, Nkosana,' added Mzingeli, his face beaming. Then he prodded Sando awake and spoke to him sharply.

'No,' said Alice. 'Let him be for a while. He will need to recover from the shock.'

Fonthill stood upright and nodded to the carcasses of the dead beasts. 'What should we do with these?' he asked the tracker. 'Just leave them for the scavengers to clear up?'

Mzingeli looked shocked. 'Oh no, Nkosi. They very valuable. Meat no good for eating, but skins good, particularly lion's tail. Fetch much money in Transvaal and Cape. Ntini and me do it now. Then we carry back to kraal.'

'Very well. I'll get Jenkins to make us some tea . . . when the poor lamb has recovered, that is.'

A fire was soon lit and a shame-faced Jenkins set their little black kettle on it, and as Alice carefully repacked her bag, Mzingeli and Ntini began to the skin the carcasses, using very sharp hunter's knives. Within minutes, the skins were stretched over bushes to dry and everyone settled down to drink strong black tea – even a woozy Sando, who kept looking at his shoulder in puzzlement.

It was, then, a peaceful scene that was interrupted by Jenkins, who looked up from his mug and murmured softly, 'Oh, shit!'

Out of the bush had materialised some ten or twelve natives. They were tall men, superbly built, with very black skins that seemed to shine over rippling muscles in the sunlight. They wore girdles of monkey's tails and headdresses of black ostrich feathers, extending over their necks and shoulders and reminding Simon of the fur tippets worn by fashionable ladies in London. Each warrior – for they seemed to be in war dress – carried a long shield of hide, like that used by the Zulus of the south, and a short stabbing assegai, except that, unlike the Zulus of the south, the blades of their spears were not silver but quite black. They moved around the edge of the clearing so that the little group was surrounded, and then stood, watching them silently.

Fonthill shot a quick glance at Mzingeli. It was the first time he had seen fear on the face of the tall man.

'Matabele,' said the tracker. 'Black blades. Bad men. Very bad.'

Chapter 2

Fonthill slowly stood. 'What do they want, do you think?' he asked Mzingeli.

'I ask. But they don't like Malakala people. Take us for slaves.' He licked his lips and spoke to one of the Matabele, who had advanced a little ahead of the rest. He wore a waxed circlet of fibre woven into his hair, like the Zulu elders, and had the air of an *inDuna*.

The man looked at Mzingeli scornfully and then, ignoring him, advanced towards Fonthill and stood for a moment, slowly turning his head to look at Alice and Jenkins before moving his gaze back to Simon. He gestured to the carcasses of the dead animals and then spoke angrily.

'He say why do we kill King Lobengula's lions and why do we come into Matabeleland without king's permission?'

Out of the corner of his eye, Fonthill saw one of the Matabele pick up Alice's rifle and then her pack. A second native moved towards Jenkins's Martini-Henry. Simon took a deep breath, then slowly bent down and picked up his own rifle, which lay at his feet.

'Pick up your rifle, 352,' he said softly. Then he sighted the long barrel over the shoulder of the Matabele chieftain and fired it into the skull of the lion, causing it to jerk. The noise of the report caused all of the natives to jump and sent echoes bouncing back from the surrounding bush. Fonthill nonchalantly reloaded his rifle, cocked the mechanism and slowly raised the muzzle until it was pointing directly into the eyes of the man facing him.

'Tell him,' he called to Mzingeli, 'to order that man to replace Alice's rifle and pack on the ground, otherwise I will blow his head off.'

'No, Nkosi.'

'Yes. Tell him.'

The tracker cleared his throat and spoke slowly. The Matabele's eyes widened for a moment, and Simon thought he detected fear in them as he regarded the muzzle of the gun, aimed so menacingly close to him. But he remained still and stood silent. At last he turned his head and nodded towards his follower. Sulkily the man dropped the rifle and the pack and Alice stepped forward to regain them.

It was a victory of a sort. Simon smiled and lowered the rifle, and nodded cordially to the *inDuna*. 'Now,' he said to Mzingeli, 'please explain the circumstances – how we were asked by your village to shoot the lions, which were attacking their herd.'

For the first time, the *inDuna* deigned to notice the tracker and stood frowning as the story was told. When he responded, it was with perhaps just a little less antagonism than before.

'He say,' said Mzingeli, 'that we should not have entered country without king's agreement.'

'Very well. Please explain that we were on our way to – what's the place that is supposed to be the guardian entrance to Matabeleland?'

'Makobistown.'

'Yes, that's it. I had forgotten. Please explain that we crossed at the Tati border and were on our way to Makobistown to gain permission when emissaries from your father's kraal asked us to remove the danger of the lions. We have skinned the beasts and were about to travel to Bulawayo to present the skins and the lion's tail to his majesty, as a gift from us.'

For a brief moment a smile flickered across Mzingeli's face before, sombrely, he translated.

The lie – probably supported by Fonthill's intransigence – was obviously convincing, for the *inDuna*'s attitude changed. He turned to Mzingeli, nodded and waved his assegai. Immediately his companions, their faces still imperturbable, squatted on the ground, their spears at their sides.

'Phew,' murmured Jenkins. 'Shall I make us all a nice cup of tea, then, bach sir?'

'Good idea. Mzingeli, ask the chief if he would like English tea.'

The tracker did so, and a brief, guttural interchange took place.

'He say no. Rather have brandy.'

'Very well. Three five two, see if you can find a drop of brandy. Not the good French, mind you. That Boer Cape stuff that you like so much.'

The Welshman made a face. 'What a terrible waste.' He shuffled across to Sando's pack and withdrew a bottle and an extra tin cup. Simon, Jenkins and Mzingeli threw away the tea dregs at the bottom of their own cups and joined the Matabele. Fonthill clinked cups with the *inDuna* and raised his mug in an unmistakable gesture. 'To King Lobengula,' he toasted. The others followed suit and the Matabele, grinning, nodded his head and joined them. Then he spoke again to Mzingeli, who now seemed to have earned his approval.

'This not good,' explained the tracker. 'He say they take us to Bulawayo to king's kraal. He say Lobengula like English. He say we should start now.'

'Oh blast! Will it be dangerous, do you think?'

'Cannot say, Nkosi. King cruel man. When some man accused of stealing his cattle, he kill him, of course. But very cruelly. He strip off skin from forehead and pull it over eyes that saw cattle. He cut off nose that smelled them. He cut off ears that hear them. He put out eyes that seen them. Then he throw man to crocodiles. Very cruel.'

'How disgusting.' Alice had joined them, after seeing to her patient, who was now fully conscious.

'Yes, Nkosana. But is true he seem to like English. Some traders stay in Bulawayo and one missionary. Other men come from other countries to try and get treaty to dig for gold and other things in ground, but king very careful. I hear perhaps he sign treaty with Nkosi Rhodes from Cape. But I am not sure.'

'Cecil John Rhodes. Ah.' Fonthill nodded his head. 'He's a shrewd devil, that one. I met him once, years ago. I wonder . . .'

His musings were ended by the *inDuna* climbing to his feet. The Matabele spoke briefly to Mzingeli then to his men, who all stood.

'I'm sorry, Alice,' said Simon, 'but it seems we are all off to Bulawayo to pay homage to the king, whether we like it or not.'

She frowned, then her face relaxed into a smile. 'Ah well,' she said. 'At least it should be interesting. Just don't get caught stealing his cattle, that's all I can say.'

Three long, thick branches were cut from the bush by the Matabele and the skins carefully draped over them. The ends of the poles were lifted on to the shoulders of six of the warriors and then they were off. As they left the clearing, the hyenas were already gathering around the carcasses of the lions.

They moved at what seemed at first to be a slow pace, set by the *inDuna*, but his loping stride was deceptive and the three British soon began to feel the heat, as they left the bush and began to traverse stony, sandy terrain. Around them, but unseen, baboons began to bark and troops of more courageous chattering monkeys formed company with them as they marched. Alice became concerned that the unremitting pace might displace some of Sando's stitches, and she insisted that the party halt, while she made a makeshift sling for the man's arm.

This attracted the *inDuna*'s attention, and he gazed in astonishment at the neat array of stitches that patterned the ugly wound in the bearer's shoulder. He demanded to know who had made this decoration, and his jaw dropped as Mzingeli explained what Alice had done. He became noticeably deferential to her afterwards.

'He think you powerful lady witch doctor,' Mzingeli told her.

'So she is,' grunted Simon. 'So she is. I should know.'

Alice aimed a playful blow at him. But her eyes were dark. 'I only wish I was,' she said.

Gradually they passed out of the mopane woodland and moved into more open country, still dotted with bush but also studded with rocky kopjes that rose from well-grassed veldt. These were interspersed with low rocks, smooth and sunburnished, that swelled up from the grassland like whales stranded on a seashore. It was obviously better country for cattle, and they passed many small kraals before stopping at one to spend the night. That evening, as they sat around an open fire eating black bread and the meat of a young duiker buck, the Matabele party, including the *inDuna*, kept well away from the British and their bearers. Fonthill, however, noticed that the Matabele were casting envious eyes on the rifles and the packs.

'Ah,' said Mzingeli, 'Matabele are thieves. Everyone knows this. We must be careful with our things.'

'Tell me about them. What sort of race are they?'

The tracker curled his lip. 'They are the conquerors of this region. Everyone afraid of them – like Zulus in south. The men think war and hunting only things for men to do. Leave everything else to their women. They take everything they see because they think it is their right.'

'I see. Where did they originate?'

'They really Zulus. They come from Zululand long time ago – maybe fifty years, maybe more – in the time of the great Zulu king Shaka. They had their own chief, Mosilikatze. He have trouble with Shaka and lead his clan north. They fight Boers in Transvaal and move north again. Come here and settle. Kill men of many tribes, including my own, and also big tribe in north, the Mashonas. Make these people their subjects and slaves. They good hunters and warriors. Everyone afraid of them.'

The flames from the fire flickered across the tracker's face. Usually passive, his features were now set grimly and his eyes were cold. 'They kill my two brothers. So I leave village as young man and cross Limpopo and go south. Work for Dutchmen on farms in Transvaal and become good tracker and hunter.'

Mzingeli fell silent, and the two men stared into the fire for a moment. Fonthill looked across the flames and saw that both Alice and Jenkins were asleep under their blankets, their heads resting on their folded outer garments, their rifles tucked under the edges of their coverings. Most of the natives of the kraal had crawled into their beehive-shaped huts, and the Matabeles from Bulawayo were stretched out on their sleeping mats.

Fonthill reached into the pack at his feet. 'A little brandy, Mzingeli?' he enquired. 'I think we deserve one, after all the fuss of the day. We call it a nightcap back home.'

The pain left the tracker's face and he gave one of his rare smiles. 'A nightcap? Ah, good word. Let us put on a nightcap then, Nkosi.'

Simon extracted the bottle and two tin cups and poured a little of the amber liquid into each. Suddenly he became aware that they were not alone.

'If there might be a drop to spare, bach sir,' said Jenkins, close to his right ear, 'then I could just be persuaded, see.'

Fonthill sighed, took out another cup, and poured a dram. 'Very well,' he said, 'but I refuse to drink with a man who is in his underpants. For goodness' sake, Jenkins, go and put your trousers on.'

Jenkins slipped away and Simon turned back to Mzingeli. 'Have the Matabele been at war lately?'

'In some ways they always at war, because they kill anyone who argues or stand up with them. But they careful with white men, because Lobengula hears about power of white men in south. He know they beat Zulus.' The tracker took a sip from his cup, grimaced and wiped his lips with his hand. 'This is problem for him. He has about twenty thousand warriors, maybe more, who have not washed their spears for long time – some of them never. They want . . . what you call it . . . honour from war and also things they take from it.'

'Plunder.'

'Yes. King must hold them back all the time. Like holding lid on boiling cooking pot.'

A trousered Jenkins had now rejoined them. 'Will they attack the Dutchmen in the Transvaal, then, Jelly?' he enquired.

'They would like to. If Matabele have guns, perhaps. But they have only a few. And Boers have many.'

Fonthill took a sip of brandy, coughed a little and asked, 'What about the king?'

Mzingeli's smile reappeared. 'He has sixty-three wives. Likes beer, brandy and champagne . . .'

'Champagne?'

'Yes. Traders bring it in for him. He drinks much. He just want to be left to his wives, his cattle and his white man's drink. He don't want war. Although . . .'

'Yes?'

'He like to kill. Bulawayo mean Place of Man Who Was Killed. My father tell me – he the one that tell me all this – my father say that Lobengula six months ago or so send *impi*, war party, to punish two villages where men defy him. They kill all the men, and the children and girls taken as slaves. Then the wives and older women made to carry all good things . . . what you say, plunder . . . back to king's kraal. Then they pushed into circle with spears and women all killed by two young warriors, who so wash their spears.'

'Miserable bastards,' murmured Jenkins.

Fonthill frowned. Then he drained his cup and stood. 'It seems we shall have to handle King Lobengula with care. Bed now, I think. Good night.'

Mzingeli put a restraining hand on his arm. 'Nkosi, it was very good shooting today. Very fine. No one afraid. And you did clever talking with Matabele. Very good.'

'Well, thank you, Mzingeli. I am just sorry that I was stupid the first time. Thank you.'

The little party made equally good time the next day, and after midday they began to climb, so much so that the three British began to gasp a little, reminding Fonthill that this country was some four thousand feet above sea level. They emerged on to a plateau, in good open country, well watered, with a smudge of high hills on the horizon to the north-east. The pace eased a little now and the party settled into a rhythm that lasted for another two and a half days. By the time Bulawayo came in sight, Simon estimated that they had travelled some eighty miles or so from the border.

Lobengula's capital was not as big as Fonthill had expected; not as large, for instance, as he remembered Ulundi, the capital of Zululand, but big enough, perhaps half a mile in diameter. The kraal was enclosed by a great thorn fence that undulated up and down the plateau and within which hundreds of wickerwork beehive huts had been erected for Lobengula's subjects. Grazing cattle – long-horned oxen, many of them distinctively black in colour, domestic cows and steers of a provenance unknown to Fonthill – were dotted on the plateau, almost as far as the eye could see. Smoke from many cooking fires arose and a distinctive smell came drifting across to them: a mixture of cooking fat, cattle manure and human excrement.

Fonthill wrinkled his nose and exchanged glances with Alice. A thought struck him. 'Do you think these fellows will say that they killed the lions themselves and will get the credit for bringing them back to the king?' he asked Mzingeli.

The tall man nodded his head slowly. 'It could be. They like that.'

'Right. Please tell them that we would like to take our skins to the king straight away.'

The *inDuna* nodded his head curtly in response. Soon they were surrounded by dozens of dogs that yapped all around them and snapped at their heels, together with troops of naked children, who looked at the white people with wide-eyed curiosity and teeth that flashed in the sun. The children were joined by two tall Matabele carrying assegais, who, on being addressed by the *inDuna*, turned and immediately ran back to the kraal as fast as their long legs could carry them.

'They go to warn the king that we are coming,' confided Mzingeli. 'They also go to prepare the praise-singers.'

'The what?'

'When king meet new people, they have to wait outside his house while they are told, in song, of how wonderful king is. It is custom. It can take half an hour.'

'Oh, bloody 'ell,' wailed Jenkins. 'I could do with a drink, see, not the chapel choir.'

They entered through a gap in the thorn hedge, where a huge pile of oxen horns had been stacked to one side. 'This to show everyone how rich king is,' whispered Mzingeli. 'All cattle are owned by him. He has about three hundred and likes to count them into cattle kraal every night and see them out to graze every morning.'

Flies were now hovering around them, feasting on the perspiration that dripped down their cheeks and the backs of their shirts. The flies intensified as they neared the king's cattle compound, now empty, and set beside a smaller enclosure within which grazed goats and some horses. Both were adjacent to the king's kraal, a separately ringed fence of thorns enclosing huts for his wives and important members of his household. The king's own dwelling stood out by its singularity in this uncivilised setting. It was a not unpleasant-looking low thatched house, one storey high, with a veranda running the length of its front, European style.

Mzingeli caught Simon's eye. 'Built for him by European trader. Man called Grant. He dead now.'

To one side of the main house and near the goats' kraal stood a round hut built of sun-hardened mud and topped with a conical thatch. It shared with the goats the intermittent shade bestowed by a tall indaba tree, whose roots twisted and curled above ground like giant pythons frozen in time. Before the hut the ground had been beaten flat by thousands of feet, so that it seemed to glisten in the sun.

'That where king has court,' explained Mzingeli. 'Gives wisdom.'

They were halted by the *inDuna* and the skins were lowered to the ground. Immediately two Matabele appeared, caparisoned in monkey skins and ostrich feathers, their faces and bodies streaked with red ochre and carrying what appeared to be fly whisks. They immediately began to chant, swaying in unison and beating time with their whisks. At once a crowd began to gather and started to repeat the words of the singers in a hypnotic ululation, stamping their feet to the rhythm.

'The praise-singers,' confided Mzingeli.

'What are they saying?' asked Alice.

The tracker listened for a moment, his head on one side. 'Silly words,' he said. 'They say that Lobengula is King of Kings, Lord of White Men, Slayer of Men, Devourer of Whole Earth and so on . . . silly words.' His lip curled in contempt. Then, as if suddenly remembering something important, he gestured to Simon, Alice and Jenkins to come close and, raising his voice to be heard above the chanting, said, 'I forget.

When you meet the king you must not address him standing. You must sit. He must always be above you. The Matabele always move before him in bent position, with hands resting on knees.'

'To hell with that,' said Fonthill. 'We would not do that for our Queen, so I don't see why we should do it for some other monarch. I suggest we just bow our heads when he approaches.'

The chanting continued for at least half an hour, while the British three stood in the hot sun, shifting their weight from one foot to the other and wiping away the perspiration that dripped down from under their hats and beneath their shirts. Eventually the singing stopped and was replaced by a roar of acclamation as a tall figure emerged from the door of the house and slowly crossed the veranda threshold. Immediately, all the Matabele sat. It was the cue for the visitors to bow their heads, although Mzingeli and his boys squatted also.

From under his eyelashes, Fonthill observed the king closely. He was about six feet tall and of massive proportions. At first glance he seemed to be almost completely naked, his skin very black. Then it could be seen that his huge stomach hung down above a narrow strip of hide that encircled what once had been his waist and from which a profusion of monkey tails dangled. His posture was erect and magisterial and his features were regular and quite handsome, with the flat nose and thick lips of the Zulu, and the Zulu elder's narrow band of fibre oiled and bound into his tightly curled hair. His eyes seemed cold until they fell upon the lion skins; then they lit up and he smiled, gesturing towards the trio with the long assegai he carried and speaking in a low, guttural voice.

Fonthill leaned down to Mzingeli. 'Can you translate for us?'

'He is asking the *inDuna* where they come from. And,' he waited a moment, 'man is telling truth.'

The king frowned for a moment, then his face split into a smile and he nodded cordially to the trio. He beckoned behind him, and a large wooden chair was brought and set under the broken shade of the indaba tree, and then a collection of goat skins were scattered before him. Lobengula lowered himself into the chair and beckoned with his assegai for the three to sit before him on the skins. Simon grabbed Mzingeli by the shirtsleeve and dragged him down beside him.

The king was speaking. 'He say that you very welcome to his home and he thank you for gifts,' interpreted Mzingeli. 'He say that lion is not hunted here for sport because animal can contain spirit of past Matabele chiefs and bad to kill him. But if lion is attacking cattle then he must be a bad chief. King thanks you for protecting cattle of his people.'

'Well that's very nice of 'im, I'm sure,' whispered Jenkins. 'P'raps 'e's goin' to offer us a drop of somethin' to drink now, d'you think?'

As if the king had heard, he turned his head and shouted an order over his shoulder towards the interior of his house. Immediately – someone must have prepared them already – gourds of beer were brought out and presented to the three Britains. Fonthill took a grateful gulp. It was similar to the Kaffir beer he had drunk in the Transvaal: made from corn, the grain from which had been left to vegetate, dried in the sun, pounded into meal and gently boiled. Cool now, and with a slightly acidic taste, it was delicious. Noticing that nothing had been brought for Mzingeli and his boys, he handed his half-full gourd to the tracker. Alice did the same with hers to

Sando and, with rather less grace, Jenkins followed suit with Ntini.

'Tell the king,' said Fonthill, 'that we are grateful for his welcome. We are sorry not to have sent ahead to ask for permission to cross into his land, but we were diverted by the people of the village near the Limpopo.'

The king waved his assegai in airy acknowledgement of the apology and spoke again. 'Why did you not come here on horse or wagons, as all white people do?'

'Because,' replied Simon, 'we left our horses and wagon at the village and set out to kill the lions on foot. We expected to return to the village but we were brought to you immediately.'

On translation, a frown immediately descended on the royal features, and then they twisted into an expression of fury. Within seconds the benevolent, welcoming monarch had changed into a despotic tyrant, hurling abuse at the *inDuna*, who bowed his head and knelt in submission, his forehead touching the ground.

'He say that the man has caused king to lose honour with white visitors by bringing you here without horses, wagon and clothes,' translated Mzingeli quietly. 'I think they take him away to kill him now.'

'Oh no. Tell him that we were so anxious to meet the king, about whom we had heard so much, that we were happy to leave our things behind. The *inDuna* must not be blamed.'

Hearing this, Lobengula's face lightened and he waved his assegai to the *inDuna* in what appeared to a gesture of forgiveness. The man sat up slowly and shot a quick glance of thanks at Fonthill. But the king was speaking again.

'He want to know if you have met Queen Victoria.'

Simon smiled. 'Tell him yes. I met her at her palace in Windsor. So too did Mr Jenkins here.' Fonthill was not lying.

Both he and Jenkins had attended investiture ceremonies at Windsor Castle when they had received the order of Companion of the Bath and the Distinguished Conduct Medal, respectively, for their services on General Wolseley's abortive expedition to relieve General Gordon at Khartoum. The king gave an expansive smile.

'He say he has written to Queen Victoria and she has written to him.'

'Ah. How . . . er . . . very interesting.'

Lobengula now broke off to give a string of orders to his attendants and then turned back to his visitors.

'King say that he will send people to my father's village to bring horses and wagon here. He also give hut for you to live in and send food. He want you to stay a while as his guest. He say he have other white people here but they have not met Queen Victoria. He say that he don't think big man in south, Nkosi Rhodes, has met queen either. But you have. He like to talk to you later.'

'Oh blimey,' muttered Jenkins. 'I don't like the sound of that.'

'Neither do I,' whispered Alice. 'I wonder what's wrong with his foot?' For the first time, Fonthill noticed that the king's right foot seemed swollen around the big toe, and remembered that he had limped as he had come towards them. 'I would say he's got gout,' Alice continued. 'Too much champagne and brandy, I would think.'

Lobengula rose slowly to his feet to indicate that the audience was at an end, and Simon and the others rose too. Fonthill bowed his head in acknowledgement.

'The king is very kind,' he said as Mzingeli interpreted, 'and my wife, servants and I would be honoured to stay for a short time as his guests. But we must return to the south soon, for we have urgent business in Cape Town. In the meantime, however, we are at the service of your majesty to give you whatever assistance we can.'

With that, the king gave a cheery smile, barked further commands to his attendants and then limped back into his house. The *inDuna* leaped to his feet and beckoned the visitors to follow him. They all walked out of the king's enclosure towards where a party of Matabele women were hurrying in and out of a large beehive hut set apart from the rest, crawling agilely on their hands and knees through the narrow opening carrying blankets, drinking vessels and other domestic utensils.

At the entrance, Fonthill paused and, with one restraining hand on the *inDuna*'s shoulder, addressed Mzingeli. 'Tell him,' he said, 'that I would like proper accommodation also to be given to you and your boys.'

The tracker shook his head. 'Thank you, but is not right here, Nkosi. We just slaves here.'

'No you are not. The British abolished slavery in 1807 and I don't recognise it anywhere. Go on, tell him. The man owes me a favour, dammit.'

Hesitantly Mzingeli translated. Simon's request was treated with a frown but the Matabele shrugged his shoulders and then nodded his head in acquiescence.

Once inside the hut, Alice spread a sleeping mat, laid a blanket upon it and sat down. 'Well, my darling,' she said with a warm smile to Simon, 'do you know, I didn't realise that you were so well acquainted with our gracious Queen. As a result, it seems you have just been appointed Grand Vizier Extraordinary to his fat majesty here, and we are doomed, it seems, to stay here while you advise him for years and years and bloody years. Eh?'

Fonthill returned her smile sheepishly. 'Well, I only answered a question.' He looked around. 'It's not exactly the Ritz, I agree, but it will serve until our transport arrives. Then we shall be off, I promise.'

That evening, a young goat was delivered to Mzingeli from the king with instructions to slay it and cook it for his master. It came with a calabash of beer, a sack full of corn and a basket containing the delicious local umkuna plums. Later, they gathered outside the hut, squatting by firelight under the stars in the cool of the evening, tearing chunks of the goat meat apart with their hands and washing it down with the beer.

'Well,' said Jenkins, inevitably, 'I'm startin' to take to this postin' now, bach sir. The old king is lookin' after us right well, I'd say.'

Their meal was interrupted towards its end by the arrival of a visitor. A portly, bearded white man, dressed in conventional slouch hat, loose cotton shirt and corduroy trousers, he stood deferentially for a moment at the edge of the light cast by the fire before stepping forward to introduce himself.

'James Fairbairn,' he said. 'I trade here. Thought I would walk over and introduce myself and welcome you to this Paris of Africa. I've heard that you came here in a bit of a rush, so I've brought you a few things you might need, toothbrushes, soap and the like. All from the store. You can pay me later,' he added hurriedly.

'My word, you are welcome', said Alice. The introductions were made and Fairbairn joined them at the fireside and helped them to munch the plums and drink the beer. He was, he said, one of a small group of traders who had made their homes in Bulawayo some years ago and eked out a not particularly profitable living. They existed under the eye of the king but they were more or less left alone, as long as they gave Lobengula presents from time to time, 'as a kind of fee for being allowed to stay,' he explained. But it wasn't a bad life. 'At least we are all our own men.'

There was, he added, a local British missionary who spoke the Matabele language fluently and who had become intimate with the king, drafting the occasional letter for him to the authorities in the Cape Colony and even, once, to Queen Victoria. The man ran a school for the children but so far had made no conversions to Christianity.

'Why are you here?' Fairbairn asked.

Simon explained the circumstances.

The trader seemed relieved. 'We are getting a lot of white visitors here now,' he said. 'Usually they cause trouble.'

'Why?'

'Well.' Fairbairn scratched his beard. 'I don't know too much about politics back home, or in Europe for that matter. And I am no mining engineer. But I do know this much – the scramble for Africa by the white man is still going on and old Lobengula's kingdom is one of the juiciest bits that is still available, so to speak. Available, that is, if you can get the old rogue to put his cross on a piece of paper and then move in and develop it.'

'Cecil John Rhodes?'

'Yes, but not just him. Look.' Fairbairn pulled a stick from the edge of the fire, snapped off its charred end and used it to sketch a rough map of southern Africa in the dust at their feet. 'Here is Matabeleland, including Mashonaland to the north, which the king controls anyway. The British are well entrenched down at the bottom in South Africa, here. The Portuguese have vast territories in Mozambique in the east and Angola in the west, right next door, so to speak. Belgium has the Congo in the centre of Africa to the north-west here. We've got the Germans, under . . . what's his name?'

'Bismarck?' prompted Alice, her chin in her hand.

'That's the chap. Yes, the Germans here, in Damaraland, to the south-west, just itching to get more land. Then, very importantly, old Kruger with his Boers in the Transvaal here, just south of the border with Matabeleland, all cock-a-hoop after rubbing our noses in the dirt at Majuba. He wants a route to the sea for his state and reckons he can best do it through Lobengula's nation. On top of all that there's the French at the top of Africa and in the Sahara who would love to put our noses out of joint by taking the king's land. Everybody thinks that there is gold here. There's a bit of mining at Tati just over the border to the south, as you know, but no traces have really been found anywhere else around here, as far as I'm aware, although the king has not really let anyone mine in his land yet. So everyone seems to be beating a path to the old devil's door.'

Fonthill smiled. 'For someone who doesn't know much about it, that's what I would call a pretty fair summing-up of the situation, Mr Fairbairn, and matches what I heard in the Cape.'

The trader looked a touch embarrassed and scratched his head. 'Well, it's important to us all, I suppose.'

'But you said that all these visitors cause trouble.'

'Yes. Everybody makes all kinds of promises to Lobengula – promises that they don't keep. He's no fool, you know. He knows the white man pretty well now. It is true that he is well disposed towards the English – mainly I think because we knocked over the Zulus a few years ago, and also because the stories of the wealth created by the British in the diamond and gold fields down south are rife here. So he thinks we are strong. But he says that all white men are liars.' Fairbairn grinned. 'And so we are, I reckon.'

Jenkins had been listening with care. Now he lifted his head. 'Tell me, Mr Fairbairn, why do people want this land anyway? It don't look much good to me, see. Lot of woodland and these big high rocks stickin' up all over the place.'

'I suppose it's the promise of gold and other minerals, as I've said, although there's good farming land around here and in Mashonaland. But Matabeleland is also the route to the north, to the big lakes up there. You've got to go through here to get there, to get to whatever they've got to offer.' He scratched his head again. 'Seems to me that the powers in Europe have gone a bit mad about all this. I can see it leading to a scrap in the end.'

The little gathering fell silent for a moment as the flickering flames lit their faces spasmodically. Somewhere far away a hyena barked and caused Fairbairn to look up. 'Bad sign, that,' he said. 'The little devils are getting more adventurous. Coming close to our huts and stealing the rubbish.'

'What about the British in all this, Mr Fairbairn?' Fonthill asked. 'Mzingeli here tells me that he believes that Rhodes from the Cape has entered into some sort of deal with Lobengula.'

Fairbairn's teeth flashed in the firelight. 'Yes, he has. In fact his people have just left, after being here for months. He got the king to put his cross on the paper what seems like ages ago, giving Rhodes the right to prospect for minerals, mainly gold, of course. In return Lobengula has been promised all sorts of things: guns, ammunition, money and so on. But nothing has materialised. That's why he says all white men are liars. At the moment, I don't think that treaty is worth the paper it is written on. The king won't really understand what he's signed anyway. But the others are still sniffing around here, to get him to let them have rights, too.'

'Who are they?'

'Well, the Dutchmen from the Transvaal are always pulling at his sleeve, but he hates the Boers so he won't do anything with them. No . . .' The trader's voice faded away for a moment. 'The worst are the Portuguese.'

'Why?'

'They think this territory is theirs anyway, because they've been next door in Mozambique for bloody centuries. But they've never really had the guts just to come in and invade and settle the land, which is what is called for. The main problem is that they are insistent. They've got a man here now. His name is Manuel Antonio de Sousa – very fancy bloke to match his fancy name. But everybody calls him Gouela. He's a slave master in his own right and a cruel bastard – ah, excuse me, ma'am.'

Alice, whose eyes had never left Fairbairn's face, nodded her acceptance.

'He has abused all the tribes in his territory to the east. He rapes and flogs, but he's got a silver tongue from what I hear and he is here to rubbish the British to the king and to get him to sign a treaty with the Portuguese. He's got silly airs and graces but the king gets taken in by all this stuff. So Rhodes ought to watch out.'

Fonthill slowly nodded his head. 'Fascinating,' he said. 'Now, Mr Fairbairn, we have just a little drop of Boer brandy left. Will you take a dram?'

Fairbairn stood. 'No, thank you kindly. I must be getting back. He looked down at the bundle at his feet. 'I will leave all this stuff with you. Take what you want and bring the rest back to the store and . . . er . . . you can pay me there. It's about three hundred yards that way, outside the outer fence. Now, I'll say good night to you all.'

After his departure, Alice drew her knees up under her chin and stared into the embers of the fire reflectively. 'I have to say, Simon,' she said, 'that I don't like the sound of all this. You must be careful not to trade on your incredibly close relationship with our Queen,' she looked up and grinned, 'because you would just be the latest in a long line of interlopers here who couldn't deliver. You mustn't be a scapegoat for Cecil John Rhodes.'

'And, look you, I don't like what I 'ear about this Portuguese chap,' said Jenkins. 'Manuel Saucepot or whatever 'is name is. I fancy 'e could be trouble.'

Fonthill rose to his feet. 'Well, I'll try and stay out of this mess if I can. But I can't see us getting out of here before our transport arrives. We are in the hands of the king, for better or worse. So let's go to bed.'

Chapter 3

The next morning Fonthill, stripped to the waist, was washing outside the hut in a bowl of cold water when he saw a strange apparition approaching. A white man, resplendent in a yellow uniform, complete with gold buttons and red braid at the shoulders and a sword at his waist, was being slowly borne towards him on a palanquin, or litter, carried by two Kaffirs. At the door of the hut, the litter was carefully lowered to the ground and the man put out his jackbooted legs, stood stiffly and inclined his head.

He said something quickly in a language foreign to Fonthill and waited for a reply. 'I am sorry,' said Simon, hurriedly towelling himself. 'You must forgive me, but I don't speak that language.'

'Of course not.' The man's English was highly accented but it was clear that he was being contemptuous. 'Why is it that you English do not speak any language other than your own?' It was not a question, more a condemnation. Fonthill studied him carefully. He was of medium height – a little shorter than Simon – strongly built and with a face that reflected a life spent in the tropics: pockmarked and yellow-tinged. Beneath the peaked cap that matched the uniform hung hair in waved ringlets. He must be, of course, the

Portuguese spoken of last night by Fairbairn.

'I am afraid that with most of us that is true,' Fonthill replied, pulling over his head the coarse shirt that Mr Fairbairn had supplied. 'Though not all of us. *Mais si vous parlez Francais, peut-être je peux vous aidez,*' he added, 'or *vielleicht wäre die Deutsche Sprache lieber*? However, I do apologise, for I do not speak any of the lesser languages, such as Portuguese.'

A distant chuckle came from within the hut. The Portuguese's eyes hardened. 'English will do,' he said. 'I speak it fluently.' He jerked his head forward. 'Manuel Antonio de Sousa, agent for the King of Portugal in Matabeleland and Mashonaland, at your service.'

Fonthill took a pace forward and extended his hand. 'Simon Fonthill. How do you do.' He shook the man's hand, an action that resembled handling a damp, warm fish, then gestured. 'I am sorry I cannot ask you inside, but my wife is completing her toilet. We had rather a long day travelling yesterday.' He indicated a log nearby. 'Won't you sit down?'

'No. Your wife is with you?' De Sousa seemed surprised.

'Yes. We were on holiday, travelling in the Transvaal, when we crossed into Matabeleland to help one of the Malakala villages, whose herd was being attacked by lions. We met up with a party of the king's men and were brought here.'

'Ah, that explains the skins. Or does it?' The sneer had returned. 'You don't expect me to believe that, do you? You are, of course, working for Rhodes.'

Fonthill felt his temper rising but took a deep breath. 'No, I am not. I have no interest in Mr Rhodes's activities. As I explained, I am on holiday. Now, Mr de Sousa, what can I do for you?'

For a moment, de Sousa's black eyes gleamed in anger. Then he laughed. 'Listen, my friend,' he said. 'When you return to your master, tell him that King Lobengula has no further interest in the false promises of the British. This is Portuguese territory and Lobengula is a Portuguese subject, and he has agreed to allow my people – *not the British* – to develop this country. Rhodes – and you – would be well advised to stay out of my way.'

Jenkins chose that moment to crawl out of the hut. He looked at the Portuguese's litter, with its two bearers standing idly by, and spoke with exaggerated concern. 'Oh, somebody ill, then? Goodness me. It must be the heat, I suppose.' Then, pretending to see de Sousa for the first time, 'Ah, good morning. Would you like to come inside out of the heat and lie down, perhaps?'

De Sousa looked at the Welshman in astonishment. Then his lip curled. 'This is your wife?' he asked with a sarcasm to match that of Jenkins.

'No,' replied Fonthill evenly, 'this is the only accommodation we have at the moment, until our wagon arrives from the border, so we are forced to share. Now,' his voice took on a harder tone, 'I do not like being threatened, Mr de Sousa, and I can only repeat once again that I have nothing to do with Mr Rhodes. As for staying out of your way, I shall go where I like in this territory, subject to the approval of the king. I know as well as you do, sir, that Matabeleland is not under the suzerainty of Portugal and remains an independent country. If this was not so, you would not be here. Your behaviour, sir, is not that of a gentleman and I would be grateful if you would leave.'

The two men remained glaring at each other for a moment, and then the Portuguese walked slowly to his litter, lay down upon it and, with a flick of his wrist, bade his bearers carry him away.

Fonthill and Jenkins watched him go with smiles on their lips. 'What a pompous bit of offal,' said the Welshman. ''E looks an' sounds like a tin soldier, don't 'e?'

'I'm not so sure about that.' Alice had crawled out of the hut and joined them. She put a hand on her husband's arm. 'You were right to tick him off, my love, but I have a feeling that you have just made a rather dangerous enemy.'

Simon puffed out his cheeks. 'I didn't have much choice, actually. He was bloody rude from the start so I had to put him down. Obviously the man is a bounder. You'll remember what Fairbairn said about him last night. And of course he was bluffing about Matabeleland being Portuguese territory . . .'

'Yes, my dear, but I believe that they have always claimed it as being . . . what is the phrase? "In their African sphere of influence." Maybe this is recognised in Whitehall. Don't forget that Portugal is supposed to be our oldest ally. So perhaps they have some sort of case. All I am saying is that you should stay away from him.'

'Yes, well, if you say so, Alice. But I shan't lose any sleep in worrying about him.'

They were interrupted by the *inDuna*, who approached them accompanied by Mzingeli. The tracker looked concerned. 'King want to see you now,' he said.

Fonthill wrinkled his nose. 'Very well. Let me just make myself presentable for his majesty. You had better come with me, Mzingeli, to interpret, please.'

This time Fonthill and Mzingeli were ushered straight into the king's house. They found him half sitting, half lying on a chaise-longue, but dressed very differently now. Despite the warmth in the dark interior, he wore a pair of cord trousers, rather the worse for wear, a dirty flannel shirt, a tweed coat and a billycock hat in which was stuck a feather. One foot was encased in a lace-up boot; the other wore an old carpet slipper with its end cut away to reveal a swollen, obviously inflamed big toe.

The total effect was incongruous and Simon bit back a smile. Instead he bowed his head in greeting as Lobengula waved him to sit on a pile of skins before him. Mzingeli squatted at his side and the king gestured to him to interpret.

'He ask,' began the tracker, 'how was Queen Victoria when last you see her?'

'Er . . . very well, thank you, sir. Ah, she is still sad, of course, because her husband died – even though this was about twenty years ago.'

'She got no other husbands left?'

'No. It is our custom only to have one spouse at a time. And she has never married again.'

'That very silly. But your business. Give her my salute when next you see her.'

'I will indeed, sir.'

The king shifted his afflicted foot slightly and grimaced in pain, but he continued, through Mzingeli: 'You know Rhodes?'

'Only slightly. I have met him once, but that was eight years ago.'

'He never come to see me. Only send his people. If he so interested in my land, why he no come and talk to me himself?'

'I don't know, sir. However, I do know that he is very busy with affairs of state in the Cape Colony. I understand that he may soon be elected prime minister there.'

'Humph. That not king.'

'No, sir. But it means he is the leader of this very big land.'

'Not as big as my land.'

'With respect, sir, it is about twice as large.' Fonthill was not sure about this, but he rather doubted if the king would be able to check the fact.

A silence fell on the gathering, only broken when a huge black woman entered, bearing a gourd of beer for Simon. She wore native dress, which meant very few garments. The king nodded towards her.

'This my sister, Nini. She not married.'

Unsure about the significance of this last piece of information, Fonthill struggled to his feet and bowed. Mzingeli, aware of the proprieties, inclined his head from the sitting position. But Nini strode forward, seized Simon's hand and shook it vigorously, an act that made her huge bare breasts sway alarmingly. 'How is you?' she asked, disdaining to use Mzingeli's interpretive skills.

'I is . . . I am very well, ma'am. I am delighted to meet you.'

'You have wife?'

'Yes, she is with me.' A look of what might have been disappointment came across Nini's otherwise happy features. 'You know Queen Victoria?'

Fonthill shifted uneasily from one foot to the other. This was all getting rather out of hand. 'Only very slightly, ma'am.'

It was clear that the king's sister's knowledge of English was being exhausted, for she now nodded to Mzingeli to translate. 'She know that Queen has sons. She would like to marry one. You help her?'

Simon gulped, quickly dismissing from his mind the irreverent vision of the portly Prince of Wales and the eighteen-stone Princess Nini attempting to copulate. 'I fear that would not be possible, ma'am. The Queen's sons are married already, and our religion and constitution allow only one husband at a time.'

The princess nodded, seemingly not disconcerted by the news. She pointed to the gourd. 'Good beer. I make. Goodbyeing.' Then, with a cheerful grin, she left.

Fonthill squatted again and, although not exactly yearning to drink beer at half past eight in the morning, took a sip from the gourd. Nini was right. It *was* excellent. Perhaps she could have made a match of it with that famous *bon vivant* Prince Edward after all . . . But the king was speaking again.

'I trust you. Anyone who is friend of great English Queen must be honourable man. Everyone I talk to from other countries want me to give them my land. They say to dig in it but I think they put their own people on it. I know that world is changing and not like that of my father. Perhaps I must give in to these strong countries, like yours.'

The king was now looking hard at his guest and his face wore an expression of . . . what? Pleading? Desperation? Simon experienced a sudden sympathy for this man, who just wished to be left alone to live as his forebears had, but who clearly saw that he must somehow move with the times. A man who realised that he must change but not knowing which way to turn. A man under great pressure.

He cleared his throat to reply, but the king was continuing. 'I say to Rhodes he can come here and dig. In return, he promise me,' and he slapped one finger after another on to his palm, 'one hundred pounds your money on first day of every lunar month, a thousand rifles with hundred thousand bullets, and steamboat for me on Zambezi. What happen? Nothing. Now, Portuguese, Germans and other English tell me I have done wrong and should sign with them. My *inDunas* say I must not sign my country away. What do I do? You honest man. You know great Queen. Tell me, what do I do?'

Fonthill frowned. What the hell to say? He took another, reflective drink from the gourd. Then, 'I am English, of course, and your majesty will think that because of that I will favour the English in my reply. But I will attempt to be objective.' He waited for Mzingeli to translate, for it was important that the tracker found the right words. Then he continued.

'You know that the British Empire is the largest in the world. It has territories that are . . .' his brain attempted to find a comparison that would be roughly accurate and also meaningful, 'a hundred, hundred, hundred times bigger than Matabeleland and Mashonaland combined. It has ships that control the wide oceans and armies that exist in fifty countries or more. I myself have fought in these armies in five countries in the last five years and seen their power. If your majesty feels he must side with one of these great nations, then I have to say that he should choose the strongest, which is Britain.

'As for the offers you are receiving from other English companies, I understand that you have already signed a treaty with Rhodes. I do not know this man well, but he is very rich and powerful – he owns many, many more oxen even than your majesty. He is a man of distinction in the Cape, and because of his prominent position, he would not – he could not – avoid keeping his word to you. So I recommend that you should put your trust in him.

'However . . .' Fonthill paused to allow Mzingeli to keep pace, but also to gather his thoughts. He found himself empathising with the king's appeal. Could he help? 'As you know, I wish to return to the Cape as soon as possible. I promise you that I will see Rhodes and explain to him your concern. I will say to him that whatever problems he has in keeping his word to you, they must be overcome, otherwise he will lose his contract with you. I hope that may help your majesty. I fear I can do no more.'

The king listened carefully, and when Mzingeli had finished, he sat for a while looking at Fonthill. Then: 'Wise words. Yes, I keep with Rhodes, but only as contract said: he can dig, but not to settle people here. Yes, please. You talk to him in Cape. I am glad you help me.'

Fonthill bowed his head in acquiescence, and as silence descended again, he took another sip from the gourd. Then, however, a further thought occurred to him.

'Your majesty has a Portuguese agent visiting you?'

'Yes. He important man.'

Simon coughed and wondered how to go on. 'I am afraid, sir, that he does not appear to me to be a gentleman. I understand that he treats the tribes that come under his command to the east very badly. Making slaves of them—'

The king interrupted Mzingeli quickly at this point: 'That is good. Some people no good for anything but slaves. I have slaves.'

Damn! Fonthill had to recover. 'Yes, sir. But you treat your slaves well. I understand that he does not. He rapes and whips them. That is not the action of a white gentleman.'

'Ah yes. It is right, you are different. But he is friends with King of Portugal. He is agent.'

'I believe that he merely has duties involving the native tribes to the west of Mozambique. But also he has threatened me this morning' – Simon felt at this point that he was behaving rather like the school sneak, betraying another boy to the headmaster, but he ploughed on anyway – 'saying that I must not interfere with your plans to give digging rights to other countries. I think you should know, sir, that I do not think he is to be trusted.'

Another silence descended, and it was clear that Lobengula was not comfortable with the accusation. Fonthill, however, refused to retract it. De Sousa had thrown down the challenge, and this opportunity for creating bad odour between him and the king was too good to be missed.

Eventually Lobengula spoke. 'King hear your words. He think about it.'

Silence once more. It seemed as though the king had something else to say but was almost embarrassed to say it, or could not find the words to do so. He stirred on his couch, and once again a grimace flashed across his face.

'Your majesty is in pain?'

This seemed to open a door of opportunity for the big man. 'Yes. My foot gives me much hurt. It is curse put on me by my enemies.' His face took on a diffident expression, as though about to seek a favour but not knowing how to ask it of this strange, highly placed white man, who had brought him gifts but had so far asked nothing of him. Then he seemed to pluck up courage.

'Your lady has power of witchcraft, my people tell me.'

'Oh no.' Fonthill smiled. 'She is no witch doctor.'

'Ah, but she heal shoulder of the Malakala man. Put back flesh torn by lion. No one get better after lion bite or claw. They die. This man good now, I hear. Could she come and take curse off my foot?'

Consternation settled on Fonthill. First he was a close friend of Queen Victoria, the most famous and powerful monarch in the world. Now he was married to a witch doctor! He thought quickly. Alice had only rudimentary medical knowledge, given to her over four days by doctors at the

Missionary Society who knew the territory and its dangers. But there was no way she could cure gout. Or was there . . . ? Perhaps she could alleviate the pain a little. To do so would put them in good standing with the king. If she failed, however, this could diminish them both in Lobengula's eyes. Anyway, he could hardly refuse the man's request.

'Your majesty will know,' he began, 'that we do not believe in curses. The problem with your foot will be a medical one . . .' He sought for simple words that would explain it. 'It will be the result perhaps of something you have eaten or drunk too much of. Or maybe a thorn that has settled deeply in the foot.'

The king scowled. The scowl was reflected in Mzingeli's translation. 'He say he know all about thorns. No thorn in his foot.'

Simon bowed his head. 'Very well, sir. My wife is not a witch doctor, but nor is she any other sort of doctor. She does, however, have some basic skills in healing that might help you and perhaps relieve your pain. I will ask her.'

The big smile returned to Lobengula's face. 'Good. Ask her come soon. Now, I give more food to you tonight. Is there more you want?'

Smiling, Fonthill shook his head. 'Only our horses and wagon from the border, sir. We are anxious to travel south.'

'My men go get them today. Is good you go soon – to see Rhodes.' Then he added quickly, 'After your lady help me.'

Fonthill rose, pulling Mzingeli with him, and they both bowed and shuffled out of the room. As they trudged back to the hut, Simon confided, 'I shall be glad to get out of here, Mzingeli. I seem to be getting deeper and deeper into I don't quite know what. But I don't like it.'

The tracker nodded. 'King is cunning. You must be careful.'

Alice herself was just returning to the hut as Fonthill approached. 'I've been to Fairbairn's store to pay him,' she said. 'I've left Jenkins up there, trying to haggle with him about the price of a bottle of whisky. The man was not exactly giving anything away last night, but I don't begrudge him what he charges. He lives behind the shop, so to speak, and I can't help feeling that he doesn't have much of a life. But it's his choice. Now, what did his majesty want?'

They both sat on a log and Simon recounted his conversation with Lobengula, beginning with the king's request for help with Rhodes.

Alice pulled a face. 'I have never met the great Cecil John,' she said, 'but he sounds a bit of a slippery customer to me. I would not like you to become too involved with him.'

'Oh, as millionaires go, I don't think he's too bad. Of one thing I am sure – he's a genuine patriot. When I met him in Kimberley seven or eight years ago, he gave me his vision of a British route to the north, with much of his map painted red. Then, he was just the company secretary of a mining outfit. I have read since that he has made two fortunes: the first in diamonds, of course, and the second from gold in the Transvaal. It's my bet that he is not really interested in Matabeleland or Mashonaland for the mineral rights. He would rather settle the land with Britishers if he could and then try and build a road, or even a railway, to the north. The king is a shrewd old cove and I believe that he suspects this is what Rhodes is up to and he is worried about it.'

Alice sniffed. 'Well on that matter, I would be on Lobengula's side. I know he is a cruel old despot, but he has done nothing to harm the British or any other Europeans, for that matter. Why can't we leave him gradually to slip into the nineteenth century in his own way and his own time? We've got the biggest blasted empire the world has ever seen. Why do we need to add a few more African acres to it?'

'I don't quite agree, my love.' Simon smiled. They had been over this ground before. Alice's radical views were familiar to him. She yearned for the return to power of William Ewart Gladstone as prime minister of Great Britain, and for a resumption of a Liberal government's anti-imperialist policies. As a war correspondent for the *Morning Post*, she had even managed to infiltrate her views into her reports for that most Tory of newspapers.

He looked around him and gestured towards the rolling grassland behind the barrier of thorns. 'I've seen enough to know that this is good land,' he said, his eyes crinkled. 'And I gather it is even better further north in Mashonaland. As it is, it is not developed at all, and the Matabele seem to know nothing about agriculture. They will never make the most of this fertile ground. I am talking about cultivating it, not digging for gold, silver, copper or whatever might be beneath these grasslands. I wouldn't mind at all farming here.' He grinned at her. 'Bit less boring than Norfolk, anyway.'

But Alice was not smiling, and remembering the king's other request, Simon was glad of the chance to change the subject and put Lobengula's plea to her.

'What?' His wife's face was a study in consternation. 'Good lord. I am not a doctor, Simon. You know that.'

'Yes, Alice. I did try and explain, but it seems you have acquired a reputation as a magnificent witch doctor after stitching up Sando's shoulder. Perhaps there is something you could do to ease Lobengula's pain?'

'I don't know. Perhaps there is something in the self-help

medical book the missionaries gave me. I will go and get my bag.' She stood to move into the low opening of the hut, but Simon held her back.

'I'll go. I need to oil the rifles, anyway.'

He crawled through the opening and stood for a moment in the dim interior, trying to accustom his eyes to the poor light, before bending down to look under Alice's bed for her bag. Suddenly a movement caught his eye. On the low wooden-framed bed by the door – *his* bed – something was moving, undulating under the blanket that had been lightly thrown there. Then, slowly, a cold-eyed flat head emerged to regard him, followed by the coils of a body.

It was a puff adder.

Fonthill felt his mouth go dry. He made to move back towards the hut opening, but the snake followed him with his head and then slipped from under the blanket on to the ground. It was cutting him off from the exit. Where the hell were the rifles? His eye caught them: the two Martini-Henrys and Alice's gun, neatly stacked against the wall – just by the entrance. The snake, of course, was between him and the guns.

He looked hard at the reptile, which had now formed itself into a tight coil, with its head held high and back, in an 'S' shape. Simon licked his lips and tried to remember what Mzingeli had told them. The puff adder was, he recalled, the most dangerous snake in Africa. Its bite could penetrate leather and its poison was extremely toxic. It could kill a man and frequently did so in this part of Africa.

The thing was now uncoiling and moving towards him slowly, hissing, its mouth wide open and revealing its fangs. Even in the semi-darkness he could see the dark bands around its eyes. Uncoiled, it revealed itself to be about three and a half feet in length. Fonthill felt the hairs begin to stand up on the back of his neck.

He took a deep breath and shouted, 'Alice. Do not crawl into the hut. There is a snake in here. It is between me and the rifles and the door. Get 352 or Mzingeli quickly – and a gun. Quickly now.'

There was no reply. He called again. Silence once more. He looked round for some sort of weapon. His hunting knife was hung up above his bed and unreachable, but even if he could have got to it, it would have been useless against the adder, which could strike so quickly. The thing was slowly slithering towards him now. Fonthill felt completely vulnerable in his lightweight cord trousers and slip-on shoes. He had even left his socks off today, of all days. What could he use to distract the snake?

He felt behind him with one hand, encountering Alice's bed. The blanket! Slowly he pulled at it until he felt it come loose and slide on to the floor. Could he hear voices now, from outside? He called out: 'Don't come in,' and pulled the blanket towards him until he had a large portion wrapped around his wrist. He took a gentle step forward towards the snake. Immediately, it coiled its head back again. With a jerk of his wrist, he flicked the blanket at the adder, so that it almost touched the square head, now held nearly upright. The snake hissed and struck at the blanket with what seemed like the speed of light. The two, slightly back-curved fangs snapped together on the frayed edge of the cloth and immediately became entangled in the coarse wool fibres.

Fonthill tugged the blanket back, but it remained caught in the snake's fangs, pulling the thing towards him. He sprang to the side, caught his leg on the foot of Alice's bed and fell to the ground. He threw the rest of the blanket at the snake and, rolling over, saw it thrashing its head under the folds of the cloth as it tried to free itself.

This was his chance. He hurled himself towards the doorway and landed on his stomach at the foot of his bed. Scrambling to his knees, he pulled his own blanket from the bed and held it as a feeble barrier between him and the snake, like some grounded matador, in the hope that he could slip through the doorway behind its cover. The snake, freed now, had followed him and struck at the blanket, tearing it from his grasp as though it was a mere sheet of paper and tossing it aside. This time, its fangs had not become entangled.

With only inches between them, the serpent and its victim stared at each other, eye to eye. Simon saw the adder open its jaws and pull back its head to strike. He held up a hand and closed his eyes.

The shot that echoed within the confined space of the hut sounded like a howitzer cannon being fired. Fonthill felt something fall across his knee and he recoiled. When he opened his eyes, he saw the body of the headless serpent twitching on the ground by his kneecap. Turning his head, he saw Jenkins lying on his stomach, halfway through the doorway of the hut, Mzingeli's Snider rifle at his shoulder. His head lay to one side and he was being sick.

Simon could hear Alice shouting from outside, 'Let me in, let me in.' He summoned up a feeble croak. 'It's all right. Jenkins has got him. We are both all right.'

At this the Welshman raised his head, vomit on his chin. 'He didn't bite you then, bach sir?' he whispered. 'The 'orrible thing didn't get you?'

Fonthill stood slowly, shaking off the body of the snake with a shudder. Of its head there was no sign, except for a red smudge of some undefined matter on the wall of the hut. Jenkins's shot had shattered it completely. He walked over to his comrade and knelt by his side, only to see the Welshman disappear slowly backwards on his stomach through the opening, as if by magic. Having pulled him clear, Alice appeared, her face ashen.

She crawled into the hut and put her arms around her husband. 'Thank the Lord you are all right.'

'Mind where you put your feet, my darling,' Simon whispered into her hair. 'I'm afraid poor old 352 has been a bit poorly. I'd forgotten how frightened he was of snakes.'

Outside, Mzingeli, Sando, Ntini and a still trembling Jenkins awaited them. Simon pulled the Welshman to his feet and regarded him severely. 'You've made a terrible mess of our living accommodation,' he said and punched him on the shoulder. 'God bless you, old chap.' He took his hand and pumped it. 'I am just so grateful that my best friend just happens to be the finest shot in the world.'

'Not with that bloody old thing he ain't, look you.' Jenkins wiped his chin and gestured towards Mzingeli's rifle. 'If the range had been a foot or so longer I would have missed. It fires up, y'see, but anyway, I was trembling so much.' He turned to Alice and wiped away the perspiration from his face with a very dirty handkerchief. 'Sorry about the mess, miss. Can't stand snakes, see.'

She kissed him. 'I don't know how many times I have had to thank you for saving my husband's life, 352,' she said. 'But this surely must have been the closest thing. My word, it must.' She turned towards Fonthill. 'I heard you shout, Simon, and immediately ran for Mzingeli, who of course had the only other gun. Then I saw dear old 352 coming down the hill.'

Mzingeli coughed and nodded towards Jenkins. 'I want to

go in because is my gun – only one outside hut – but he say no. He best shot. I think he right.'

Fonthill shook his head again. 'Right. Let's clear up inside and get rid of what's left of the brute. Three five two, get yourself a whisky. You are relieved of duty for at least ten minutes. Then we must all talk.'

Later, the six of them squatted on the beaten earth outside the hut. 'Now,' began Fonthill, 'I want to ask you something, Mzingeli. Could that snake have crawled in through the doorway of the hut on its own?'

The tracker shook his head. 'No. Snake don't like people, although it will attack when people come close.' He gestured with his arm. 'Too many people here. Snake never live in village. Out in woods and stony holes. Not here.'

'That's what I thought.'

'What?' asked Alice. 'You don't think it was planted, Simon, do you?'

'I don't know.' He struggled to his feet. 'Excuse me for a moment.' He was back within a minute. 'As I thought, someone has cut a hole in the wickerwork at the back of the hut and closed the gap with a large stone. The snake was obviously slipped though the hole. The noise outside the entrance would probably have stopped it from escaping that way. By the time I got inside, it was a rather angry snake, I would say.' He turned to Mzingeli. 'Did you or either of the boys see anybody approaching, perhaps, say, carrying a sack?'

The question was translated but received no affirmative reply.

Fonthill frowned. It had to be de Sousa. The bastard! He looked ruefully at Alice. 'You were right. I *must* have upset him. Must be very sensitive people, these Portuguese. What a nasty piece of work!'

'What are you goin' to do about 'im, then, bach sir?' enquired Jenkins in a low voice. 'Let me nip over with me knife to where'e lies on 'is fancy bed, like.'

Fonthill shook his head. 'No. The king obviously respects the man for some reason. I certainly don't want to have blood on my hands while I am in his kraal – and neither did de Sousa, for that matter. That's why he used the snake. A very African way to kill a European, don't you think? He wouldn't have been suspected.'

He mused for a moment. 'I think I will let the matter rest.'

Jenkins's black eyebrows almost met his moustache. 'You don't mean lettin' 'im get away with it? 'E will just try again, won't 'e – an' keep tryin' till he gets you.'

'He might, but that's a risk we just have to take.' He looked at them all in turn, resting his eyes last on his wife. 'We must all be on our guard.' He rose to his feet. 'Anyway, we shall be getting out of here soon, when our transport arrives. I would give it only a few days now. It's not far from the frontier.'

'Yes,' said Alice glumly. 'And I have become the Royal Physician. I must get my bag and bone up on gout, or whatever it is that's wrong with the old boy.' Her face fell further. 'What if it's syphilis, or something like that? I shall be a bit stumped then. What the hell would Florence Nightingale have done?' She rose to get her bag, then, at the hut opening, paused for just a moment.

'Let me go first,' said Fonthill hurriedly. 'I'm sure there is not another one in there. But if there is, don't worry. I can fight snakes single-handedly now. Just give me a blanket. Oh . . . and perhaps Jenkins with a rifle.'

With a grin, he crawled in and Alice followed him.

Chapter 4

Three days later, they were on their way to the border, relieved to be rid of the hothouse atmosphere, the ever-present scent of danger, that characterised Lobengula's kraal. The king's men had arrived with their wagon and horses remarkably quickly and the monarch himself waved them off, shouting, 'You come back,' as they rode away. The sun sent shafts of welcoming light across the plain and it was pleasant as, blessedly on horseback again, they followed the faint trail across the veldt. Mzingeli loped on ahead, his Snider over his shoulder, with Sando at his heels and Ntini handling their team of oxen from his seat on the wagon at the rear.

Alice, riding a little behind Simon, allowed her mind to dwell on the last three days. She had visited the king twice, on successive days, and she grinned as she recalled the details. She had been apprehensive about her ability to make a correct diagnosis, but she need not have worried. There was no thorn or broken bone under that cutaway slipper that protected the swelling – and how had that cosy item of Victorian domestic footwear come to be worn by an African chieftain? – but a significant clue was provided by the pile of empty champagne and brandy bottles that glittered in the corner of the hut.

Gout, it had to be! Her little handbook on African diseases made no mention of this malady, but her father had suffered a little from it. Too much meat, port and red wine was the cause, the local general practitioner had lectured. A balanced diet was the cure.

She had alleviated the pain on both visits by administering a little morphine into the naked bottom of the monarch as he lay on his couch. Lobengula had taken it well and had called in his *inDunas*, wives and children to witness his bravery. They had all applauded when he waved airily to them as the needle entered the great rump. But he had taken less well Alice's injunctions to give up the white man's drink, reduce the amount of beef he ingested and eat more berries and other fruits. She knew that it would take more than the homilies of a white woman to change these indulgences, so she had visited Fairbairn to ask him to refuse to sell the bottles to Lobengula. The trader had smiled, waved his pipe and delivered his own lecture on the inadvisability of him telling the King of the Matabele how to live. 'He's God around here,' he had explained. 'If he wants champagne and brandy, then by golly I've got to sell it to him.'

So Alice had shrugged and taken her bag away. On the morning of their departure, however, the king had summoned her and given her a bottle of splendid French cognac, vintage 1880. Whatever his vices, the man had good taste – and a sense of humour. 'For your man,' he had boomed, pressing the bottle into her hand. 'Be careful he don't get goot.' She had decided that she liked the old ruffian. And oh how the little children had gasped, laughed and applauded as he presented his buttocks to the needle. . .

As she summoned up their laughing faces, Alice's eyes filled with tears. Sniffing, she blew her nose, gulped and then gently urged her horse forward until she rode side by side with her husband.

'Our son would have been four just the other day,' she said.

Simon nodded his head, looking straight ahead but gripping her hand tightly. 'I know,' he said. 'The day we shot the lions.'

They rode hand in hand for a few minutes, lost in their own thoughts. Intuitively Jenkins had let his own mount fall back a little as soon as he saw their hands meet. His godson, their son – George Jenkins Mustapha Fonthill – had lived only a few minutes after his birth at their farm in Norfolk, back in 1885. The pregnancy had been difficult and Jenkins had always had his doubts about the survival of the babe. Perhaps its unconventional conception in the sands of the Sudanese desert, amidst the trauma after their escape from the Mahdi's camp, might have had something to do with it. He sighed. It was rarely spoken of now and it was clear that their attempts to have another child since had failed. He knew that the two people he loved most in the world carried with them this constant sadness, and he in turn was sad for them. Time to cheer them up.

He kicked in his heels. 'What about a nice cup of tea?' he called. 'My mouth feels like old Lobengolly's armpit. But if you don't want a *nice* cup of tea, *I* can make it.'

It did the trick. 'Perish the thought,' said Alice. 'But let's stop for a minute.'

They did so and stretched their legs, standing to drink from their tin mugs near a large kopje.

Mzingeli threw away the dregs and moved close to Fonthill. 'We are followed,' he said quietly.

'How long?'

'Last hour, perhaps. Now people ahead. Behind kopje. They watch us from top.'

'How many?'

'Do not know. Perhaps six, ten. Perhaps more.'

Fonthill nodded and took a last reflective drink from his mug. Thank goodness for your splendid eyesight, Mzingeli. Have you any idea who they might be?'

'Just Kaffirs, I think.'

'Very well.' He paused for a moment and walked to his horse on the pretence of adjusting the saddle cinch. From under his hat he scanned the top of the kopje, which was perhaps a quarter of a mile away and some sixty feet tall. He could see nothing. His gaze swept around. They were still on the plateau, although its undulations would have made it easy for them to have been followed and then overtaken. There was no sign of any other living thing.

Softly, he called Jenkins to him. 'Mzingeli tells me that we are being followed by natives who are armed,' he said. 'They have been observing us from that kopje up ahead – no, don't look! I am surprised, because I thought that if we were going to be attacked it would be when we were in the bush. But these people obviously didn't want us too near the security of the border, in case we made a break for it.'

'Is it that Portuguese swine, bach sir?'

'I can't think of anyone else who might want us dead. De Sousa must have learned of our mission to meet Rhodes and wants to stop us. The Matabele wouldn't attack the king's friends – and particularly his doctor.' He gave a grin to show a confidence that he did not feel. 'Now, the trail takes us quite close to the kopje. It is my feeling that they will attack us from its cover. So we will not give them that chance. I don't want them to know that they have been seen, so we will gently change course to take us away from the kopje, and then they will have to break cover to attack.'

'Do they have horses?' he asked the tracker.

'Not seen any, Nkosi.'

'Good. Tell Sando to climb into the wagon with Ntini. Alice, into the wagon too, please, with your rifle ready.'

Alice opened her mouth to protest, but he held up his hand. 'Only one general here today, my love,' he said. 'You must obey his orders. Hitch your horse to the side of the wagon away from the kopje, so that it is protected. Mzingeli, stay leading us from the front on foot but drop back a little, and as soon as the attack comes, get into the wagon quickly and fire from there.'

Jenkins frowned. 'What do we do then, bach sir?'

'We will act as a sort of cavalry screen. Drop back a little on the kopje side and I will do the same. They will have to run across open ground to get anywhere near us – I am gambling that they don't have horses and that's why they wanted to attack from the kopje. As soon as they leave cover, we charge at them, halt, fire two rounds and then gallop back to the wagon. We throw our reins to Ntini and then we climb aboard the wagon and fire from there. It will be our fortress.'

'Humph.' The Welshman's eyes lit up. 'You will probably fall off.'

'If I do, you will just have to pick me up.'

The tracker's face carried a faint smile as he tried to follow the exchange, but Alice's features were grim. 'Surely it is best to stay in the wagon, Simon? Make it a fortress, as you say.'

'No, my love. We can break them up at short range as they run towards us. Kaffirs can't shoot well and they certainly won't be able to do so on the run. They may not even have guns. No. We will do as I say. Make sure that your rifles are loaded, but do so surreptitiously. I don't want them to know that we are on to their game.'

He swallowed hard. His brain worked smoothly in assessing the situation, as that of a soldier should, but he knew that they were outnumbered and in great danger. No one in the little party betrayed open fear, not even the native boys, but he could see that faces were drawn and chins set determinedly. Everyone realised that they would need calm nerves and straight shooting – or perhaps a miracle – to survive the coming attack.

They mounted and set off again. This time Mzingeli led them slightly off to the right. Leaving the track was no hardship, for it was only faintly defined and the grassland was dry and the going firm. Fonthill put a handful of cartridges from their ammunition box into both his pockets, and he and Jenkins drifted out to the left. He tried not to eye the kopje too suspiciously, but he caught a flash of light as the sun reflected off . . . what? It wouldn't be an assegai head, for the natives this far north had blades of beaten black iron. A rifle barrel? Possibly.

They had drawn level with the kopje, although not far enough away from it to satisfy Fonthill, when the first shot rang out. It came from the base of the rock and was the signal for a stream of spearmen to emerge at a fast trot and fan out and run towards them. Simon was reminded briefly of that terrifying moment at Isandlwana when the Zulu impis had poured down from the escarpment and spread out to surround the British camp. Except that this time there were fewer attackers – but even fewer defenders.

He saw Mzingeli and Sando climb into the wagon. He nodded to Jenkins, and the two of them galloped towards the natives. Good, they were not carrying rifles! The charging men were dressed exactly like Matabeles – monkey-tail adornments, ostrich feathers and little else – and carrying, in their left hands, the long hide shields behind which, in Zulu style, would be clutched a handful of throwing spears, and in their right, the short, stabbing assegais. They looked formidable enough and seemed completely unfazed by the approaching horsemen.

Fonthill reined in, steadied his horse and raised his rifle at a range of about two hundred yards. Jenkins, however, was even quicker, and his shot brought down the leading native. Simon's own missed. Cursing, he rammed another round into the breech and took careful aim, this time spinning round the third man in the line and bringing him down. Jenkins's next shot tore through the shield of the second man, whirling it away and causing the native to stumble. Then a puff of smoke came from the base of the kopje and a bullet whistled between the two horsemen. As the smoke began to clear, Simon saw a small figure in yellow behind it.

'Back to the wagon,' yelled Fonthill, pulling round the head of his horse.

They galloped back, wheeling around to the far side of the vehicle, where Alice's horse was already tied, and, throwing their reins to Ntini, scrambled aboard. Alice and Mzingeli had now lowered the white canvas canopy and were kneeling, their rifles levelled across the wooden side pieces of the wagon.

'Don't waste ammunition,' cried Fonthill. 'They will circle around us until we are surrounded and then run in. That's when we will need every bullet. We shall have to reload very quickly. I don't think they have realised yet that we have two Martini-Henrys. Old Gouela must have gambled that we only had light hunting rifles. But keep your heads down – he has a rifle himself and is taking shots from the kopje, although I think he's too far away to be effective.'

The natives now formed a loose ring around the wagon and stood for a moment, raising their spears and chanting.

'They not Matabele, not Zulus,' grunted Mzingeli.

'I don't care who they are, bach,' answered Jenkins grimly. 'I've just counted twenty-five of 'em left, an' if we let 'em close enough to come aboard, I'd say we're done for.'

'They're out of range of anything but the Martinis,' said Simon. 'See if you can pick off a couple before they charge, 352, and I'll do the same. When they come in, you fire over to the right, Alice. Jenkins, you go over the oxen to the front – it's the most difficult shot. Mzingeli, you take the rear and I will fire to the left.' He nodded to the tracker. 'Tell the boys to stand ready to fight with their spears if anybody gets through.'

The last was a superfluous remark, because Ntini and Sando were crouching by the wagon side boards, their spears at the ready. Their faces, however, showed the fear they felt. But that seemed to disappear when Mzingeli spoke quickly to them.

Fonthill raised an enquiring eyebrow. 'I tell them that these just Hottentots from the east, not Matabele,' grunted the tracker. 'Make them feel better. They afraid of Matabele.'

Further discussion was halted by the crack of Jenkins's rifle. Immediately, one of the natives crumpled. 'Good,' said the Welshman, reloading. 'Just in range.' He shuffled on to the driver's seat and sighted again. ''Ere. 'Ave another one, lads.' A second man in the ring staggered and fell, clutching his shoulder.

Fonthill now fired, and a spurt of dust sprang from just

ahead of his target. 'Elevate, elevate, for goodness' sake,' cried Jenkins.

'Sorry, Sergeant,' murmured Simon. He adjusted his sights and fired again, this time hitting his man. This seemed to be the signal for the attack, for the rest raised their spears, stamped their feet and then began running for the wagon.

'Hold fire until I give the order,' cried Fonthill, then, in a lower voice to his wife, 'You all right, my love?'

Alice was nestling her cheek against the butt of her Westley Richards. She replied without looking up, 'I'm all right. Good luck, Simon.'

'Fire!'

The four guns spoke as one, and three of the attackers fell. Jenkins, closely followed by Fonthill, was the first to reload, and their second bullets also found their marks. Simon realised that Alice, firing from the right, was either out-ranged or her accuracy was wanting, so he added his firing to hers, but he could not leave his flank completely unprotected and it was difficult to switch position and fire accurately. Nevertheless, it was the Martini-Henrys, of course, that had the greatest firepower, and the warriors seemed to sense this, for they veered away from the guns of Jenkins and Fonthill and ran towards the weaker sides, those manned by Alice and Mzingeli.

It became clear to Fonthill that these 'Hottentots from the east', whoever they were, seemed to possess the courage and warlike skills of both the Zulus and the Matabele, and he took up his position at his wife's side, firing as fast as he could inject the single cartridges and jerk down the cocking lever behind the trigger guard. The bravest and fastest of the attackers had now reached within range of the wagon to launch their throwing spears, and one buried itself into the breast of the already injured Sando, who sank to the floorboards, feebly clutching at the assegai. Ntini plucked it out and threw it back, all in one movement.

'Nkosi!' The cry came from Mzingeli, whose slow-loading Snider was now being used as a club as he tried to fight off two natives who were stabbing at his feet and trying to climb into the rear of the wagon. Fonthill shot one and then stabbed the muzzle of his rifle into the face of the other, pushing him to the ground, where the thrown spear of Ntini penetrated his breast.

'Behind you, bach.' Simon whirled and saw a tribesman climb over the side of the wagon behind Alice, who was now kneeling to tend to the prostrate figure of Sando. He swung the stock of his rifle towards the man's chin, but this one was made of sterner stuff. He bowed his head to take the butt of the gun on his tightly curled hair, shook his head as though to get rid of a fly and then gave a short-arm stab in reply. The blade grazed Fonthill's thigh and its point stuck for a moment in the side of the wagon, giving a slight advantage to Simon, who brought the barrel of the gun strongly down on his adversary's neck. The crack could be heard above the firing and the screams of the attackers, and the man slumped to the floor of the wagon.

'They're goin'! They've 'ad enough.' Jenkins's cry came from the driver's seat, where he was standing, waving his rifle.

Fonthill wiped the sweat from his eyes and looked around. It was true. The remnants of the attacking force – now reduced to a dozen men – were running back towards the kopje, one of them limping. Behind them, in a ring surrounding the wagon and stretching back towards the kopje, lay the inert figures of those who had fallen.

'Alice, are you all right?' whispered Simon as he knelt by her side, putting his arm across her shoulder.

'Yes thank you,' she replied. 'But I am afraid Sando is not. I think he has gone. Oh Simon . . .' and she turned and buried her face in his chest, her shoulders shaking in sudden reaction. He swayed with her, gently patting her back and kissing her hair. Then the soldier in him reasserted itself. 'Any more casualties?' he called.

'No, sir,' said Jenkins. 'All present and accounted for. I can't understand why they didn't spear the oxen or the horses. Why d'you think that was?'

'They too valuable.' Mzingeli was now squatting on the floor of the wagon, wiping his brow with the tail of his shirt. 'Take them back to Mozambique and sell them. Make money.' He looked sadly at Sando and shook his head. 'He good boy. Bad thing, this.'

Simon felt suddenly shamefaced. Still holding Alice, he said, 'I am so sorry, Mzingeli. This was not your fight. I don't know . . . I am so sorry.'

The tracker looked up. 'Ah, it was our fight. If we don't kill them, they kill us. But why this man attack us?'

'It's a long story. Here.' Tenderly Simon put Alice away from him. 'Are you all right now, my love?'

She nodded.

'Good. Jenkins?'

'Sir.'

'You stay here just in case there is another attack, although I don't think for a moment there will be. They have clearly had enough.'

'Where are you goin' then?'

'Yes, Simon.' Alice's eyes were wide. 'Where *are* you going?'

'Mzingeli, break out our two horses and come with me. I may need your tracking skills. I am not going to let that Portuguese bastard get away with this. If I catch him, I will bring him back here and we will hang him. A bullet's too good for him.'

'I'll come with you, bach sir.'

'No. Do as you are told. Stay here.'

Fonthill dipped into the ammunition box, filled his pockets with cartridges once more, scrambled over the side of the wagon and mounted his horse. Waiting only for Mzingeli to join him, he set off at a gallop for the kopje. The remaining tribesmen had long since disappeared, but he paid no heed, setting his horse towards the side of the rock opposite to that from which the attack had been launched, in the hope that he could cut off the Portuguese if he was retreating.

They found nothing except a few empty cartridge cases at the base of the rock on the other side of the kopje.

Fonthill grunted. 'The man's a coward as well as a murderous swine. He set his men to attack but wouldn't join them. Now, which way have they gone?'

The tracker pointed to the north. Together they galloped to a rise and then stood in their stirrups peering ahead. The retreating group could clearly be seen, the warriors on foot gathered around a solitary horseman, who was setting a fast pace.

Mzingeli shook his head. 'I think, Nkosi, we do not follow. Still too many for us two. Kill him another day.'

Fonthill shot a sharp glance at the tracker. Then he relaxed. 'I suppose you are right. I think they have had a lesson and will not attack again. Anyway,' he shook his head, 'we should not leave the wagon. Even if he gets reinforcements from Bulawayo, I doubt if he can overtake us before we reach the border. And he would not dare to follow us into the Transvaal.'

He looked to where the trail wound around the kopje. 'Mzingeli,' he said, 'we all owe you a debt. If you had not seen them on the kopje we would have been unprepared and they would have swung round here and overwhelmed us before we could bring our guns to bear. It was quite a clever ambush, actually. Thank you.'

He held out his hand and the tracker shook it, a little self-consciously.

'Why this man hate you?' he asked.

'He thinks I am in the pay of Rhodes, in the Cape, and that I will stop him from signing a treaty with Lobengula to overturn the agreement the king has already made with Rhodes. Well. . .' he shifted in the saddle and looked again for the retreating figures, now almost out of sight, 'that's exactly what I now intend to do. After his two attacks on us, I intend to stop that man being involved in the development of Matabeleland. Come on. Let's go back.'

Back at the wagon – to Alice's great relief – Fonthill allowed his wife to fix a dressing on his grazed thigh,and he then joined the others in digging one shallow grave, into which they tipped the bodies of the attackers. Mzingeli gathered up all their assegais and looked at them carefully.

'They dress like Matabele,' he said, 'but they come from Mozambique border. Look.' He pointed at the spear heads. 'These from Portuguese land. They want us to think them Matabele. Strange.' Then he shrugged his shoulders. 'But they just as dead.'

Tenderly Sando's body was wrapped in a blanket and placed in the back of the wagon. 'Where does he come from, Mzingeli?' asked Alice.

'My father's village. My village. I know his mother, father. Sad.'

It was indeed a sad little group that set off to the south, Ntini cracking his long whip over his oxen and the three other men ranging out on horseback to the rear, right and left to ensure against another surprise attack. They camped that night without incident, and continued for another two and a half days along a track that had become a miserable mixture of rough stones and deep spruits with precipitous banks until eventually they entered Mzingeli's village. At first they were greeted with happy cries, for the carcasses of the lions had been found, of course, and their killings confirmed by the Matabele who had arrived from Bulawayo to collect the horses, wagon and oxen. Then, however, as Sando's body was lowered to the ground, a wailing began, soft at first and then growing in grief and intensity.

The party spent only two nights in the village, for Fonthill felt uncomfortable there: guilty, of course, for being responsible for Sando's death, however indirectly, and frustrated that he could not explain it to anyone's satisfaction, least of all his own. He was glad then when they said a muted goodbye to the *inDuna* and made for the river crossing into the Transvaal. Once across, the open veldt helped to restore a touch of tranquillity to them all, and they made good progress under the snowy-white balls of cloud that chased each other across the sky.

'What now, then?' asked Alice, as she rode companionably with her husband, Jenkins following alongside Mzingeli and Ntini at the rear.

Fonthill eased his buttocks in the saddle. 'Back to Cape Town, I think. I should pay my respects to Lamb.' Major General George Lamb, CB, the recently appointed army commander-in-chief at the Cape, had been the man who, as a colonel and chief of staff in Cape Town, had sent Simon on his first mission, to the camp of the Zulu king, ten years ago. He had then become his mentor in the second Afghan War on the North-West Frontier. Lamb had been away, up country in Natal, when Simon had called on their arrival in the colony.

Alice nodded. 'Of course. But then what do we do?'

'I must see Rhodes.'

'Do you have to? He's a strange character, as you know. He can ensnare people.'

'Oh come along, Alice. I'm no bloody rabbit.'

'I know that, darling. But, well . . .'

'I gave my word to Lobengula. Besides which,' he frowned and screwed up his eyes to focus on a distant kopje, 'I have a debt to settle. I want to do everything I can to make sure that the Portuguese and that blasted man de Sousa do not talk the king into giving them his country.' He turned in the saddle and looked directly at his wife. 'You know, Alice, once Matabeleland is settled, I wouldn't mind at all buying a tract of land there, up in the north, perhaps, where they say the country is magnificent for farming.'

Alice remained silent, so Fonthill hurried on.

'We would keep Norfolk, of course, but that almost farms itself these days. It would be good to come out here in our winter, get some sun, sport and so on. We could well afford it, you know . . .' His voice trailed away as Alice's frown deepened, and then it became more plaintive. 'It would, well, make life more interesting, don't you think?'

She gave him a quick, rather forced smile. 'If that's what you want, then of course.' Slowly the smile faded. 'But I can see a lot more trouble developing before Lobengula gives away his land to us, the Portuguese or anyone else for that matter. He's no fool, you know.'

'That's true. But Rhodes does have an agreement with him, so that must be a head start. Anyway, it will be interesting to see what Lamb says about it all. He's no fool either.'

The five of them rode on in silence, some thinking of the sadness left behind in the village; others steeling themselves for the challenge that lay ahead.

Chapter 5

A little over three weeks later, Simon found himself waiting in a small anteroom outside the impressive office of Major General Lamb in Cape Town. He and Alice had dropped off Mzingeli and Ntini at their huts in the Boer farm in the southern Transvaal where they had first employed them. The parting had been unemotional, as befitted the bearing of the dignified tracker, but Mzingeli had gripped Fonthill's hand and said in farewell, 'You call, whenever. I come.'

The door into the inner office was suddenly thrown open and Lamb exploded through it. Fonthill grinned and stood. Nothing had changed. Energy seemed to fizz and spark from the general's every movement, and now he bounced rather than walked towards Simon, his hand outstretched.

'Damned glad to see you, Fonthill. Knew you would call. Sorry to have missed you last time. How are you? Tell me, how are you?'

'Fit as a fiddler's fox, thank you, General. And you?'

'Couldn't be better. Come through. Sorry to have kept you waiting.' Then, over his shoulder, 'How's old 473?'

'Three five two, sir.'

'Dammit. Never could remember his number. Sit down. Sit down. Cigar?'

Fonthill regarded Lamb with interest. The general was diminutive – hardly more than five feet two inches – and his complexion, a ruddy nut brown, gave testimony to his years spent in India. They had last met outside the gates of Kandahar, after General Roberts's comprehensive victory over the Afghan army. Simon and Jenkins had played a not insignificant part in that victory but Fonthill's refusal to rejoin the army at Roberts's request had soured his relationship with the general. Lamb, then a brigadier, had tried to be ameliorative, but Simon had left the Frontier under a cloud. His relationship with Lamb, however, had remained one of mutual admiration.

The general walked from behind his desk to light Simon's cigar. 'Delighted to see you awarded a CB after the Sudan. Joined the club, eh?' Fonthill nodded behind the cloud of blue smoke. 'My God, for a young chap you've moved around since we last met – Sekukuniland, that terrible Majuba business, then Egypt and the Sudan.' The general's bright blue eyes twinkled. 'For a feller who didn't want to rejoin the army, you've done a fair bit of soldiering, I'd say.'

Fonthill shifted uneasily. 'On my own terms, though, sir. But I should congratulate you on your promotion and appointment here.'

Lamb puffed at his cigar and shrugged. 'Not bad for an old India hand, I suppose. Lucky to get it under Wolseley, I have to confess.'

Simon grinned. The rivalry between the two best generals in Queen Victoria's army, Roberts and Wolseley, was well known. Lamb had always been a Roberts man, which meant that with Wolseley at the Horse Guards in London as adjutant general, he should have been doomed to spend the rest of his career in India, where Roberts was commander-in-chief. Somehow he had slipped through the net.

'Now.' Lamb leaned across his desk. 'You've been in Lobengula's kraal, I hear.'

Fonthill lifted his eyebrows. 'How did you know that? We only returned yesterday.'

'It's my business to know these things. Seen Rhodes yet?'

'How did you know I was going to see him?'

'I didn't, but I know that he wants to see you.'

'Why should he want to see me?'

Lamb pushed his chair back and let a spiral of blue smoke curl towards the ceiling. 'Several reasons. Firstly, you have become almost famous, my dear fellow, with your exploits in various parts of the Empire, and Rhodes would admire that. He is, as you must know, first and foremost an Empire man.'

'Yes, I do know that. I met him in Kimberley some years ago.'

'Did you now? Secondly, Rhodes is always trying to recruit bright young men into his own empire – and my word, that empire has become almost as large as the Queen's. He owns all the diamond mines in Kimberley now, of course, and most of the gold strands too.'

'So I understand.'

'But the third reason is the most important. I think he has a job for you.'

'For me? Well, I'm not at all sure that I would want to work for him, thank you very much.'

'Ah!' Lamb let the silence hang after the word for at least twenty seconds. Then he waved his cigar and looked up at the ceiling. 'But my dear Fonthill, both Wolseley in London and I here rather hoped that you would, you see.'

'What, work for Rhodes? Why should you want that?'

'Well, here's the background.' The general let his chair crash to the floor. 'You know that Rhodes believes he has done a deal with the King of the Matabele . . . what's his name again?'

'Lobengula.'

'Yes, that's the feller. Rhodes's agreement gives him permission to dig for mineral rights in Matabeleland and Mashonaland. Now, young Cecil John – dammit, the man can't be much older than you – would certainly want to pick out all the gold and silver that those two territories have, but he is really after settlement. He wants to open up the route to the north, beyond Mashonaland, and the best way to do that, he knows, is to settle the land. Let pioneers in. Of British stock, of course.'

'But that's not part of the contract with Lobengula, is it?'

'It certainly isn't, and from what I hear of the king up there, the old blighter would never agree to it.'

'Yes.' Fonthill put his hand to his mouth pensively. 'In fact, Rhodes is in some danger of losing the contract he has anyway.'

'What? Why is that?'

Fonthill proceeded to explain the mission he had been given by the king, and also the presence in Bulawayo of de Sousa and his own brushes with the Portuguese agent. 'I gather,' he went on, 'that the Germans, the Boers and other, independent British companies are all sniffing around the king's kraal, trying to persuade him to drop Rhodes and let them in. Bit of a mess really. But what's the British government's view of all this?'

Lamb smiled. 'Where Her Majesty's Government is involved, my dear boy, nothing is straightforward, but I will try and explain. The Government does not wish to venture into any further expensive acquisition of territory in Africa. It has enough on its plate as it is down here and with the

Russians across the border on India's North-West Frontier. It certainly would not wish to become involved in another war with the natives – another Zululand, if you like.'

'Would it try and stop Rhodes, then?'

'On the contrary. Despite what I have just said, the idea of settling the country north of the Transvaal – *at no cost to the Government* . . .' Lamb emphasised the phrase heavily, 'is quite attractive, because it could open up the north and even facilitate Rhodes's dream of a transcontinental railway from Cairo to the Cape, which, again, HMG would rather fancy if someone else pays for it and it doesn't involve another bloody great war. You talked about the hangers-on in Bulawayo. We would rather have the king locked into a firm and legal agreement with Rhodes than with anyone else.'

Fonthill wrinkled his brow. 'So what is the problem, then?'

'Ah. It is the character of young Rhodes, d'yer see? He is damned impulsive and even more damned ambitious. His riches give him great resources, and the Government and Wolseley – the AG because the army will almost certainly become involved if Rhodes gets into trouble – are worried that the bloody man will use force if necessary to take Matabeleland and Mashonaland. All those wet knickers on the Opposition bench in Westminster will raise hell if he invades the territory willy-nilly and causes Lobengula to unleash his army and let his men wash their spears. It could be another Isandlwana all over again – and we've only just got over paying for that lot.'

'I see. Well, I think I see. But what I don't see is how I fit into all of this.'

Lamb stubbed out his cigar, as though he was trying to push it through the bottom of the ash tray. 'Wolseley knows you well and he has huge respect for your capabilities. I had picked up the rumour that Rhodes wants you on his team, and reported this to the AG. As a result, Wolseley has asked me to beg you to accept whatever Rhodes is about to offer you – if this can possibly be made to work into whatever your own plans are down here – and see if you can exert a calming influence on the man. Don't let him antagonise Lobengula. You know the king and Rhodes does not. You will have influence as a result of this if nothing else.'

A silence hung heavily in the smoke-filled room. Fonthill shifted on his chair. 'Well, I don't exactly know what I—'

The general interrupted him. 'I don't mind admitting it's an appeal to your patriotic sensibilities, Fonthill. Look,' he leaned forward across his desk, 'this country – and I don't just mean the Cape Colony – is on the verge of something rather extraordinary. Our colonies here are going to become some of the most influential in the whole of the Empire. Dominion status is just around the corner. We are rich in mineral, agricultural and labour resources, and as these are developed, we shall be able to provide leadership for and set an example to these cock-eyed little states that the great powers of Europe have set up in the middle of the continent.' The blue eyes twinkled and then hardened. 'We don't want Rhodes going over the top, upsetting the apple cart and raising Europe against us.'

Simon opened his mouth to speak, but Lamb raised his hand. 'Rhodes loves to have able and promising young men around him, and we know that he listens to them, more, much more than to old warhorses like me, or, for that matter, to anyone in Whitehall – whom he calls, derisively, "the Imperials". You, with your comparative youth and your magnificent record in various parts of the Empire, will be just the sort of fellow that Rhodes will take notice of – not least because you have never toed the party line, so to speak, in imperial circles. You have always been your own man. Rhodes will like that.'

'I am not sure that doing what you and Wolseley ask is exactly being my own man, but . . .' Fonthill thought for a moment. 'Have you any idea what Rhodes wants of me?'

'No. I heard in the club that he had been singing your praises and that he had heard of your return to Cape Town. Knowing his interest in Matabeleland, I cannot see him not wanting to contact you.'

'Hmmm. From what I have read of Rhodes, and from what I remember of my meeting with him, I can't see him being nursemaided by anyone.'

Lamb rose to his feet, a touch of exasperation in the action. 'Of course you can't be his nursemaid. But if you feel that he is being impatient, for instance – and this is his abiding failing – then you can counsel caution. I rather fear that the fellows he has round him at the moment are caught under his spell and have become a bit sycophantic. He will respect someone who stands up to him. But you must judge for yourself how to act. Just stop the blasted man from charging in with guns blazing, if you possibly can. We can't exactly offer you a salary, by the way.'

'I don't want money.'

'Good. In any case, Rhodes has the reputation of rewarding his people well. Often in kind – land, for instance, in the new territory.'

Fonthill raised his head. 'Land?'

'Yes. Could you be interested? This is fine country.'

'Ah. I don't know. I must consult Alice, my wife.'

'Dammit! I knew there was something I had forgotten.' The little man extended his hand to Simon. 'You married that remarkable lady Alice Griffith. Congratulations, my dear fellow. Belated, I know, but sincere none the less.'

Fonthill stood and the two shook hands. 'Thank you very much, sir.'

'Yes, well, of course you must consult your wife. Call me if you need anything while you are here. I am completely at your service. But let me know what you decide as soon as you can. I have a feeling that Rhodes is very much on the march, so time could be of the essence.'

'Thank you. I certainly will.'

Fonthill chose to walk back to their hotel, his brain working hard. What could Rhodes want with him? He was intrigued, despite his cautious reaction to Lamb. The chance to work with a man who within a decade had risen from comparatively humble beginnings as a sugar farmer in Natal to become the most influential figure in the whole of South Africa and, if rumours were to be believed, the next prime minister of the Cape Colony was intriguing, to say the least. It would be a new experience after four years of farming under the grey skies of Norfolk. And if it carried with it the possibility of acquiring new land of his own in this vibrant new colony – ah, now *that* could be of distinct interest!

Treading with a jaunty new step, Fonthill realised how much he was relishing this visit to South Africa. The business in Matabeleland had been disturbing, to say the least, but also exciting. It was good to be in action again after the sad, fallow years since the death of his son. Good to be here with Jenkins, too, reviving that unique comradeship that had been forged in danger and tempered under attack from so many different enemies. A gentle smile crept across his face as he reflected that even Alice, whom he loved more than life itself and whom he would never consciously put in harm's way, had subtly changed when the time had come to defend the wagon. He recalled her calmness in firing at the lion as it charged and the cool determination with which she had reloaded her rifle at speed and kept firing at the Portuguese Kaffirs. He gave a little shrug. Perhaps not so strange, though. She was a soldier's daughter, after all. But this country, with its wild, indigenous people, its wide vistas and its changeable, challenging climate, could well suit her.

He looked around him at the bustling streets. Cape Town was just his sort of place. In some ways it reminded him of Bombay: so many faces, so many characters and so many colours. The dark skin of the locals, with their bare feet and scraps of clothing; the scurrying Indians, wearing turbans and a determined air, as though anxious to get back to their stalls to make another couple of shillings; the patrician white men, aloof under their pith helmets – quite unnecessary headgear here, where the breeze from the Atlantic cooled the heat of the sun, and worn more as a sign of class; the mixed bag of sailors from the docks; and the black-bearded Boer Dutchmen from the high veldt, striding along on legs bowed by years in the saddle and looking as though they had just strayed from the pages of the Bible. Yes, this was a vibrant port, a city of empire and, undoubtedly, the gateway to a land of promise.

Alice was standing by the reception desk in the modest hotel into which they had booked. 'Ah, my dear,' she said. 'I am so glad you have come.' Her face was clouded.

'What is the matter?'

'Well . . .' Her voice trailed away. 'It's 352. I asked him if he would go to the post office to see if we had mail. It is only ten minutes away and he went off quite happily, but he has been gone about three hours now. I called at the post office to see if he was there, but he was not. I picked up several letters. It looks as though Jenkins has not been there at all.'

Fonthill sighed. 'Oh dammit all. He's gone drinking.'

'Yes. That's what I thought.'

Fonthill kicked himself for not realising that the Welshman would be building up for a thirst-quenching run ashore as soon as they had booked into their hotel. The problem was that one or two drinks would not be sufficient to wash away the dust in Jenkins's throat. Once the familiar taste and tingle had entered his system, he would continue until he was completely drunk – or left for dead in an alley with a knife in his back.

Simon turned to the Indian receptionist. 'Where would I go if I wanted to drink myself senseless?' he asked.

The man's jaw dropped. 'You would not wish to do that, sir, surely?'

'Yes, I would. I want a street with rough bars in it.'

'Ah, goodness. Well. Let me think. The docks, I think, sir. Turn left at the door here and walk—'

'Yes, thank you. I will find them. Alice, you stay here. I might be some time.'

His wife opened her mouth to argue, but Fonthill was gone before she could do so, whirling on his heel and heading towards the clouds of black dust billowing into the air from where several freighters were re-coaling. Between the black columns he caught a glimpse of the blue Atlantic.

The harbour, when he reached it, seemed vast and he realised that his search would be more difficult than envisioned. The first bars he met seemed comparatively respectable, with white traders in creased cotton suits, merchant navy officers, their peaked caps tipped to the back of their heads, and port officials drinking whisky. Jenkins would not feel at home here. He would want beer and the company of off-duty soldiers and sailors.

Eventually Fonthill reached a narrow street off one of the quays where every second doorway seemed to be the entrance to a bar. He turned into the first, where the atmosphere reeked of tobacco smoke, beer and cheap gin. It was crowded but there was no sign of the familiar black moustache and stubbled hair. In the second, he approached two British soldiers of a line regiment and, describing Jenkins, asked if they had seen him.

'Yes, mate. It was 'im all right. Drank about three pints, bought us one and then said that'e was on 'is way to the post office. Welsh bloke, old 24th, wasn't 'e?'

Fonthill nodded his thanks and continued his way up the alley. He doubted if the post office would have seen Jenkins that day, although he had certainly left his mark in six bars, where he was warmly remembered by the clientele. Simon gritted his teeth and continued the search. He knew the pattern. Jenkins would be affable to begin with, and then, on the slightest provocation, the Mr Hyde in his nature would surface, fuelled by the pints he had put away, until he would become argumentative, truculent and then violent – and violence in this quarter almost certainly meant the use of knives.

Leaving the seventh bar, he paused. This was proving pointless. The man could be anywhere in this thriving but seedy port. Perhaps he really had put down the last glass and made for the post office. Then he heard a crash and shouting from an open door under a swinging inn sign. He ran to it and turned inside.

If Landseer had painted the scene, he might have entitled it *Jenkins At Bay*. The Welshman, his shirt torn and perspiration pouring down his face, was holding a broken, jagged-ended pint glass and backing away to a corner of the bar. Facing him and moving irrevocably towards him were two large men in dungaree trousers and vests. Both were coal-stained, and under the black smudges it appeared that one was white and the other coloured, perhaps a Lascar. It was clear that they were stokers from the coaling freighters, and it was also clear that they were intent on causing serious harm to Jenkins, for they both had knives in their hands. Around the sides of the bar pressed a bedraggled crowd of onlookers, loose grins on their faces in anticipation of seeing blood shed. Two smashed tables were strewn on the sawdust floor, and beside them lay a third stoker, blood streaming from his nose and a cut above his eye. He appeared to be unconscious.

'That's enough!' Fonthill's voice cut through the anticipatory buzz and he strode forward. 'The police will be here in a minute. Give me those knives.'

'Ah, good to see you, bach.' Jenkins nodded in greeting. His eyes were rheumy but alert. 'Now don't you worry about this,' he said. 'You don't need to get involved, see. I can' andle these gentlemen all right on me own, thank you very much.'

'Don't be ridiculous. Put down that glass. You men, give me your knives before someone gets hurt.'

At first his strong, upper-class voice and his air of command made the two men pause, glaring over their shoulders at him. Then the white stoker spoke, slowly and with a strong Scandinavian accent. 'Stay avay, out of dis. We cut oop this man. We cut oop you as vell if you interfere.' He gestured with his knife.

Jenkins, with the experience of a dozen or more barroom fights behind him, sensed that this was his moment. Taking advantage of the Swede's confrontation with this unexpected stranger, he leapt forward and smashed the bottom of his pint glass on to the man's head, then, swaying to his right, swept a left hook into his stomach. In doing so, however, he left his back unprotected, and the Lascar swung back his arm to bury his knife into it.

Instinctively, Fonthill launched himself into a low rugby tackle and caught the Lascar behind the knees, crumpling him so that the man collapsed on top and then away from him, his knife spinning into the crowd. For a moment the two lay winded on the floor, and Simon felt the taste of sawdust in his mouth. Then he threw himself on to the Lascar's back, fighting to thread his arms beneath the man's shoulders to lock him into a half-nelson, dimly remembered from his wrestling days in the school gym. But the stoker was a quarter as big again as Fonthill, and with one convulsive heave he threw him off his back, as though he was tipping a sack of coal into the hold of his ship.

Simon cracked his face on the planking of the floor, sniffing the sawdust again and landing at the feet of the onlookers. Immediately many hands raised him, and with a cheer, he was pushed back to meet the giant Lascar, who advanced on him now, both hands outstretched, seemingly to embrace and then crush him. Involuntarily, Fonthill grabbed the shirt of the man in the crowd nearest to him, whirled him round and sent him crashing into his opponent. The stoker was huge but he was also ponderous, and clutching the onlooker to him, he fell backwards. Simon leapt forward and kicked his boot into the stoker's face. It seemed to have little effect, however, for the man merely shook his head and rose to his feet.

Fonthill advanced and put three successive jabs with his left hand into the face of the Lascar. Cheers rose from the crowd, but he might have been hitting the wall for all the damage he caused the big man; he was merely a mosquito stinging an elephant. The stoker lumbered forward, his arms outstretched once more, and Fonthill ducked under the attempted embrace and hit the man as hard as he could in the stomach. The wheeze that the blow produced showed that the man was not as invulnerable as he seemed, and Simon danced in again to repeat the blow, but the bloodstained sawdust was no place for fancy footwork and, inevitably, he slipped. Immediately his hair was seized and he was locked into a bear hug, his nose pressed to the dirty grey vest. His senses became overwhelmed by the smell of stale beer, perspiration, cold dust and then fear, as his chin was pushed back by the palm of the Lascar's right hand, while the left arm held him tight and exerted pressure on his vertebrae. The bastard was trying to break his neck!

Fonthill knew that it would be only a matter of seconds before the giant would relax his grip on his chin and then jerk it up and under, so snapping his neck. In desperation, he wriggled his left arm down the Lascar's abdomen until he felt the softness of the man's testicles. His fingers sank in, then, with almost his last breath, he squeezed and pulled. The big man shrieked and relaxed his hold, allowing Simon to slip out of his grasp.

Sucking air into his lungs, Fonthill staggered away, gasping and holding his throat, as the Lascar doubled up in pain. He was dimly aware that one section of the crowd was screaming 'Unfair!' while the other was whistling and cheering. But they had not yet seen enough blood spilt, for someone threw back the Lascar's dagger, which the coloured man caught in one giant fist before advancing on Fonthill again.

''Ere, mate,' another shouted. 'Let's make it a fair fight.' And a second knife curved through the air and quivered in the floor at Simon's feet.

He picked it up. It was a knife fight now. He dared not spare a moment to see how Jenkins was faring, but it seemed clear that he would have to see this through on his own. Kill or be killed.

Fonthill realised that he was completely outranged by the Lascar's reach and that his only hope would be to use his greater mobility. The big man was holding the knife blade down, as a dagger. That meant that he would have to bring it upwards before slashing down – perhaps there would be a fleeting moment of opportunity there, if Simon could get close enough to thrust himself. His brain raced. Close enough, yes, but how to get in under the man's guard?

Then he remembered a technique he had seen Jenkins use many years before when the Welshman had been confronted by a giant Zulu. Simon took two quick steps forward and then pretended to slip, going down almost on one knee, except that the bent leg remained balanced on the ball of his foot. His left hand went to the floor, and as the Lascar stepped forward and raised his knife, he picked up a handful of sawdust and threw it in the coloured man's face, causing him to blink and turn his head away for a second. Almost in the same movement, Fonthill brought his own knife hand upwards and thrust the blade into the other man's forearm, twisting it and pulling it away as the blood spurted.

The giant howled, dropped his own knife and grabbed his arm, sinking to one knee. At almost the same moment, Simon glimpsed the bloodstained face of Jenkins materialise behind that of the Lascar, as he lifted a chair leg and brought it down with a thud on the man's head. For a moment the big man teetered, and then, like a forest giant felled by a woodman's axe, he toppled to the floor and lay still.

'Blimey,' said Jenkins, 'why did you choose the big one?

You could 'ave 'ad my bloke, though come to think of it, 'e wasn't so small either. Eh, you all right, bach sir?' He threw away the chair leg and, frowning, inspected Fonthill. 'Blimey, your nose is bleedin' a bit . . .'

His voice tailed away as he saw the look of fury in Simon's eyes. 'Yes, well, sorry, bach sir.' His manner now was abjectly apologetic, and he fumbled to put a very grimy handkerchief to Fonthill's nose. 'I only slipped away for a minute, see, to 'ave one or two 'alves. Sorry if you've been . . . er . . . inconvenienced like.'

'Inconvenienced!' Fonthill staggered to his feet and looked around. There were three stokers on the barroom floor, two of them now stirring and the third, the Swede, sitting and holding his head. 'You've broken up a bar, nearly killed three men, as far as I can see, and almost caused me to have my neck broken. And you call it *inconvenience*!'

'Ah well, yes, I can see what you—'

The Welshman was interrupted by a very large barman, who advanced on them carrying what seemed to be a Zulu knobkerrie. 'Now, man,' he addressed Jenkins in the guttural tones of an Afrikaner, 'I want paying for two broken tables and three chairs. And you're not going till I get my money.'

A look of intense indignation alighted on Jenkins's sweat-stained face. 'Hey, bach, I didn't start it, look you. It's these three bastards you should get to put their 'ands in their pockets. I only . . .'

Fonthill put his hand on the Welshman's shoulder. He pressed a white five-pound note into the bartender's hand and tossed the knife he was still holding on to the floor. 'That should cover it,' he said. 'And if it doesn't, you'll just have to get the rest from these bruisers. Come on, Jenkins. I've had enough of this place.'

If the barman had thoughts of arguing, they were dispelled by the looks on the faces of the two men, who were given a rousing cheer from the onlookers, now pushing furniture back and lifting the wreckage of broken chairs and tables, attempting the impossible task of fitting the shattered pieces together again.

Outside, Fonthill pushed his own handkerchief to his nose to staunch the bleeding and seized Jenkins's arm. 'I know this sounds out of character,' he said, 'but I could use a drink. Is there a bar here that you haven't wrecked and is not full of ruffians?'

Jenkins's face broke into a grin and he attempted to push the remnants of his torn shirt beneath his waistband. 'What a good idea, bach sir. Yes. I think the first one I popped into might suit. Bit quiet it was. Down 'ere, sir.'

Once seated, Simon placed a pint of ale and a whisky chaser in front of each of them, took a deep draught of the beer and then sat gazing at his comrade in silence. At first Jenkins grinned happily and half drained his glass. Then he realised that the genial forgiveness that seemed to be linked to the drink was not, in fact, going to be on offer, and he began to shift uncomfortably in his chair. He sniffed and ran the back of his hand under his nose.

'Look, bach sir,' he began. 'I really am sorry, honest.'

Fonthill held up his hand and the Welshman fell silent. But Simon kept looking at him, his face expressionless. In fact, he was attempting to weigh up how it was possible for someone only five feet four inches tall to take on three men, all much bigger than him, without the slightest trace of fear. How was Jenkins able to do it – particularly having consumed enough alcohol to sink a battleship? He had laid out two of the stokers, and although it was difficult to conceive that he would have survived without Simon's arrival, it was quite possible. Fonthill shook his head, and Jenkins took the kind of tiny sip of whisky that would not been out of place in a rectory and looked up at the ceiling, waiting for the storm to break.

But Fonthill was still trying to analyse the kind of fighting machine that had been at his side for the last decade. In idle moments in the past, watching the huge hands of his servant stitching back a button or ironing a shirt with dainty precision, he had wondered at the dual nature of the man. Not only patient batman/servant and disciplined infantryman, but also fierce barroom brawler, as good with his fists or a wrestling stranglehold as with a knife. Why did he always come out on top? Well, he was magnificently strong, of course, with the courage of a lion. Then he was light on his feet and always seemingly unaffected by the drink he had taken. He also possessed a very low centre of gravity, which enabled him to take on much taller men. Simon shook his head and gave up. Over the years, he had benefited hugely by his comrade's ability to fight in any situation. Best to be thankful for it and regard it as a credit on the balance sheet of a very complex character.

He leaned forward. Jenkins's eyes now switched to the floor apprehensively. 'I suppose I was able to help . . .' Fonthill began.

'Oh, you did, bach sir, you did.' Jenkins jumped in thankfully. 'And I'm very grateful, indeed I am. My word, I couldn't see much of what was goin' on because I 'ad me 'ands a bit full, like, but from what I could see you was fightin' a lovely dirty fight. Not like an officer at all, see. I was very proud . . .'

Fonthill held up his hand with a sigh. 'But I would have lost out to that brute in the end, because he was too big for me. So thank you for knocking him over the head. Anyway.' He raised his glass to his comrade. 'If I did help a bit, then it came no way near to matching what you did in that tent with that damned snake. So, my dear old 352, thank you and cheers!'

Jenkin's jaw dropped for a moment, and then, with a relieved grin, he downed his whisky in one gulp. 'Cheers, bach sir. Shall we 'ave just one more, then?'

'No, we will not. And I want your word that you won't go on another drinking rampage while we are in Cape Town.' Fonthill shook his head and sighed. 'You must stay out of trouble for the rest of our stay because by the look of it we may have some work to do again before long.'

The Welshman's eyes lit up. 'Oh really? An' what would that be, then, bach sir?'

'I don't know yet. But I shall soon. Now drink up – although God knows where you will put it all. We must get back because Alice will be concerned.'

Chapter 6

The expected invitation came from Rhodes the next day. It was amazingly informal: a page seemingly torn from a cheap notepad and covered with strong, forward-sloping handwriting. It read:

> *My dear Fonthill,*
> *We met in Kimberley some time back. Could you spare me an hour or less tomorrow? Come to breakfast at my rooms. Best bacon and eggs in the Colony. Shall we say 8 a.m.?*
> *Yours, Cecil J. Rhodes.*

As an afterthought, Rhodes had scribbled the address of his apartment on the back of the page.

Fonthill grinned and passed the note to Alice. She read it with a frown and passed it back. 'Well,' she said, 'at least we can say that there are no frills about this particular millionaire. It seems he doesn't employ a lady with the new typewriting machine. Will you go? How stupid of me. Of course you will go.'

'Yes. Of course I will. I have a message to deliver to him,

and in any case, I am bursting with curiosity to know what he wants of me.'

'Very well, but Simon, do be careful. Don't be bullied or blackmailed by Lamb and Wolseley. You have served your country well enough now not to owe it any more.'

Fonthill bent and kissed her brow. 'Have no fears, my love. The great ensnarer will not catch this rabbit – unless he wants to be caught, that is. In any case, I love bacon and eggs and this hotel does a miserable breakfast.'

Fonthill arrived a little early the next day for his appointment and found that 'The Richest Man in Africa' lived in second-floor rooms in one of the busiest streets in the middle of Cape Town, accommodation typical of a youngish bachelor of moderate means. The rooms were wood-panelled and cosy, those perhaps of a don at the University of Oxford. Rhodes himself answered the door and led him to a table of some polished dark African wood set for breakfast.

'Sit down, my dear Fonthill,' he said. 'My man will have breakfast for us in five minutes or so. That gives me the chance to ask you about Gordon. I knew him well, you know. But you must have been the last white man to have seen him. Tell me about him.'

Fonthill studied the great man with interest. Rhodes had put on considerable weight since last they had met. He must now weigh about fourteen stone, but he carried it well, for he was tall and broad-shouldered. He was dressed carelessly in an old tweed jacket and cream cricket flannels, and the air of an undergraduate was enhanced by the auburn hair, now touched with grey, but flung loosely over his forehead. His eyes were bluish grey, dreamy and kindly and rather bulbous. They seemed to be those of a country parson – Fonthill remembered that he was indeed the son of a clergyman – and they certainly betrayed no trace of ruthlessness or commercial avarice. The moustache had been allowed to droop either side of his full lips, and his voice was high-pitched and had risen to a squeak at the mention of General Gordon. His appearance and demeanour were far from those of a determined businessman and political schemer.

'Ah, Gordon,' said Simon. 'I did not know you knew him, sir.'

'Indeed. We were great friends. Worked together in the early eighties when we were both members of the Losses Commission set up to decide compensation for those Basutos who had remained loyal through the rebellion at that time. Big difference in our ages, but we got on well and Charlie asked me to join him in the Sudan. But I was about to come on to the Cape Cabinet and had to decline. Tell me what happened at the end.'

Fonthill described the voyage of the two steamers sent up the Nile ahead of Wolseley's expedition in a desperate attempt to relieve the general in a besieged Khartoum, and their arrival just two days too late. To his surprise, Simon saw tears well up into Rhodes's eyes.

The big man fished out a red handkerchief and blew his nose noisily. 'Disgraceful,' he said. 'Disgraceful and tragic. I wish I had been with him. I do, you know.'

The awkward silence was broken by the arrival of a beaming black man carrying two tureens on a tray, which he placed on the table. 'This is Tony,' said Rhodes. 'Been with me for years. Couldn't do without him. Tony, meet Mr Fonthill, a great man of the Empire.'

To Simon's surprise, the servant gave a half-bow then extended his hand. Rising, Fonthill took it and they exchanged hearty handshakes before the man retired.

Rhodes took off the lids of both tureens. 'You know, Fonthill,' he said confidentially, 'these Kaffirs are great people. I like and respect 'em. When I was farming in Natal years ago, I lent a great deal of money to them when it was hut tax time, and they always came and worked if off for me. Kaffirs are really safer than the Bank of England. Two eggs or three?'

'Er . . . two, please.'

Rhodes busied himself with adding bacon, tomato, black pudding, mushrooms and sausages to Fonthill's plate, and Simon realised why the man had put on so much weight since last they had met.

'Now, Fonthill. You have just returned from Lobengula's kraal, I hear. Tell me about him and conditions there.'

'I have, and indeed I have a message for you from the king.'

'Oh.' Rhodes looked up sharply. 'Pray tell me.'

Fonthill put down his knife and fork and first described the situation in Bulawayo – the supplicants at the court of the king and in particular the pressure being applied by de Sousa on behalf of the Portuguese.

'Ah, Gouela. I've heard about him. But what's the king's message?'

'It seems that in return for the king's signature on a concession allowing your company to develop the mineral rights in Matabeleland and Mashonaland, you would deliver to Lobengula a monthly retainer of a hundred pounds, a thousand Martini-Henry rifles with a hundred thousand rounds of ammunition and a steamboat with guns suitable for defensive purposes on the Zambezi river. But the king says that none of these promises have been met, and, to put it politely, he will consider the contract to be null and void unless he receives these payments soon.'

Rhodes nodded his head slowly and removed a tureen

cover. 'Do have another egg, Fonthill. They come from my house up towards Table Mountain outside the city. I have a little farm there.' He nodded towards the pale blue flowers arranged in a bowl on the table. 'Plumbago. My favourites. They're from there too.' He ladled an egg. 'Come along. I insist.'

Fonthill sighed and accepted the egg.

Helping himself to bacon, Rhodes nodded his head again. 'All true, my dear fellow. All true. Incidentally, how is the king's gout?'

Shifting uncomfortably on his chair, Simon resisted the temptation to cry, 'Oh do get on with it,' and carefully explained Alice's treatment of the king and of her champagne diagnosis.

'Quite right. Best thing is to give it up. I only drink moderately, you know. Much too much to do. Now, turning to the king's message . . .' He pushed his plate away from him and, turning his head, shouted, 'Tony. Toast and marmalade, please.' He fixed his big grey eyes on Fonthill. 'Yes, the payment. As you can imagine, my dear fellow, it has not been exactly easy to get together the contingent parts of that. But I have done so. At least, the steamer on the Zambezi is certainly not there yet – and more of that later – but the gold, the guns and the ammunition are all now gathered together and are waiting in Kimberley to go north.'

'I am glad to hear it, sir. Why do they not go now?'

'Because, Fonthill, I am waiting for you to lead the expedition to take them to Bulawayo. It will not be an easy journey – particularly in view of what you tell me of de Sousa and his behaviour, although I had already had some indication of the man's determination to undo my treaty. No. It needs a person of great resource and qualities of leadership, with knowledge of the country, and yes, someone I could trust. My dear fellow, you would do me a great service if you could take this precious cargo to Lobengula and secure from him his confirmation that he will accept a party of my people, who will march north to Mashonaland to develop the land. I had heard you were somewhere in South Africa, and knowing of the fine reputation you have earned since last we met, I have waited until we could meet here and I could explain to you my plans and beseech your help.'

Fonthill's eyebrows rose. 'Well, sir, you certainly flatter me. But I don't know . . .'

Rhodes silenced him by raising his hand and standing. 'Let me first of all fill in some all-important details. Do come over here, there's a good fellow.' And then, over his shoulder: 'Tony, where's the toast and marmalade? Stir yourself, lad.'

They moved to a large table set against the panelled wall and covered with documents. Selecting one of them, Rhodes untied the red tape that bound it and smoothed it flat with his hand. 'Here you are,' he said. 'One of the three original copies of the treaty of friendship that I persuaded the British Government to enter into with Lobengula last year. This is important because it precludes the making of any other treaty or ceding of land with any other foreign power. Got it?'

Fonthill smiled as he remembered from their first meeting the staccato questions that so often ended Rhodes's statements. He nodded. 'Got it.'

'Good. Now.' Rhodes threw aside the document and unrolled another one of similar size. 'Here's the treaty the king signed with me. Look, see, there's Lobengula's cross and his great elephant seal. It gives me, as you say, the right to prospect and dig for minerals on his land.'

'Quite so, sir. But has the British Colonial Office seen this and approved it? If so, I am a bit surprised that it was happy to arm the Matabele with rifles. You know that these people are fierce warriors, and I understand that a law was passed here some years ago prohibiting the provision of arms to the natives.'

Rhodes threw back his head. 'Ah, that only applied to the Basutos. And don't worry about the Imperials back home. The deal was done before they'd adjusted their pince-nez and I got them to rubber-stamp it, though they looked down their noses at it a bit. These rifles won't make the Matabele an armed force, because there's no one to train 'em to use 'em. But Lobengula wants them to frighten the Boers, who are his main worry in terms of invasion, and they will probably do that, which also helps our cause, y'see. Old Kruger in the Transvaal would love to get his hands on Matabeleland and Mashonaland, and these guns and this document will stop him, or at least make him pause, because the treaty has legal viability.'

Fonthill gave a half-smile. 'But not, of course, if Lobengula renounces it on the grounds that you have not carried out your side of the bargain.'

'Exactly. By Gad, Fonthill, that's where I need you. And not just in terms of delivering the cash and the hardware, although that's vital.' Rhodes seized Simon by the shoulder. 'There's two other vital things that I want you to do for me and your country. Firstly, I want you to get the king's permission to allow a column of my men to go through Matabeleland – in fact, I intend to skirt it more or less, but that's a detail – to Mashonaland to start prospecting . . .'

'Is there gold or silver there?'

'There may be, but it's important to get men on the land up

there. Once they are there, nobody will get 'em off. Occupation is the thing. Got it?'

'Yes, but what's the point of occupying the land? What do you want the men there for, if not to dig for minerals?'

Rhodes pulled from the table a map of South Africa, extending from the tip of the Cape to the great lakes north of Mashonaland. 'A road to the north, and homes, my dear Fonthill, homes. Mainly for the British, but I don't mind providing for the Cape Afrikaners too, if they want to go north – although not those dull Boers of Kruger's in the Transvaal.' He spread his hand across the northern part of the map. 'I would like to see all of that red.'

He began to pace the room and his eyes took on a gleam that Fonthill again recalled from their first meeting. 'I contend, old chap, that we are the first race in the world, and that the more of the world we inhabit the better it is for the human race. I contend that every acre added to our territory provides for the birth of more of the English race who otherwise would not be brought into existence.' He stopped abruptly and stared sharply at Simon.

'You've fought in more wars than I have been near to. Do you favour wars, Fonthill? Do they serve their purpose, despite the cost?'

'Absolutely not, sir . . . well, not most of the time.'

'Absolutely right, my boy. I quite agree. The absorption of the greater portion of the world under our rule simply means the end of all wars. A road and homes, Fonthill, a road and homes. Not more wars.' He walked back to Simon, and his messianic tone left him for a moment. 'Do you know, I believe that every man has his price. At this moment in Bulawayo, as you know, there is a veritable foreign legion trying to bribe Lobengula to renege on his treaty with me, including your nasty Portuguese piece of work. Ah. Thank goodness. Here's the toast and marmalade at last.'

Fonthill tried another tack. 'Lobengula seemed rather perturbed that you hadn't been to his kraal to negotiate directly with him. Wouldn't it be easier for you to talk to him personally? Every man has his price, as you know.'

'Can't get away.' Rhodes shrugged his shoulders. 'Just can't do it. I am the only man who can drive these company purchases on and I have to be here to do it. And I also have to be in the Cape Parliament.' He dropped his voice and growled. 'Something coming up there that will involve me. No. Just can't get away. I need you. Come and have some toast. Marmalade's made on my land too.'

Fonthill smiled slowly. The sheer energy, drive and brutal honesty of Rhodes appealed to him, he had to admit. It was like being in the presence of a charming steamroller. He joined his host back at the table and buttered some toast, as much to gain time to think as to satisfy a hunger long since sated.

'Rhodes,' he began, 'you mentioned that my task would not just be delivering the rifles and persuading Lobengula to confirm the treaty. There was something else . . . ?'

'Indeed.' Rhodes, his mouth already half full, inserted another piece of toast and marmalade under his moustache. 'Look.' And again he was on his feet, walking to the map on the table. 'See here.'

He stabbed a finger on to where Mashonaland was marked, rather indistinctly. 'Once my pioneers are there, it will take time for them to develop the land to feed themselves, so every damned thing,' he paused to wipe his moustache with a finger, which he then put into his mouth to remove an errant fragment of marmalade, 'will have to be carried overland, probably from the Cape, as near as dammit over a thousand miles. I must find a path to the sea, to the east, so that I can supply them that way. If the Portuguese would let me, we could perhaps do it by steamer up the Zambezi, but they control the river mouth and I don't see the blighters letting me go that way into country they claim as their own. And I am not even sure that the Zambezi is navigable that far to the west – which is another reason, of course, why Lobengula has not had his damned steamer, although I did promise him five hundred pounds to compensate him if I couldn't manage it.'

'So . . . ?'

'So, when you have settled things with the king, I would like you to explore to the east. Find a way through to the coast there, see if the tribes are friendly, then come back and meet up with the pioneer column that I intend to send off as soon as I hear from you that Lobengula has given his consent.'

'I see. I have to say, Rhodes, that that is quite an undertaking.'

Rhodes fixed Fonthill with his protuberant grey eyes and spoke earnestly. 'Indeed it is, but I know that you can do it, Fonthill. You were undoubtedly one of the finest scouts ever used by the British Army. You would be instrumental in opening up this vital route to the north, in extending this remarkable empire of ours and spreading the beneficial rule of the British to that huge unclaimed interior, the great plateau of the continent, stretching from the north of the Transvaal up to the equatorial lakes and then the Sudan. Think of it, Fonthill, cool under the equator, good farming land, a country for white men.'

Rhodes's eyes were now ablaze. 'Up in the north there is something to make up to England for the loss of the American states. He who holds the north holds the balance of the map. The north is the trump card, the key position, the bulk of the shares. If Kruger gets the north, he holds a solid block of claims from the Orange river to the Zambezi. If he gets the gold of Witwatersrand, he could build his Delagoa Bay railway, which would make him independent of the British in South Africa.'

He made a dismissive gesture with his arm. 'I don't want gold. But I want the promise of it to lure people in and occupy the land. Remember what the great East India Company did? In India there was trade to bring people in. Here it could be gold. If the north was occupied by a British company, it must then become a British colony. The north would be in British hands, and one might therefore federate South Africa on British lines.'

In his head, Simon heard again the words of Lamb: 'Dominion status is just around the corner . . .' but Rhodes was continuing.

'This would be a wonderful opportunity, my dear fellow, to make your mark on history. You would virtually be treading in the footsteps of Livingstone and Stanley – opening up a vast territory.' Then suddenly the visionary disappeared and the pragmatic man of business replaced him: 'And of course you will be paid: ten pounds sterling for every day you are away and three thousand acres of good farming land in Mashonaland.'

Fonthill's mind raced. The task would be prodigious. Hauling the guns and the ammunition to Bulawayo would be daunting enough, especially with Gouela lurking on the edges of the expedition. But exploring a route to the sea, through – what sort of terrain? Probably jungle and swamp. He had heard that the country to the east of Matabeleland was a breeding ground for the tsetse fly and goodness knows what else, and of course it was probably all claimed by Portugal anyway. What on earth would Alice say? He looked closely at Rhodes. The man's eyes were still alight with his vision of developing the whole of southern Africa for the British and spreading the enlightenment of the Empire. Was he mad? Merely a fanatic aiming to stretch personal power further from his base here in the Cape? Or was he a man of his time, perhaps even ahead of his time, a genuine visionary who would bring a balanced rule to vast territories under the sway of barbarians? Simon remembered his own embarrassment at being formally introduced to Rhodes's black servant, and the man shaking his hand is a gesture of equality. Well, Rhodes was clearly no conventional, black-hating white colonist. A liberal? Perhaps in some ways, and yet in others he was a prototypical exploiter of land and people. Whatever he was, he was undoubtedly different. No wonder he was treated with suspicion in Westminster and Whitehall. The politicians and the diplomats in London would almost certainly see him as some sort of rogue elephant crashing through the under-growth of southern Africa – a wild and rich entrepreneur who could do harm but perhaps some good, as long as he was kept on a leash. Yes, a leash. Had the British Government already slipped some sort of harness around him?

Fonthill cleared his throat. 'Well, sir, I must confess that it all sounds fascinating. But let me tell you now that if I did agree, I would not wish to be paid. I have private means, and I would wish to preserve my independence – although I would expect you to meet all reasonable expenses, and I must add that the land grant could interest me.' His thoughts turned quickly to General Lamb's injunction. Would Rhodes rush into Matabeleland with all guns blazing? 'However,' he went on, 'I am anxious to know under what authority you would mount what would seem to be virtually an invasion of Lobengula's land.'

'Yes. A fair question. Here, look at this.' Rhodes returned to the table and picked up yet another sheaf of documents. '*I would not be marching into the king's land*,' he said. 'A pioneer column would be entering Matabeleland under a charter – a *royal charter* – signed by the Queen herself, allowing the British South Africa Company, my company, to do so under the terms of my original agreement with Lobengula.' He waved the document. 'This is the charter. Once it has the Queen's signature – and I am informed reliably from London that it will be forthcoming very soon – the chartered company can make treaties, promulgate laws, preserve the peace, maintain a police force and acquire new concessions. Here, read it if you like.'

He thrust the document forward, but Fonthill shook his head. 'I will take your word for it, Rhodes,' he said.

'Very well. These powers are wide-ranging.' Rhodes resumed pacing around the room. 'We can make roads, railways and harbours,' he went on, 'or undertake other public works; own or charter ships; engage in mining or any other industry; make land grants; establish banks and carry on lawful commerce, trade and business. In fact, my dear fellow, this gives me all I want, virtually the panoply of a modern state under British law.'

Fonthill frowned. 'But does British law apply to Matabeleland?'

'Given that I have the king's original agreement, it does. We are a British company, answering to British courts if there is a contravention in any way.'

The frown stayed on Fonthill's forehead. This didn't sound

a very effective leash. 'Are there no restrictive clauses?' he asked.

'Oh yes, usual sort of stuff. Freedom of worship and protection of native rights, of course – the Aborigines' Protection Society have a strong lobby in Westminster. But I don't mind that. I wouldn't dream of exploiting Kaffirs. As I've said, on the whole they are fine people. The Secretary of State for the Colonies has limited rights of supervision, and after twenty-five years, or sooner if the company abuses its privileges, the charter can be revoked. No, Fonthill, once Her Majesty has signed this piece of paper – and she will, I am assured – it will give me all I want. And it will be legally and morally watertight.'

Rhodes replaced the document and extended his arm expansively. 'The capital of the new company will be fixed at one million pounds in one-pound shares. I can tell you now that subscribers will pour in.' He smiled. 'But, my dear fellow, it all depends upon you. Lobengula has given me the right to develop the land, yet I must have his permission – however informally – to enter it with my men and start road-building. I need you to get it for me.'

Fonthill nodded slowly but did not speak. The silence seemed to present itself as a challenge to Rhodes. He spoke again, but softly this time. 'My greatest worry, Fonthill, is the Portuguese. Oh, the Boers of the Transvaal are anxious to move in, and they hate us after Majuba. Lobengula is afraid of 'em and detests 'em, so I doubt if he will listen to them. But the Portuguese are on the spot and have always claimed suzerainty over Matabeleland. De Sousa, the man who tried to kill you, will probably be pouring poison into the king's ear this very moment. Once the king has accepted the rifles and ammunition, though, and given you his word, I am sure that the old buster will not go back on it. I don't want the Portuguese to have this country, Fonthill, and the Matabeles will not be able to keep it for themselves. Better me than de Sousa. Don't you agree?'

Simon cleared his throat. 'Would you . . . er . . . attack the Matabele?'

'Of course not. Not unless I was unreasonably provoked.'

A silence hung over the room. It was broken, of course, by Rhodes. 'Do have some more toast and marmalade, my dear fellow.'

Fonthill grinned at the banality. He could not help liking the open roguery of this strange man – the reference to de Sousa was a sly piece of blackmail. He shook his head. 'No thank you, sir. You are quite right. You do serve the best breakfast in the Cape, but I have had more than my fill. Now, I would welcome a little time to think this over and to consult with my wife. How long can you give me?'

'Oh, plenty of time. Shall we say twenty-four hours?'

'Good lord.'

'I must get on, Fonthill. These great events don't wait upon the ponderings of men, you know.'

'Very well. I will give you my decision by tomorrow morning.'

'Good. Think carefully, my dear fellow. Much depends on your decision, for I have no one who could do this as well as you. So weigh my proposition very carefully. Oh, and give my regards to your wife.'

'I will, sir. Goodbye.'

Once outside, Fonthill took a circuitous route back to the hotel, to give him time to think before meeting Alice. Jenkins must be involved, of course, in making the decision, but he would go along with whatever Alice and Fonthill decided.

Simon's own mind was already made up. The challenge was too great to resist. The chance to be in at the birth of a great country; the pleasure of ruining de Sousa and his government's plans for Matabeland; the call to find a route to the eastern coast – they were all too strong and compelling to evade. He and Jenkins had been lying fallow for far too long. It was time to set off again and to follow their star.

He grinned at the thought. Then his features hardened into a frown, as he remembered his promise to Lamb. It would not be easy to keep Rhodes on that leash. And Alice, of course, would not be pleased. There was naturally no question of her accompanying them on this mission. It would be far too dangerous, and in any case, it was far from certain that she would approve of the purpose of it all. It was clear that she carried no banner for Rhodes and that she categorically disapproved of empire-building. She was wont to quote Gladstone's words from his Midlothian campaign – words that she had reported for the *Morning Post* – of his 'shame' in thinking of 'the events which have deluged many a hill and many a plain with blood' in pursuit of Britain's colonial ambitions in Africa. Would she not see a danger of this happening again if Rhodes was allowed to release his column of pioneers to 'develop' Matabeleland? And was Simon himself not being incredibly selfish anyway in proposing to leave her again to go adventuring? He sighed.

Alice, of course, was waiting for him at the hotel, as was Jenkins, who was cleaning shoes in his room, nursing a ripening black eye.

'Sit down, my dear,' she said, her eyes sharp, 'and tell me what the great man has offered you. Was it the throne of some mountain kingdom in the hinterland, or merely a seat in the Cape Cabinet?'

'Now don't tease, Alice. This is quite important.'

'Oh, I'm sure it is. Shall I pack now?'

Fonthill sighed. It *was* going to be difficult. He cleared his throat and began to tell her, as accurately as he could remember, all that Rhodes had related. She interrupted him almost at once to call in Jenkins to hear the details, then listened impassively and without further question until the end. Then: 'You have accepted, of course?'

'Certainly not. I told him I wished to talk it over with you.'

'Good. That was thoughtful. How much time did he give you?'

'Er . . . twenty-four hours.'

'*Twenty-four hours!* How very considerate of him.'

Fonthill squirmed in his chair and caught Jenkins's eye. 'Now don't be unfair, my dear. You know yourself that Lobengula is becoming very restive. Time is of the essence.'

'And you wish to go?'

'Well yes, subject of course to your approval. I do consider it the most remarkable opportunity—'

She interrupted him quickly.

'And what do you think, 352? Do you wish to go exploring in deepest Africa?'

Jenkins screwed up his discoloured eye. 'Well, you know, Miss Alice, I'll go anywhere the captain goes.'

'Not quite *everywhere*, I trust.' Her tone was acerbic. 'Good. Then that's settled. I'm afraid we can't set off immediately, my dears, because I need at least one new pair of breeches. My present ones are virtually transparent. But I will only need a couple of days . . .'

Fonthill set his jaw. 'No, Alice. That is out of the question. I am afraid you cannot accompany us. This will be far too dangerous for a woman. You have seen already how de Sousa likes to play things, and goodness knows what other dangers will lie in wait once we start to head to the east. Please, my dear, stay here in the Cape and—'

'And do my knitting and embroidery while you two are having fun in the bloody jungle? Certainly not. No. I shall have work to do.'

'Work? What on earth do you mean?'

She leaned forward, and Simon realised that her eyes were gleaming in anticipation. To the side, he caught a glimpse of Jenkins grinning. 'Simon,' she said, 'this will be a damned good story, don't you see? I shall cable Cornford, the editor of the *Morning Post* immediately. I'm sure he will take me on again. The birth of a new nation, or at least a new colony, that sort of stuff. Those damned jingoes back in London will lap it up, and I shall have an exclusive.'

'You can't do that. What would Rhodes say?'

'To hell with Rhodes. The man can't operate in a vacuum. The world outside should know what he's up to. Oh, when his column starts to invade – and that is what it means, a bloody *invasion* – the correspondents for the nationals down here will be on board, I expect, so I shan't have that to myself. But they won't be coming with you first, my darling, taking your guns and bullets up to the dear old king, but *I* shall and I shall tell the world, from deepest, darkest Africa.'

'You can't. There are no cable facilities up there.'

She sighed. 'What sort of journalist do you think I am, my love? I have been solving those kind of logistical problems for years. The cable in the north begins from somewhere in the Free State, if I remember rightly, and I shall instruct a bearer to take my stuff back to be sent from there. I shall arrange all this myself with dear old Mzingeli. I presume that you will take him with you?'

'Well, I don't know . . .'

'Then I shall take him myself.' She turned round and gave Jenkins the sweetest smile. 'Does all that sound logical and sound to you, 352?'

'Well, Miss, I must say that—'

'Oh for goodness' sake be quiet, Jenkins.' A scowl was now firmly settled on Fonthill's face. 'Alice, it is dangerous and you will be a hindrance. This will be no place for a woman.'

'Oh, really?' The scowl was reflected in Alice's features. 'And who was it that treated old Lobengula's gout? Who fired the shot that stunned the lion when it charged? And who took part in the defence of the wagon? Was I a hindrance then? Come along, my dear. Was I?'

Fonthill bent his head for a moment in silence, but when he looked up he was smiling. 'Of course not. You were and are the bravest woman in the world. What do you think, 352?'

'Well I must say, Miss Alice seems quite determined.

'You would say that. Very well, my darling, you will come with us. But for goodness' sake, don't criticise Rhodes in your dispatches. If you do, he might well recall us.'

She beamed at him. 'Oh my love. He might recall you two but he has no power to recall *me* – and if he did abort your mission I would just have to tell the world about it, wouldn't I? Now, if you will excuse me, I must send a cable and buy a new pair of breeches. I won't be long. While I am away, why don't you two find a nice little bar and start another war with the locals?'

Chapter 7

It was not, in fact, until three days later that Fonthill, Alice and Jenkins were able to set off for Kimberley. There was no train link north to the Transvaal, but Rhodes insisted that they take a ship round the Cape to Port Elizabeth, where a rail network had been established between that port and Durban and from which a line north was being built to Bloemfontein in the Free State. It had only reached as far as the northern Cape border, but it would still be much quicker than going by wagon or horseback overland from Cape Town. Fonthill sent a message to Mzingeli at his farm asking him to meet with them at the Kimberley headquarters of the de Beers diamond mining company of which Rhodes was chairman. He then went shopping with Jenkins to acquire two more up-to-date Martini-Henry rifles and a brace of revolvers, before meeting with Rhodes for a final briefing.

The meeting was disconcertingly vague. Firstly, Rhodes mentioned – almost in passing – that the number of rifles and cartridges awaiting Fonthill in the diamond town had been halved, to five hundred and fifty thousand respectively. 'All the promised money is there, my dear fellow,' he explained, 'but it's been damned difficult to find all the shooters, et cetera, in the time available. But don't worry. Old Lobengula will never notice, and if he does, just explain that this is the first down-payment on account. Anyway, this will lighten your load. The original consignment would have been dashed difficult to manage in one go.'

Rhodes was also less than precise with his instructions about finding a route to the eastern coast. 'Just head east. See if you can come to an agreement with the tribes out there – get a treaty of friendship between the chiefs and the company. We may have to build a road through to the coast eventually. Take plenty of gifts for the chiefs – lengths of cloth, hatchets, mirrors, that sort of thing. You can get all this from old Fairbairn up in Bulawayo. Don't let him overcharge you. But he knows the territory a fair bit and he could be helpful all round. I have used him before. I have given instructions for you to be able to draw on the company's account in Kimberley. Use the de Beers office as a means of communicating with me. They can telegraph me from there. Got it?'

On the day before their departure, Alice received an enthusiastic cable from the editor of the *Morning Post* agreeing to her proposal, and Fonthill felt it honourable to inform Rhodes that she would be accompanying him and of her journalistic role. He seemed remarkably sanguine about it all. 'I'm open about what I do, Fonthill,' he said. 'Nothing to hide. As for her alerting the opposition, by the time she gets her reports back to London, you should have settled the whole business with the king, eh, what? Oh, and tell her to use my name in full, Cecil John, there's a good fellow. It's just a small vanity I have, you know.'

It only remained for Fonthill, this time with Jenkins, to pay a farewell visit to Major General Lamb. The little man had heard, of course, of Simon's decision – was there nothing that escaped his attention in Cape Town? – and he showed his pleasure also at meeting Jenkins again. The last time we met, 384,' he reminisced, 'was on the ramparts at Sherpur, just outside Kabul, when the Pathans were attacking. I remember you had blood pouring down your face then. Now you've got a black eye. Where'd you get it, eh?'

'Walked into a door, General.'

'Lord, the same old barrack-room excuse. Well, good luck to you both, and God speed. Remember, Fonthill, curb the beast as best you can.'

'I will do my best, sir.'

And so they set off the next day, just the three of them, for Alice was not the sort of woman to employ a lady's maid on a journey such as this. Within two and a half weeks they were in Kimberley, thanks to the new railway. The town had changed a little since Fonthill's last visit nine years before. It still sprawled out on to the veldt in surprisingly orderly rows of single-storeyed wooden shacks, with their sad veranda *stoeps*. But the centre had become more sophisticated, with two- and even three-storeyed buildings predominating, many of them now made of brick and offering financial and other commercial services. Most of these were set around the large market square at a crossroads, big enough to turn an oxen team without it outspanning, and which seemed to be an open-air meeting place for an eclectic mixture of dust-covered miners, bearded Boer farmers and barefooted Kaffirs in overalls. The de Beers headquarters, however, seemed exactly the same: an unpretentious low wooden building, set, like most of those in Kimberley, under a corrugated iron roof. There was nothing to indicate that the company now handled ninety per cent of all the diamonds mined in South Africa, or that its chairman could airily promise to launch a steamer on the upper Zambezi for a native king to play with.

Fonthill booked them all into a modest hotel, then, with Jenkins, hurried to the de Beers office. He was half hoping to find Mzingeli waiting for them, but realised that the tracker would have to make his way by foot for perhaps three hundred miles to reach the diamond town. He would need more time yet.

The two were ushered into a dark, gloomy office and greeted by a small, fastidiously dressed man who addressed them in perfect English, overlaid with a slight German accent. 'Alfred Beit,' he said. 'I have been expecting you.'

Fonthill regarded Beit with interest. He knew little of his background, except that as the son of a Hamburg Jew, he had been sent to Amsterdam to study the diamond business and then out to Kimberley to work as a diamond merchant. What he had heard, however, was that Beit and Rhodes had set up a warm and informal business relationship and that the big man now trusted the little Jew implicitly. Beit, in fact, had become Rhodes's right-hand man, although he avoided the limelight whenever he could.

'You have, gentlemen, taken on quite an assignment,' he said, favouring them both with a distant smile. 'But Mr Rhodes tells me that he has complete confidence in you, and of course I shall give you all the help I can.'

'That's very kind of you, Mr Beit. Can you tell me how far advanced are the preparations for my departure?'

'Indeed. Everything is ready. The rifles, ammunition and gold for King Lobengula are locked away in one of our diamond vaults, and I can assure you,' his smile became more affable, 'that nowhere could be more secure than that.'

He began to enumerate points, with one finger dropping precisely into the palm of his other hand. 'The rifles are packed into ten wooden boxes, which are sealed and locked with steel bands, fifty rifles to each box. The cartridges similarly are carried in two boxes, with the rounds wrapped in greaseproof paper in batches of twenty-five each. The money is in gold sovereigns and is carried in one smaller but stout box. I will require you to inspect them all and give me a receipt for them before you leave. I have provided five Cape wagons for you, which I suggest should be sufficient for the load you carry and your own travel requirements. Each wagon will be pulled by six oxen, and another ten oxen have been supplied to accompany you as reserves.'

Fonthill began to open his mouth to deliver a question, but Beit, the accountant supreme and master of detail, was well into his dry delivery. 'I don't believe that you will need mules, for oxen are the most reliable form of locomotion in the territory you will cover. However, there are three good horses for yourselves and, ahem, your wife, plus two reserves. They are all salted against the tsetse. Your personal belongings, of course, will be carried in the wagons. These include four serviceable tents and, of course, cooking utensils.'

'Men?' Simon was able to interject.

Beit nodded. 'Yes. I have provided five good Kaffirs to drive the wagons and another five to carry out whatever tasks you require from them on the journey. You may well become bogged down in drifts and need – what shall I say? – direct muscle to push and pull you through, although it should not be too bad at this time of the year.

'Of course you will need an overseer, and I have hired a man for this purpose and another to act as his assistant. They are British and have had some experience, I understand, of taking wagons to and from the gold fields on the Rand.' The little cough came again. 'They are a little what you might call rough and ready,' he smiled, 'but I think that will be an advantage on your journey.'

Fonthill frowned. 'Do they know the nature of the cargo – in fact, do any of the men know the nature of the cargo?'

'No. They know that the boxes contain gifts for the king, but I have deliberately had it put about that these are the usual knick-knacks that we have given to natives in the past.'

'Hmm. Won't they be rather puzzled that we have bound knick-knacks in stout boxes with steel bands?'

Beit waved a well-manicured hand. 'Oh no. A wagon could well overturn crossing a dry donga or whatever, and it is important to protect these things from rough treatment. The men will know that. You will meet these people at whatever time you wish. Perhaps tomorrow?'

'Yes please. If all is in order, I would wish to set off as soon as possible.'

'Of course. Now, let me think if I have overlooked something. Ah yes. Do you have rifles?'

'Yes. Do the overseers?'

'No. Do you think it might be necessary?'

'If they are trustworthy, yes.' Fonthill had a quick mental vision of de Sousa's Portuguese Kaffirs streaming round the base of the kopje. 'There are those in Matabeland who have a vested interest in seeing that we do not reach the king with our cargo.'

Beit raised his eyebrows. 'Really? Well, Mr Fonthill, these are unsettled times, and certainly you are going into territory that has no conventional rule of law, to say the least. I will provide rifles for your two overseers, whose names, by the way, are Murphy and Laxer. May I enquire as to your route?'

'Yes. We will take what I understand is the now reasonably well-established northern road through Bechuanaland, paying King Khama a courtesy call at his capital at Palapye, before continuing up through the Tuli Block between the Shashe and

Macaloutsi rivers and crossing into Matabeleland at Tuli. There is a little gold mining there, I understand?'

'Umph, yes. It's been going on for some time, before the recent finds on the Rand. But it's small and not very profitable. When last I looked, Tuli gold was worth about four pounds per ounce. But a word about King Khama.'

'Yes?'

'I have not met him, but by all accounts he is a civilised man and an enlightened ruler. However, he hates the Matabele. His people are peaceful and non-aggressive, all the things the Matabele are not, and Lobengula's men still raid into his territory, even though Bechuanaland recently became a British protectorate. In fact you could say that a state of war exists between the two countries, so I advise that you keep the contents of your cargo secret. It would not do for you to be seen taking weapons through his country to give to the King of the Matabele.'

Fonthill nodded. 'I take your point, Mr Beit. Tell me about the area just south of the Tuli crossing. I understand that it is a bit of a no-man's-land, lots of cattle stealing and that sort of thing.'

'Indeed it is. It is really a disputed territory, but no one is actually prepared to go to war to possess it. It has the reputation of being a rather lawless place – although, indeed, one could say that everywhere north of here fits that description.' The gentle smile had returned. 'Mr Fonthill, this may be . . . what shall I say? . . . a not exactly incident-free journey you are about to undertake. But I know of its importance and I do wish you well.'

'Thank you, sir. Perhaps I could see the overseers at eight tomorrow? Ah. Just one other point. I am expecting a tracker – a member of the Malakala tribe, named Mzingeli – to arrive here to join me within the next couple of days. I would be grateful if you would direct him to our hotel. Oh yes. He will need a tent, please, and a good rifle.'

Beit's eyebrows rose again. 'A tent and a rifle for a Kaffir?'

'Yes. This man will be vital to me on this trip. Now, may I see the cargo?'

'Of course.' Beit rang a small handbell on his desk and gave instructions in German to a young man who entered. 'Hans will show you. Please let me know if there is anything more you need.'

There were no signs of diamonds in the diamond vault but the boxes were as described: made of stout timber, with two bands of strip steel strengthening them, and padlocked. The young German gave them two keys and Fonthill unlocked the boxes and examined and then counted the contents. It was, of course, all in order. The Cape wagons waiting outside were new and of sturdy construction, the maids-of-all-work in South Africa upon whose stout axles most of the transport in the southern colonies rested.

Early the next morning, Fonthill, Jenkins and Alice visited the de Beers offices again to meet Murphy and Laxer, the two men who would be virtual managers of the expedition while on trek and overseers of the natives.

The first impression was less than favourable. Murphy, the senior of the two, was in his middle forties and carrying a full black beard and a stomach that hung well over the belt that held up his woollen trousers. His face was pockmarked but his eyes were bright enough. Laxer, a dark-countenanced man with a strong Cockney accent, was younger, small and thin, but seemed wiry and energetic. Both men were burned by the Transvaal sun and they were dressed, Boer style, in wide-brimmed slouch hats, check shirts and lace-up boots.

'Have either of you been to Matabeleland before?' asked Fonthill.

'No, your honour.' Murphy had kept his Irish accent. 'But we've bin just about everywhere else in this godforsaken land. Down in the Cape, in Zululand, 'ere in the Free State an' through the Transvaal.'

'Doing what?'

'Drivin' most of the time. We can 'andle any size of team you can yoke up. An' we're used to 'andlin' the blacks and can speak the Bantu lingo.'

'Fine. Have you seen the oxen and the Cape carts?'

'Sure enough. Good beasts an' well-found wagons.'

'And you've agreed terms with Mr Beit?'

'Yes, your honour. 'Appy about that.'

'There is one point.' The two men's heads turned towards Alice in some surprise at hearing her intervene. 'We do like to treat our boys well, you know,' she said. 'There will be no beatings or anything of that kind. Is that understood?'

The two exchanged glances and this time Laxer spoke. 'Well, missus, I'd 'ave to say that in our experience a touch o' the whip is what's needed to get the black fellers movin' properly. We've bin at this lark a long time, see, an' they're a lazy lot. I don't care where they come from.'

'Well, Mr Laxer, whatever your experience, there will be no whipping on this trip. Is that clear?'

'Er, yes, mum.'

'Good.' Fonthill spoke again. 'We shall be trekking through Bechuanaland and then north through some rather wild territory. Can you handle rifles?'

'Oh aye, governor. We've 'unted all our lives.'

'Good. There is a possibility that we may be attacked at some time by unfriendly natives who will be ... er ...

covetous of our cattle. So you may be expected to help us defend ourselves. Do you have a problem with that?'

'Oh surely no, sir.' Murphy's accent seemed to have grown during the course of the meeting, as though he was curbing it deliberately at first. 'We don't mind pottin' at the black fellers at all, at all. Ah, that is, missus, when they're out of order, that is. An' only then, bless you.'

Fonthill nodded. 'Very well,' he said. 'I am hoping to leave just after first light tomorrow, if, as I hope, my native tracker arrives in time, so I will expect you to inspan before dawn and for us to be fully loaded by then. We have a long way to go and I don't want to waste any further time.' He shook hands with them both. 'Let's hope it's a safe and uneventful journey. You can expect bonuses if you perform well. Jenkins and I will be here to help you load the cargo.'

The two men nodded, touched the brims of their hats with their forefingers and shuffled away. Fonthill, Jenkins and Alice exchanged glances.

'What do you think?' Simon asked them both.

'I could have wished for more congenial travelling companions,' said Alice, 'but I suppose we must take what we can get. At least they seem experienced enough.'

Jenkins made a face so that his black eyebrows seemed almost to meet his great moustache. 'Tough birds I'd say, bach sir. Not completely to be trusted, either. Let's hope they can do their jobs. I will keep a close eye on them, look you.'

'Oh goodness.' Alice smiled. 'I do hope that doesn't mean punching them in the eye, my dear.'

'Oh no, miss. Unless they deserve it, that is, see.'

Fonthill's last pre-departure worry was removed when, just after noon, Mzingeli arrived. He came in covered in dust and riding a decrepit mule, so that his bare feet nearly touched the ground on either side of the animal's flanks. Behind him, grinning widely, walked an equally dishevelled Ntini. 'Sorry, Nkosi,' said Mzingeli. 'Long way. Am I late?'

'My dear fellow, no, not at all,' said Fonthill, pumping his hand. 'I am glad to see that you have joined the cavalry.'

The tracker allowed himself a faint smile. 'Too far to walk. Where we go?'

In his message to Mzingeli, Simon had merely said that he must be prepared to be away for at least a year and that they would journey to the north. He knew that the tracker could not read and that the message would have to be conveyed to him by the Afrikaner upon whose farm Mzingeli had his home. He therefore felt it prudent to betray as little as possible of their destination.

'Well, I'm afraid that it is back to Bulawayo to begin with . . .' the tracker let his face signify faint disapproval, 'and then exploring out to the east, towards the coast.' He explained the reason for the trip, and Mzingeli's expression lightened a little at hearing of the contents of their cargo.

'King will be pleased,' he said. 'But not Gouela, I think.'

'Indeed. I fear that we may be attacked again and we must keep a very keen watch. That is one of the many reasons I am glad you are with us.'

'Ah. I bring rifle.'

'Good, but perhaps Ntini can be taught to use it. I have a modern army rifle for you – and it will be yours to keep. Oh, and the pay will be higher this time because Rhodes is providing everything.'

Mzingeli allowed one eyebrow to rise and his mouth to twitch a touch to show his pleasure. 'Thank you. Good.'

It was after dawn before the column set off. Although the

Kaffir drivers and herdsmen seemed competent, the oxen were not fully broken in to the yoke and it took a little time – with many curses from Murphy and Laxer – before they could be inspanned. Fonthill had begged an extra horse for Mzingeli to ride, which did not set well with the two overseers, who had been allocated seats in the wagons when they were not required to walk with the oxen and the boys. The mule was handed down to Ntini.

Eventually the party set off in a cloud of dust that rose and then hung sparkling in the rays of the early sunlight. Fonthill rode ahead, his compass in his pocket, for the trail to the north out of the town was clearly defined. By his side rode Alice and Jenkins. In the leading wagon sat Murphy by the side of the senior Kaffir driver, who handled his oxen team well. Behind them, under the white canvas sheeting that protected the cargo from the sun, sat the tents and the paraphernalia of camping. If there had to be a trial crossing of a particularly difficult-looking river or donga, Fonthill reasoned that this load was the one that could most easily be risked, so it should lead. The second wagon, the most heavily laden, carried the guns and ammunition boxes. Then came the gold sovereigns, secured in one box, although Fonthill had procured other similarly bound containers, filled with stones, to sit around it to mitigate whatever attention might be prompted by one box being carried in singular state. The fourth wagon contained their personal belongings and half a dozen barrels of water, plus a similar number of light *fatchies*, or water bags. The last wagon was used to spell the Kaffirs who were herding on foot the oxen and extra horses at the rear. Laxer – at least to start with – was walking with these boys, ensuring that no animal was allowed to wander. Set out ahead of the column at angles of forty-five degrees, like probing horns, rode Mzingeli and Ntini as scouts, each equally proud of his new mount.

It was, felt Fonthill, looking around him, a well-equipped, well-organised convoy, and, he reflected grimly, it needed to be. Their route lay over untrammelled territory that bristled with danger. Despite the sunshine and the crispness of the morning, he felt a sense of foreboding.

The first day was uneventful and easy riding, in that the veldt surrounding Kimberley was a huge plain, level and virtually featureless, even boring. The air was good but the country was dreary: the plain broken only by small, flat-topped hills, with a few thorny mimosa and a little wild jessamine poking through the thin sandy soil. Away from Kimberley, this land was arid and empty, as though it had never been farmed or occupied, and so unlike the prosperous, burgeoning town that they had just left behind them.

And so it continued for the next ten days or so, until they were well into the kingdom of King Khama, where the land became dry and arid, with the surface terrain coloured a dark red and the fresh water sources becoming few and far between, forcing them to rely on their carried reserves. The travellers met no one. It was as though they had discovered a new land, undefiled by human beings or other living things.

While they were still within a couple of days' riding of Kimberley, Fonthill had set a surreptitious watch during the hours of darkness to ensure that the precious cargo remained untouched. He, Jenkins and Mzingeli took it in turns to remain awake under their blankets for three hours at a time, keeping the boxes under surveillance, until, on the second night, Alice insisted on being added to the rota. Neither Murphy nor Laxer, nor any of the Kaffirs, however, showed the slightest interest in the cargo, and after a week Simon ended the guard duty.

The two overseers, in fact, displayed every competence. They took it in turns to spell the native drivers on the wagons' hard benches and they supervised the workers genially and managed the daily tedious outspanning and inspanning rituals with efficiency. When a little game showed itself on the plain as they neared the heart of Bechuanaland, Murphy hunted down a duiker buck and took it with a shot fired from the saddle. That night they ate boiled rice and fresh meat, the latter roasted by means of a sharpened stick thrust through it and extended over the fire, the stick leaning on the V of a forked branch pushed into the ground. They drank Kaffir beer purchased from one of the native villages that had now begun to appear. The consistency of very thin gruel and a pinkish colour, it was made from local corn, the grain of which had been left to vegetate, dried in the sun, pounded into meal and gently boiled. Jenkins pronounced it excellent – sweet, he said, 'with a slight acidity in the finish, like'. Bowing to the knowledge he had acquired as mess corporal in the 24th Regiment, they accepted his wisdom and bought several *fatchies* of it to supplement their water supply.

Alice had come to an agreement with Mzingeli that Ntini should take her dispatches back to Kimberley, from where they could be cabled to the *Morning Post* in London. It seemed that the young man knew where the cable office was – he had been employed similarly by a London businessman anxious to keep in touch with share values while on a hunting trip led by Mzingeli in the Transvaal. He was also reliable and anxious to earn the extra money that Alice promised him for providing this service. If it became necessary for her to cable while Ntini was away, she was resigned to relying on her ability to acquire a similarly trustworthy runner from local sources.

She had filed a preliminary story from Cape Town describing the purpose of their journey, the nature of their cargo and the route they would take. It was, she confessed, only a 'colour story', with little hard news. But it was a necessary preliminary sketch for what she hoped would follow.

After three and a half weeks of slow but not unpleasant progress, they reached King Khama's capital. It was little more than a collection of shacks made of mud and some timber and peopled by several hundreds of the king's rather unprepossessing subjects.

Observing them, Fonthill could well understand why the Matabeles treated them with derision. They showed little of the northern tribesmen's fine physique and posture, being smaller and diffident in bearing and not at all warlike. Their king, however, was obviously made of a different fibre. In the past, as a comparatively young man, he had fought both his father and his brother and banished them, ruling ever since with justice and kindness, while showing a bold front to Lobengula, who ever looked for an opportunity to raid into Khama's kingdom.

On arrival just outside the dusty little town, Fonthill sent a respectful message to the king, asking for his permission to camp in his capital and to pay a visit. The next day, a tall, slim, white-haired black man strolled unaccompanied into their camp. His high-cheekboned face featured a clipped beard and moustache, and he wore a well-cut European jacket, impeccably creased trousers and a wide-brimmed black hat, around whose high crown a white cloth had been wound. Khama, King of the Bechuanas, could not have cut a figure more different than that of Lobengula, King of the Matabele, had he worn the uniform of an admiral of the British fleet.

'Good morning,' he said to Fonthill. 'I am Khama. I heard that you were on your way. I trust that you have had a pleasant and safe journey,' and he extended his hand in greeting. 'I believe that you are on your way to Bulawayo?'

Simon, who had been oiling his rifle, hurriedly wiped his palm on a piece of rag, shook hands and allowed his face to slip into a momentary frown. Did *everyone* in Africa know his business? He composed himself. 'That is true, sir. Please, sit down, and may we offer you coffee or perhaps some tea?' He pulled forward a camp stool.

'Oh, I am quite happy to squat on the ground, you know. I am very much an African, you see.' He sat cross-legged on the beaten grass and, awkwardly, Fonthill sat beside him. 'But I would very much like a cup of tea. You do not have Darjeeling, by any chance, do you? I have quite acquired a taste for it, you know.'

'Darjeeling?' Simon was just able to prevent his jaw from dropping. 'I think we might be able to oblige you, sir. One moment, please.' He scrambled to his feet and called to Alice. She immediately assessed the identity of their visitor and, quickly adjusting her hair, strode forward to be introduced.

'Darjeeling?' she repeated. 'Of course, your majesty. It is our favourite. It will not take a moment.'

A minute or so later, the three sat together on the ground, drinking their tea and discussing the weather, as though they were in a vicarage garden on a sunny morning in England. Then came the question that Fonthill had been fearing.

'May I ask what it is you take across my land to the King of the Matabele?'

Simon drew in his breath. He had decided long ago that he

would not lie to the man, but he knew that to reveal that his cargo contained rifles could well bring a refusal from Khama to allow him to continue his journey through Bechuanaland, so adding many days to the trip. What to say?

'I hope your majesty will forgive me if I do not reveal the contents of my cargo,' he said. 'They are items agreed by Mr Rhodes and King Lobengula as part of the treaty recently signed between the two, and I must respect their confidentiality. However, I give you my word, sir, that these cases will not be broached during our passage through your land and that their contents will have no adverse effect on your relations with the King of the Matabele.'

He inwardly winced at the dissembling, but clutched to himself Rhodes's assurance that the Matabele army would be unable to use the rifles effectively without the sort of training that would be unavailable in this part of Africa.

A frown settled on the king's dignified features. Alice hurriedly stepped in. 'May I refill your cup, your majesty?' she asked.

'Thank you. Yes. Excellent tea.' A silence descended for a moment. Then: 'Very well. I accept your word as an English gentleman that whatever is contained in those wagons will not be used against the Bechuana people.' He gave a wistful smile. 'You know, Mr Fonthill, that we are a rather poor country, with few mineral resources, in that most of our land is a kind of desert. My people are not aggressive and, unlike the Matabele, do not take easily to fighting. We are pastoral, not warlike. I would not wish to have the uneasy balance between these two countries swing unfairly towards our militant neighbours.' The smile deepened. 'I am sure you understand me.'

Fonthill felt a wave of sympathy towards this urbane man.

He also felt guilty. Could he relieve Khama's fears, at least slightly, without compromising his position? 'I quite understand, your majesty,' he said, 'and I echo your sentiments. As I understand it, if this cargo has any significance outside Matabeleland, it would lie mainly towards the Transvaal.'

'Mmm.' The king did not look exactly mollified. 'Excellent tea,' he said again to Alice. 'Thank you very much.' He stood. 'You may proceed, and I wish you a safe journey.'

'Thank you, sir.'

'There is, however, one further point on which I fear I can offer no indulgence.'

'Sir?'

Khama nodded, and his face was grave. 'Yes. Alcohol. We make our own very good beer, Mr Fonthill, but one must drink a substantial amount before it affects the senses, and on the whole it does not produce drunkenness in my people. This is not true, however, with the white man's spirits. It is against the law here to sell such substances to the native people of Bechuanaland. It corrupts their health and their behaviour. Do you follow?'

Fonthill inclined his head. 'Of course, sir. We do carry some whisky and a little Cape brandy, but I will ensure that while we are in Bechuanaland it is consumed only by us – and then moderately.'

'Good. Now tell me the route you expect to take.'

'We shall follow the north road towards Tuli and cross there.'

'Umph. Dangerous country. Keep a good watch.'

'So I have been told.'

'Come and say goodbye before you leave.'

'We will, your majesty. Thank you for your visit.'

The tall man bent down and brushed a few strands of grass

from his trousers, then he looked around, gave a cheery wave of his hand to the company and sauntered away.

'Wow,' said Alice. 'What an interesting man. He would grace any drawing room in London.'

Fonthill nodded his head. 'I feel a bit of a cad for misleading him – if I did, that is. I am sure he knew we were carrying rifles.'

'Well, you didn't tell him any lies and I think he respected you for that. We'd better be sure that Messrs Murphy and Laxer don't slyly sell the odd bottle of whisky, though.'

'Oh I think we can trust them now, but I will warn them of course.'

That evening, after sharing a customary dram, Fonthill told his overseers of the king's request, and although the two exchanged glances, they seemed to accept the situation well enough.

The little party stayed for one more day in Palapye, resting the oxen and horses, replenishing their water containers and buying reserve stocks of biltong, the strips of dried meat that sustained natives and whites alike on long journeys throughout South Africa. Before leaving, Alice and Simon called on the king, but he was away from the capital. They left a scribbled note of farewell, together with their remaining bags of Darjeeling tea.

'I've only met two African kings so far,' mused Alice to Simon as they rode off to the north. 'One likes the finest French wine and the other the best Indian tea. Strange. Do you think they're all like that?'

'Why not? Why shouldn't they share the benefits of civilisation? Why should it be only English devils that sing the best tunes?'

As the little cavalcade journeyed further north, it became

clear that the terrain was becoming drier, with the few watercourses they crossed completely bereft of any form of liquid. So on the second night after leaving Palapye, they made their camp early, near a small village that had settled around a waterhole. Here, Fonthill ordered Laxer to replenish a couple of their *fatchies*.

The little man had been gone more than half an hour before he returned, carrying the bulging water bags and, incongruously, a small elephant tusk under his arm.

'I bought it orf the black fellers, missus, fer 'alf a crown,' he explained to Alice. 'Not bad tradin', I fort, eh?' And he grinned, showing blackened teeth.

'Bloody good,' agreed Jenkins. 'Let's 'ave a look, then.' He took the tusk and scratched it with his thumbnail. 'Seems genuine all right,' he said, handing it back. 'Worth about thirty quid back in the Cape, I'd say.'

Shortly afterwards, as Fonthill was attempting to light a fire under some carefully husbanded dried oxen dung, Jenkins squatted down beside him. 'I thought so, bach sir,' he said. 'There's a whisky bottle missin' from the store.'

'What? Are you sure?'

'Oh, it's gone, right enough. I counted this mornin' an' we're one down since then an' we 'aven't pulled a cork today. That little bastard Laxer must 'ave pinched one and took it into the village to trade for that bit of ivory. 'E knows its value well enough. I thought 'is shirt was bulgin' a bit as 'e walked off. 'E's a sneaky piece of work, that one, look you.'

'Right. Come with me.'

Together they strode to where Murphy was pegging out the tent he shared with Laxer. The little Cockney was inside, unrolling their bedding.

'Laxer,' called Fonthill. 'Come out here.'

'Yes, guv.'

'How much did you say you paid for that ivory?'

A hunted look came into Laxer's face. 'Two an' six, guv.'

'No it wasn't. It was a bottle of whisky, wasn't it?'

'No, I promise yer. On me mother's deathbed. It woren't me.'

Fonthill sighed. 'Don't lie. Bring out that damned ivory. We will go together and take it back and recover what might be left of the whisky. I told you that on no account must we sell spirits to the natives.'

'Well, your honour,' Murphy interjected, 'I 'spect old Jim 'ere thought that just one little bottle wouldn't 'urt, so far out 'ere in the bush, bless you. We was goin' to share the proceeds o' the sale of the ivory with you all when we got back, sure we was.'

'Of course you were. Don't you bloody well lie to me as well. I'm not a fool. Now, Laxer, bring out that damned tusk and we will go to the village this minute, before the contents of that bottle has gone.'

They returned ten minutes later, a half-emptied bottle in Fonthill's hand. He threw it to Jenkins. 'Put it back in the store, 352.' He turned to the two overseers. 'I just hope the king doesn't hear of this,' he said, 'otherwise we'll be thrown out of Bechuanaland long before we reach the northern border. You have jeopardised this journey and I shall be taking ten pounds each off your wages at the end. Don't step out of line again on this expedition. Do you understand?'

Sullenly, they both shook their heads.

That evening, as the flames from the fire flickered across their faces, Fonthill took counsel with Alice, Jenkins and Mzingeli.

'With respect, bach sir,' said Jenkins, 'I don't think we can trust these two to stand by us if we run into trouble, see.'

Alice frowned. 'What do you mean by trouble?'

Jenkins squirmed on his buttocks and cast a quick apologetic look at Fonthill. 'Well, not *real* trouble, like, just if old de Sousie tries 'is 'and again, when we get into Matabillie land. O' course we can see 'im and 'is black fellers off quickly enough, but it might be a bit easier if we 'ad a couple more 'ands to back us up. Though, look you, there's not much point in 'avin' 'em if they're goin' to bunk off, is there now?'

'But it wouldn't be in their interests to flee if we are attacked, would it?' Alice looked at Simon. 'I mean, we are miles from anywhere. Where would they go?'

Fonthill sighed. 'Well, although they say they've never been here before, they've knocked about this part of the world for years and I would say that they know how to look after themselves. Anyway, they might be rogues, but I doubt if they would desert us. This is the first time they have fallen out of line. What do you think, Mzingeli?'

The tracker looked up, his face quite impassive. 'These white men no good,' he said and lapsed into silence again.

'Well,' Jenkins broke the silence, 'this Portuguese bloke – 'ow's 'e goin' to know that we're comin'? It's still bloomin' miles till we get to the border. 'Ow would 'e know we're on our way, like?'

Fonthill gave a sad grin. 'I'm afraid everybody in Africa seems to know where we're going and why, old chap. I think de Sousa will have picked up the vibrations by now. Anyway,' he sighed, 'I don't think we have much of a choice. We must soldier on but keeping an eye on these fellows.'

The next two days passed uneventfully, but progress was slow, for the wagons were now being forced to cross more and more dongas, where everyone – even Alice – was needed to manhandle them up and down the steep sides of the dried-up watercourses, as the oxen strained and pulled up ahead. The party was quite defenceless at these times, but Fonthill believed that they were too far away from the border – even from the Tuli Block – to expect trouble. Even so, he instigated a night watch, with all the white men taking it in turns to stand to throughout the hours of darkness.

Shortly before dawn on the fifth morning after leaving Palapye, Fonthill was shaken awake by Jenkins. 'They've 'opped it,' said the Welshman.

'What?'

'Both of 'em, gone, an they've taken two 'orses an' the mule with 'em.'

'Have they taken anything else?'

''Aven't looked yet.'

'Damn.' Simon pulled his shirt over his head. 'If they've taken the mule, it must mean that they have stolen part of our load. Oh hell. I shouldn't have put them on watch on the same night. Stupid of me.'

Together they ran to the wagons. The full complement of boxes containing the rifles and the cartridges remained, but two were missing from the wagon containing the gold. A slow smile crept over Fonthill's face.

'The fools have taken boxes containing nothing more than stones,' he said. 'Oh, I would love to be there when they open those.'

Jenkins returned the grin. 'Very clever of you to mix 'em up. But are you sure they've not taken the right one?'

'No.' Fonthill showed him a faint mark on the back of what seemed to be an identical box to the others. 'This one carries the gold sovereigns. They obviously thought they were all full of coins – as they were supposed to – but couldn't take the lot with just one mule. So they took just two to set themselves up for life. Well, well, well . . .'

'They'll be miles away by now, bach sir. Best to let 'em go an' good riddance, eh?'

Fonthill shook his head. 'They can keep their precious stones, but I'm damned if I'm going to let them get away with two horses, two rifles and old Mzingeli's mule. I'm going after them. Wake the others up, I don't want to waste a minute.'

'Right, I'll come with you.'

'No. I want you to stay here to protect the camp. I will just take Mzingeli – I may need a tracker.'

'Oh blimey . . .'

'No arguments, Jenkins. There is precious cargo here of all kinds. I want you here to protect it. I think we are too far away from the border to be in danger, but you never know. Put the wagons into a laager and keep a good watch.'

Fonthill and Mzingeli stayed just long enough to fill their water bottles, stuff biltong into their pockets and drink one cup of coffee each before they kicked their heels into the flanks of their mounts. The sun tipped the flat horizon and sent their shadows long over the red earth as they rode away.

Chapter 8

It was not difficult to follow the trail, for the hoofprints were clear on the soft earth of the desert, and Mzingeli's skills were needed only when patches of rock and the occasional spread of dry, wispy vegetation made the ground unreceptive.

'How far ahead are they, do you think?' asked Fonthill.

Mzingeli shrugged. 'Maybe two, three hours. But they don't go fast. Look.' He pointed to the smaller spoor of the mule. 'Mule heavy loaded. Sink into ground. Slows them. Maybe we catch up when sun is at highest. They stop then, I think, to eat.' He shot a quick glance at Fonthill. 'They know we come after them. Yes?'

Simon frowned. 'I don't know. It depends, I think, if they have been able to break open the boxes. If they do and they find just pebbles, then of course they will be furious, but they may well think we would not bother to track them, so they won't be on their guard.' He urged his horse on. 'But I think they will have difficulty in opening the cases, so we must be careful on our approach when we do catch up. They both have good rifles and Murphy, at least, can shoot.'

They rode on during what Fonthill felt must surely be the hottest morning of the journey so far. The heat forced them to allow their horses to find their own, plodding pace and perspiration dripped down from the sweatband of Simon's hat, making it difficult to see very far ahead. His head was down and his horse had almost collided with that of Mzingeli before he realised that his companion ahead had halted with raised hand. The tracker pointed to the ground. Small spots of blood, not yet dry, lay on the earth, melding in so well to the soil that they could only be discerned by a man with Mzingeli's skill.

'They worried,' he said. 'They want to go faster. They beat my mule. Near now, I think.'

'If they are hurrying, that means that they are expecting to be followed.' Fonthill stood high in his stirrups and concentrated on looking ahead. He could see nothing. 'Can you see them yet?'

The slim man raised himself similarly and shaded his eyes. For a moment he did not speak, and then, 'Ah yes. I think. Maybe half a mile or more. I think they stop.'

'Good. In that case, let us dismount so that there is less of a profile of us on their horizon.' Fonthill pulled out his compass and took a rough bearing. 'I would like to get round them while they are eating, so that we can approach them from the south. They will not expect us to come that way.' He looked hard at the black man. 'Mzingeli, I do not want to harm these men if I can help it. But if they do resort to violence, then we must both shoot to kill.'

The tracker nodded his head slowly but said nothing.

'Right. Let's go. I will rely on you to keep them in sight – but only just. I don't want them to know that we have caught up.'

They dismounted, slipped a round each into their Martini-Henrys, and set off at a tangent, leading their horses. It took them nearly an hour before Mzingeli nodded and pointed back to their left. 'They back there,' he said. 'I think they lie down under some sort of shade.'

'Good. Perhaps we can take them while they sleep.'

The two mounted and urged their horses into a quiet trot. It soon became apparent to Fonthill that Murphy and Laxer had indeed used their tent awning to provide them with shade from the midday glare. His lip curled as he noticed that the poor mule had been left tethered in the sun with the two heavy boxes, still unopened, strapped to its back and hanging down on either flank. The horses stood close beside the mule. As they neared, Simon could see two pairs of boots sticking out from under the awning. The overseers appeared to be asleep.

But they were not. At about one hundred yards away, Mzingeli pointed. The boots were unattached to human limbs and merely propped up against the edge of the awning. The whereabouts of their owners became clear as two shots rang out from behind the horses, where Murphy and Laxer had been taking cover. The bullets sang over the heads of the approaching horsemen and Fonthill made an immediate decision.

'Don't fire,' he cried. 'We'll charge at them while they are reloading. Go quickly, NOW!'

Remembering a technique used by Jenkins years ago, Simon let out a penetrating shriek and dug his heels sharply into his mount's flanks. Heads down, the two galloped towards the little group of horses, mule and men, with Mzingeli screaming his own tribal cry, dredged up, Fonthill presumed, from distant days when the Malakala were more warlike. The combination of the gunshots, the shrieks and the thunder of the hooves bearing down on them had the effect of causing the overseers' horses to rear and scatter, knocking the two men to the ground and sending spinning away their rifles and the cartridges they were clumsily trying to insert.

Fonthill reined in and pointed his rifle at the men as they tried to scramble after their guns. 'Stay down or I will fire,' he cried. 'Lie flat, I say.'

Murphy looked up over his shoulder. 'Don't shoot, your honour,' he cried. 'We're not armed.'

'I said lie flat. Go on. Faces on the earth.' Fonthill's voice was emotionless. 'You are liars as well as thieves.' He seemed now to address Mzingeli. 'Best thing is to put two shots in their spines and just leave them to the vultures. Save both of us a lot of time and trouble. No one is going to miss scum like this.'

'Now, now, sor.' Murphy's voice was high-pitched. 'That wouldn't be the action of a gentleman, so it wouldn't. You couldn't do that, now. I admit we did you wrong but we didn't cause you harm. Sure, we only took two o' the boxes now. We left you the rest, did we not?'

'You only took two because you couldn't carry more. I'm not a fool. Stay down! Faces to the earth. That's better. Mzingeli, get their rifles and bring back the horses and the mule.'

As Mzingeli busied himself with retrieving the horses and the mule – none had gone far, and the poor beast of burden had only trotted a few yards – the little tableau in the desert was maintained for five minutes or more, with the two overseers lying spreadeagled, faces down on the hot ground, and Fonthill remaining in the saddle, keeping the men covered with his Colt as his mount shuffled in a half-circle and then back again. Eventually the tracker returned, leading the horses and the mule, with the Martini-Henrys lying across his saddle. He looked expectantly at Simon, with a faint gleam of amusement in his eye.

'We kill them now, Nkosi?' he enquired.

'No, mate.' Laxer's voice was a whine, as he spoke with his nose pressed against the red soil. 'Don't shoot us. We never meant no 'arm, honest.'

Murphy's plea was almost a shriek. 'Don't shoot, your honour. I'm sorry, I really am. We're white men like you, so we are. You can't kill us in this terrible country. It would be an unchristian act, so it would.'

Fonthill grinned across at Mzingeli. 'Oh, very well.' Slowly he dismounted and gestured to the two with his revolver. 'Get up. You, Laxer, go and get your boots. Cover him with your rifle as he goes, Mzingeli, and if he moves sharply shoot him.

'Now,' he addressed Murphy. 'Do you have full water bottles?'

'What? Oh yes, your honour. More or less.'

'Right. We will top up your bottles from our reserves. Do you have knives?'

'Oh yes, sor. We have knives.'

'Good. You may need them if you are attacked, because I am taking back the rifles, your horses and the mule, of course. They are not your property anyway. I don't think this is lion country, but I know the beasts are about just a mile or two north, so you had better be prepared when you sleep. Oh, you can have your tent, of course. It will be a long walk back to Palapye, but if you keep the sun on your backs more or less, you will keep going south and you can follow our tracks. They are not going to be washed away by rain, that's for sure.'

Murphy wiped his brow with the back of his hand. 'Aw, yer

not goin' to leave us unprotected in lion country, are yer? Yer can't do that, man.'

'Oh yes I can. If I give you the rifles, you could well come after us. No, my friend. As I said, I don't think this is lion country, but one or two could well come this far south. So thread the tent up tightly at night.'

Fonthill grinned. 'Got the boots? Good. Mzingeli, top up their water bottles, there's a good fellow, and give the horses, and particularly the mule, a drink from your hat.'

Five minutes later, Mzingeli linked up the three animals on a leading rein and slowly walked them away to the north. Fonthill mounted his own beast and looked down at the overseers.

'You've been dishonest and stupid,' he said. 'If your greed hadn't taken over, you would have been well paid for this journey. As it is, you won't get a penny. Now, start packing that tent.'

The two men looked up at him with hatred in their gaze. Laxer was about to say something but, seeing the steel in Fonthill's eyes, decided against it, and the pair trudged back to the tent and began striking the awning. Without a backward glance, Simon rode away after his tracker.

The black man gave him one of his rare grins. 'You would not kill them, Nkosi?' he asked.

Fonthill smiled grimly. 'Only if it turned into a gun fight. Then there would have been no alternative. No, I just wanted to frighten them. I think it worked.'

'Oh yes. It worked. They frightened.'

It was after dark when the two returned to the camp to find a fidgety Jenkins on guard and a relieved Alice tending a fire within a loose circle made by the wagons. The oxen had been put to graze on whatever vegetation they could find on the unpromising earth, with a boy to watch over them.

'Why didn't you leave the boxes with the stones?' asked Alice.

'Because we may just need them again, to serve the same purpose.' Fonthill turned to Jenkins. 'We will need to stand guard from now on, 352,' he said. 'I don't think those two will bother us again, but you never know, and it won't be long before we are back in lion country, and our oxen and horses are precious.'

He turned to Mzingeli. 'Can we put Ntini in charge of the boys, do you think?'

The tracker nodded.

'Good. Then tell him he must put the boys on a guard rota for the animals through the night, and we three will do the same for the camp.'

'Not three,' said Alice over her shoulder. 'Four.'

Fonthill sighed. 'Very well. Four it shall be.'

The next few days proved uneventful as they resumed their journey north. The guard watch was maintained each night, with Alice taking her turn (and Fonthill struggling to stay awake on her watch to ensure her safety), and Mzingeli circled the camp each morning to look for signs of nocturnal visitors. It became clear, however, that the overseers had decided to leave well alone, and as the days rolled by, they felt able to relax their guard a little.

The going was now much more difficult. As they neared the Sashe river, which for a short way formed the border between this part of Bechuanaland and Matabeleland, the semi-desert gave way to more broken country, with tall kopjes standing up like broken teeth from terrain that had become more verdant, and thorny plants hindering their progress. Particularly annoying were the wagt-jen-betges, or 'wait-a-bit', a generic name for plants that had double thorns, one slender and outward-pointing and the other curled backwards from it. They caught and held the clothing and often reduced it to rags.

Fonthill's mind had been occupied for some time with de Sousa. Given the way news travelled in this barren country, it was likely that the Portuguese knew of their coming. Would he make an effort to stop the arms reaching Lobengula and so cementing his treaty with Rhodes? It was highly likely, and after the first reverse, he would probably bring more men with him to attack this second time. Once across the river, the expedition would enter the densely wooded country of southern Matabeleland, and this would be the most likely place for the Portuguese to strike. Simon confided as much to his companions.

'We know that country,' he went on, 'and it's difficult to see through the bush for a hundred yards. I think that's where he will hit us if he does. What do you two think?' He nodded towards Jenkins.

'Well, bach sir, the thinkin' bit is your department, but that sounds about right to me.' The Welshman frowned. 'What worries me is that now that them two rascals 'ave gone a-walkin', like, we're a bit light-'anded in the fightin' department, see.'

Fonthill nodded. 'True. Mzingeli, can Ntini use a Martini-Henry, do you think?'

'Not good yet. Perhaps Nkosi can teach?'

'Good idea. Better Jenkins than me, though. Can you teach him, 352?'

'Certainly. Would you care to join the class, bach sir?'

'That will be enough of that. What about any of the boys, Mzingeli? Could we trust them to use a rifle properly?'

'Only one. Boers call him Joshua. Lead driver. Good boy. He has fired the Snider. Give him lessons too.'

'Very well. See to it, Jenkins. I think we are safe until we are across the Sashe.'

But they were not. On the sixth day after losing their overseers, Mzingeli, who had ridden on far ahead as usual, could be seen in the distance galloping back towards the wagons. Reining in, he called to Fonthill: 'Tree across track further up. Not blown down. Cut down by axe. Fresh marks on stump. Could be . . . what you call it?'

'Ambush?'

'That is word.'

'Did you see anybody?'

'No.' He used his hands to gesture. 'Two kopjes close together, like this, about mile away. Trail narrow down. I see tree down on other side of kopjes. Other side is plenty bush. I think men hide there but I don't see.'

'Did they see you?'

'I think no. I get off horse long way off and take look, very careful. Keep hidden.'

'Good.'

'I think they expect us to ride through, stop at tree and then they come back and front, all around. We . . . ah . . . strung out. They kill us easy.'

'Mzingeli, you should be a general. Now, get Joshua to circle the wagons here in the open, and have Ntini get the boys to drive the oxen and horses inside the laager. It's going to be very crowded with the cattle in here, so we will have to space the wagons out a little and somehow fill in the gaps. We must be quick. They will come at us immediately they realise that we have sensed what they are up to, and we don't want them down upon us before we've laagered. Alice . . . yes, what is it?'

His wife had taken out her notebook and her pencil was

poised. 'Exactly how many are there of us to fight now?' she enquired.

'Er . . . ten boys, Mzingeli, Ntini and the three of us.'

She scribbled in her book. 'And how many rifles?'

'Why do you need to . . . Oh well. We have five Martini-Henrys, the Snider and your hunting rifle.' Alice wrote down the figure.

A touch of exasperation now crept into Fonthill's voice. 'Since you are so interested in our firepower, perhaps you would break out the ammunition and distribute the spare rifles. Jenkins, you come with me.'

'Where're we goin', then? To fight 'em single-handed?'

'Not quite. If there are many of them, we could have our hands full keeping them off, given that our firepower has been sadly reduced. But I have an idea.' Fonthill looked around carefully. 'It's good that we're in a nice open spot, before the bush begins. Come on, we've got to work quickly.'

He strode towards the wagon that housed the bedding and tents and extracted from under the cargo two small kegs of powder. They had been taken along as an afterthought in case the expedition needed to manufacture its own cartridges. So far they had not been opened. Fonthill rummaged again and produced a small bottle of lamp oil and then a bottle of Cape brandy. Quickly he twisted out the cork and threw away half the brandy.

''Ere' bach,' wailed Jenkins. 'Steady on. That's good stuff.'

'If it is, it may save our lives.' He unstoppered the lamp oil and, again, threw away half its contents. Then he took two of their tin cups and filled one with brandy and the other with lamp oil, before pouring the contents back into the wrong bottles so that each contained a mixture of brandy and oil. He then tore his handkerchief in half, poured a little of the mixture on to each half so that it was thoroughly soaked and laid them to one side. As a puzzled Jenkins watched, Fonthill then withdrew the cork from one of the powder kegs and poured a little powder into each bottle so that it was completely full. His last act was to screw up the wet pieces of fabric and twist them into the tops of the bottles as substitute corks.

A slow smile spread across Jenkins's face. 'Ah,' he said, 'bombs, is it?'

'Not as such. I am not sure that they would explode when I want them to, or if the explosion would be effective. But I am damned sure that they will burn for a short while, and that's all I want. Pick up the kegs and come along.'

Down from the wagon, Fonthill pointed to the edge of the scrub, which stopped some two hundred yards from the trail and ran parallel to it on both sides of the camp.

'The oxen have beaten out all the vegetation from the trail to there,' he said. 'So a fire wouldn't cross these strips either side of our wagons. But it would take hold deeper in the bush. I want you to spread a thin trail of powder just inside the edge of the vegetation all the way round the camp in a rough circle.'

Jenkins frowned. 'What are we doin' with the bottles, then? You can't 'ave wasted good grog for nothin', surely?'

'No.' Fonthill looked ahead down the trail. It twisted a little over ground that undulated, so that the distant twin kopjes could not be seen. 'Good. It looks as though they didn't spot Mzingeli. That means they're still waiting for us and we've got a few more minutes yet. But when we don't turn up, they'll send scouts out to look for us and then they'll attack. But at least we can face them in the open.'

'Yes, that's all very well, but what are we doin' with the bloody bottles, look you?'

'Don't worry about them. That's my department – until I call you in, that is. When you cross the open space, across the trail itself, make sure that you continue the powder line so that there's an unbroken circle of the stuff.'

Jenkins nodded. 'Just inside the edge of the bush, then?'

'Yes. Off you go, there's no time to lose.'

The Welshman pulled a face and, keg under each arm, set off. 'With respect, bach sir,' he called back over his shoulder, 'I do not approve of the use of alcohol in this way – even though I don't know what you're goin' to be doin' with it. It could set a bad example to the natives.'

Fonthill watched him go and then turned to observe Mzingeli directing the formation of the laager. The boys were cracking their long whips, and slowly, agonisingly slowly, the five wagons were being pulled into a small, very irregular circle within which the oxen and the horses were now being herded. It was becoming clear that there were not sufficient wagons to form a tight circle big enough to enclose the beasts, and as the oxen were freed from their traces, Simon rushed to help Mzingeli tie the long boom of each wagon to the rear of that in front to extend the perimeter of the ring. Even so, a space had to be left between some of the wagons and the booms to stretch the ring and accommodate the animals.

'We have to fill these gaps,' he called to Mzingeli. 'Get some of the boys to cut thorn bushes and pile them under the booms and in the spaces. Bring bedding and whatever else they can carry.'

He turned and noted that Alice had carefully laid out the Martini-Henrys, her own hunting rifle and Mzingeli's Snider at intervals around the ring, with piles of cartridges beside each one. Her action, however, had only underlined the paucity of their firepower. Seven rifles – two of them of doubtful efficiency – against ... how many? He shrugged. Out in the bush, Jenkins had almost completed his circle. Well, they would soon find out how effective his plan would be.

He walked back to the wagon from which they had taken the kegs and picked up the two bottles. Carrying them carefully, he strode out into the bush and located the powder trail at an angle of ninety degrees to one side of the flattened circle formed by the wagons. There he found a thorn bush of the size he was seeking and which was just a touch away from the powder line. He smeared dust over the bottle so that it would not reflect light from the sun and would be, if not invisible, then at least difficult to distinguish. Gingerly he placed the bottle at the base of the bush and partially concealed within it. With his knife he cut away a large branch and wedged it at the top of the bush, so that it stood out clearly. Running now, he took the remaining bottle into the vegetation on the opposite side of the wagons and repeated the same operation.

Back inside the laager he met Jenkins, smelling of gunpowder. 'Brush those trousers, for God's sake,' he said. 'If you get a misfire on your rifle, you'll go up in smoke.'

'Blimey, yes. Very good, sir.' Jenkins shielded his eyes from the sun and looked northward. 'Can't see a bleedin' thing,' he said. 'Nothin' movin' up there, as far as I can tell.' He turned back to Fonthill, brushing his breeches with a soiled handkerchief. 'Maybe old Jelly was mistaken, eh? You said yourself that these blokes wouldn't come at us until we were in Mattabellyland. Perhaps that tree just fell down because these bloody ants that creep under my blanket 'ad a go at it. What d'you think, bach sir?'

Fonthill shook his head. 'Mzingeli has a sixth sense for these things. I think they have come to get us here – if they are de Sousa's men, that is, and I think they are. He's crossed the river because we are in that disputed area of no-man's-land where nobody is going to worry about a fight. If he attacked us in Matabeleland, he could well upset the king, given the nature of our cargo. No. They are out there all right.'

He looked around. The formation of the laager was almost complete. Inside the ring, it was ridiculously crowded. The cattle and horses were pressed together into an almost solid mass. How would they react when the shooting began? He had read somewhere that oxen never stampeded, and the sensitive horses had been put in the middle of these placid beasts. But fire? Smoke and flames?

An additional thought struck him. 'Where the hell is Alice?' he cried.

Jenkins pointed. 'In that wagon. Writin' somethin', look you. Dunno what, though.'

Frowning, Fonthill pushed his way between the milling oxen and climbed into the wagon. 'What on earth are you doing, darling?'

She looked up, her pencil between her teeth, her fair hair straggling down from under her wide-brimmed hat. 'What the hell do you think I'm doing?' She glowered. 'I'm writing my story, of course.'

'Oh, lord!' Then he grinned, a touch soulfully. 'I wish I shared your confidence that we shall come through this so that you can write a piece about it all.'

She knocked back her hat so that it hung down her back, held only by the thong around her throat. Then she smiled and leaned across to plant a kiss on his chin. 'Of *course* we shall come through this, my love,' she whispered into his ear.

'We are led by those two Great Indestructibles, Fonthill and Jenkins, Soldiers of the Queen and Heroes of the Empire. And if we don't, I personally shall be very annoyed, because I have the germ of a great story here. What's more, it is exclusive and I am setting the scene for it now.'

He stayed silent for a moment, looking at her. Then he cupped her chin within his hands. 'Oh, Alice,' he said. 'I am so sorry to put you in this danger.'

She thrust his hands away. 'Rubbish. Simon, you really must stop treating me like a china doll. It's true that I haven't gone through as many scrapes as you and 352, but there have been a few now and I have every confidence in you, my love. Now, kindly leave me to finish the first part of this masterpiece. But rest assured that I shall not be scribbling when these people attack.' She smiled up at him. 'I have my rifle here and, look, a pile of cartridges. I shall play my part in the defence.'

He seized her hand, kissed it and jumped down from the wagon. Some of the boys were tying the last boom and others were milling about among the oxen, pushing their way through, talking softly to each beast and scratching their ears as if to reassure them. Fonthill called Mzingeli.

'Do the boys without rifles have assegais?' he asked.

'Yes, Nkosi. But they frightened of Matabele.'

'Yes, I thought so. Please tell them that if we are attacked, it will not be by the Matabele. These will be Bantu from the Mozambique border, slaves of the Portuguese who are being pushed into this by their master. They are not warriors. The boys must fight with us. Spread them out to stand with their spears by the thorn bushes between the wagons. Those that fight well will be given an ox each when we reach Bulawayo. I promise that.'

Mzingeli nodded his head slowly. 'A good thing—' he began. But he was interrupted by a shout from Jenkins.

''Ere they come at last, bach sir.'

Simon jumped on to a wagon boom and looked northwards along the trail. At this distance they appeared merely as a black blob, but as he focused his field glasses, he realised that – whatever he had told his own Kaffirs – these were indeed warriors. Each man carried a large shield, and he could see plumes nodding above them. They were too indistinct to count and he could catch no glimpse of any European amongst them, nor whether they carried rifles. But as he watched, they began to fan out on either side of the trail, trotting Zulu style, quite quickly. There were clearly enough of them to surround the ring of wagons.

He turned to shout to Mzingeli, but the tracker was already walking among the Kaffirs, quietly talking to them and dispatching little groups in turn to gather their assegais and man the gaps between the wagons where the thorn bushes, mattresses and boxes had been wedged to form very insubstantial barriers. He let the man be and turned to Jenkins, now at his side.

'Right, old chap.' He pointed to where a tall branch on either side of the laager marked the sites of the two bottles. 'See those branches?'

'Yes.'

'At the base of each bush I have hidden my fire bottles. When I give the word, I want you to fire at the base of the bushes – it will probably take a couple of shots or more – to hit the bottles and set them afire. I am gambling that they will fall on to the powder trail, spark if off and so set the bush alight. But it is important to wait until sufficient of the blacks are between us and the trail, so that the blaze will spring up behind them and put the fear of God into them.'

Jenkins's eyes gleamed. 'Ah, now I see. But 'ang on. What if I can't see the bleedin' bottles for the black fellers in between?'

'Then you must get into a high position on top of one of the wagons where you can see and fire downwards.' He grinned. 'You keep telling me that you were the best shot in the British Army. Hit the bottles and I will give you an ox for each one.'

'Oh thank you very much. What would I do with a bleedin' ox?' But he was already clambering up on to the side board of one of the wagons. He called down. 'It might just work.'

'Good.' Fonthill climbed up beside Jenkins and looked north along the trail. The approaching warriors were now running and spreading out further to encircle the wagons. He made a quick estimation: about fifty, perhaps fewer, but still no sign of rifles being carried. They had about four minutes.

He jumped down. The boys were now carrying their spears and running to the thorn bush barriers. He called to Mzingeli: 'Bring Ntini and Joshua here and interpret for me. Alice and Jenkins, join me here, quickly.'

The little circle gathered around him. 'Alice has already spread the rifles,' he said. 'Each of you take up position in one of the wagons, where you will find the rifles. Alice, I leave it to you whether you use Mzingeli's Snider or your own hunting rifle.'

'I will use my own,' she said. 'I will be more accurate with that.'

'Very well. You will each have a wagon. Pile up whatever you can find to fire behind. They may have rifles. I will stay more or less in the centre to reinforce whichever wagon is under most pressure. Do not fire until I give the order, and then ... shoot to kill. Oh, Mzingeli. Perhaps it might be a good idea to put two of the boys in among the animals to quieten them if things get ... er ... hot. Yes?'

Mzengili, ever economical with words, nodded, interpreted for Ntini and Joshua and then ran off to find two herdsmen from the boys manning the gaps in the wagons. As the group broke up, Simon pulled Alice back. 'I will be right behind you, my darling.'

She gulped but regarded him steadily. 'Yes, thank you,' she said. 'I may just need that.'

Fonthill thrust a box of matches into his breeches and then climbed up again on to one of the booms and watched as the warriors halted, spread out across the track, some two hundred and fifty yards away. He could now see that they seemed to be wearing full warpaint, and that they had monkey's or cow's tails attached, garter-like, just below their knees and elbows and, from what he could see behind their shields, more across their chests, suspended from neck-laces. They stood in silence, perhaps waiting for orders. Simon could see no European, nor any evidence that the warriors were armed with anything other than spears, although these were not black-bladed like those of the Matabele, but shone silver in the morning sun.

'Who are they, Mzingeli?' he called. 'Where are they from?'

The tracker climbed up beside him. He was silent for a while. Then: 'Not sure. Not Matabele. Maybe Zulu.'

Fonthill's heart sank. Although they had been finally defeated by the British at Ulundi eleven years before, the Zulus remained among the finest fighting men in Africa. They were the bravest of the brave. 'They can't be, can they?' he pleaded. 'Their homeland is about eight hundred miles away.'

'Yes. You right. Not Zulu. Perhaps Swazi.'

Simon gulped. That was no improvement. The Swazis were fierce enough and he had seen how well they fought when they had joined forces with Wolseley to defeat the Sekukuni tribe some nine years before on the Transvaal border with Portuguese East Africa. But they too would have been forced to travel a vast distance to link up with – and be paid by – de Sousa. Unlikely.

His supposition was interrupted by a great cry as the warriors lifted their spears and shields and stamped their feet.

Mzingeli did not change his expression but spat. 'Not Swazi cry,' he said. 'Minor tribe from east. Look good but not fight well.'

It became clear that the cry was some form of salute, for Fonthill saw their front rank open for a moment and a pale figure in a familiar yellow uniform push through. He stood still for a moment as he surveyed the pathetic little laager before him, his outline reduced by the tall warriors flanking him.

'Can you see him?' Fonthill called softly to Jenkins.

'Just about, bach sir. Shall I try?'

'No.' Then into Simon's mind's eye came the image of the puff adder, poised to strike. He did not hesitate. 'Don't try,' he called. 'Kill the bastard.'

The shot rang out clearly and de Sousa staggered for a moment, clutching his shoulder, before the ranks closed around him once more. The warriors raised their shields and assegais again and shouted their war cry. Yet it seemed more a gesture of defiance than a signal to attack. They remained standing, waiting for something.

'Hold your fire,' shouted Fonthill. 'Wait until I give the

order.' Then, quietly to Mzingeli, 'Back to your post, old chap. Quickly.' He gave a reassuring grin to the boys crouched under him behind the thorns, and remained standing on the boom. If there were rifles among the warriors he wished to draw their fire. No answering shot came, however, and he frowned as he looked at the ranks ahead of him, still bunched together. It was not an overwhelming force, but his worry remained that they would fan out completely, surround the wagons and then attack all at the same time. With one gun per wagon, and only three reasonable shots among them, it was highly unlikely that a concerted attack could be withstood. If, however, the natives attacked in a tight bunch on one side only, relying on overwhelming force concentrated on one target – which was a usual tactic – then he might be able to reinforce the attacked side.

He shouted to Jenkins: 'If they bunch and attack just one side, leave your post and join me in firing from that side.'

'Very good, bach sir.'

Then he heard a cry from among the line of warriors. It was not delivered in the normal guttural deep bass of the Bantu. More a high-pitched shriek – Portuguese? It was enough, and the warriors immediately broke into a loose run towards the north-facing wagon, in which crouched Alice. His heart in his mouth, Fonthill waited for a moment to see if the attacking line would deploy to spill around the little circle, but it did not. It came straight for Alice's wagon.

'On the north side, 352,' shouted Simon. 'FIRE!'

A ragged volley ensued and Fonthill rushed to the side of Alice's wagon. It brought down just two warriors, but that was enough to trip up another. 'Reload,' shouted Simon. 'Wait ... FIRE! This time three attackers fell, and then Fonthill realised that Mzingeli was at his side. 'Reload,' he ordered, and then, again, 'FIRE!' This time the range was considerably shortened and four warriors fell, showing that Alice, too, was causing damage.

It was enough to halt the attack, and the line stopped at a distance of about one hundred yards as the warriors faltered and then stood, undecided, waving their spears and shouting. Fonthill tasted again that familiar acrid powder on his lips and smelled the cordite as it entered his nostrils. The old elation of battle, first savoured – albeit for only a tragically brief moment – at Isandlwana returned, and he grinned as he thumbed another cartridge into the breech. 'Let's give them another while they're standing,' he screamed. 'FIRE!'

It was impossible to miss at that range, and the line immediately broke, turned and fled, leaving ten bodies on the dusty ground, two of them slowly attempting to move. The boys at the thorn bushes raised their assegais and hurled derision at the retreating warriors.

'Are you all right, Alice?' Fonthill called.

'All is right in this wagon, sir. Although I have to say that this gun smoke is ruining my hair . . .'

'Good girl. Anyone hurt, Mzingeli?'

'No, Nkosi. They not really near enough to throw spears. Next time perhaps.'

'Hmm.' Would they come again? They had lost about a fifth of their number, and if they had any sense, they would spread out and attack from all sides at once. It depended upon whether there was leadership in their ranks. Had Jenkins finished off de Sousa?'

He called up to the Welshman. 'Good shooting, 352. It looks as though you got the Portuguese.'

'Oh yes, bach sir, I got 'im all right, but only in the bloody shoulder, see. It was a bit long range to be accurate an' he was partly covered by the black fellers either side of 'im. I wish 'e would do somethin' brave, like, an' lead a charge.'

'Fat chance of that.'

'Will they 'ave another go, then?'

'Oh yes. I think they will. But they might spread out the next time and come at us from all around. That will make it difficult.'

'Do you want me to shoot the bottles?'

'Not yet. Only if we're hard pressed. I am worried about the cattle if we start a blaze. But we will if we have to. Can you see the bushes?'

'Just about.'

'Good. Wait for the command. Mzingeli . . .'

'Nkosi.'

'If the attackers reach the spaces between the wagons, do you think the boys will stand up to them and fight?'

The tracker's face remained expressionless while he considered the question. Fonthill marvelled once more at the man's imperturbability in the face of danger. He was, after all, not a fighting man, and this certainly was not his war. He had not even asked why they were being attacked.

'They not warriors, Nkosi,' he replied. 'We will see. At least oxen behind them means they cannot run.'

It was a point. Even if the attackers broke through, they would have precious little room in which to move. Unless . . .

'But will these warriors kill the oxen?'

Mzingeli allowed the nearest that he ever came to a smile to steal across his features for a moment. 'No. Cattle are precious. Oxen not as good as breeding cows but still worth much. They want to take them when we are killed. They don't kill them—'

He was interrupted by a cry from Jenkins. 'They're doin'

what you said, bach sir. They're spreadin' out to encircle us.'

'Right. Cross to the boys in the wagons on the other side. I'll stay on this side to support Alice.'

He saw the Welshman make his way through the oxen and climb into the wagon of first Ntini and then Joshua. Each was crouching, his long Martini-Henry balanced on the edge of the wagon side boarding. Jenkins patted each boy on the shoulder and grinned at them. They both smiled back, albeit distinctly nervously. Fonthill was not sure how effective they could be, even with Jenkins to back them up, for they had not been subject to the first attack. They would be tested now, though. And he thought again of Alice.

He called across to Mzingeli. 'Ask one boy at each of the thorn bushes to get into a wagon to help fight off any natives who get through.'

The tracker lifted his rifle in acknowledgement, and Fonthill felt some reassurance as he saw the boys, smiling broadly and waving their assegais, climb into the wagons. At least *they* seemed confident enough. But was this very thin line enough to resist an attack from all sides? He looked at the cattle. The oxen had been seemingly unfazed by the gunfire and were standing, heads down, quite passively. Even the horses in their midst were trying to graze in the tiny space allowed to them. The warriors were taking their positions now, spreading out on the edge of the bush, with the powder trail behind them. No, he could not afford to wait.

'Time to shoot the bottles,' he called across to Jenkins.

The Welshman waved his rifle in acknowledgement and climbed on to the side planking of his wagon, situated next to that of Joshua. There he paused, wobbling for a moment as he wrapped an arm around one of the steel roof hoops, now bereft of their canvas covers. He raised his rifle to his shoulder . . . and paused. 'Can't see the bleedin' bush on this side,' he shouted. 'These bastards are in the way.'

'Damn! try when they start running. I'll do the one on this side.'

'All right. 'Ere they come again.'

Balancing at the end of his wagon, Fonthill raised his rifle to find the bush with the tall branch, but Jenkins was right. The attacking warriors gave him no sight of it. Forgetting the need for translation, he shouted, 'No volleys. Fire at will. FIRE!'

Once again gunfire rang out from the wagons, but on the word 'Fire', the warriors had immediately plunged to the ground, so that the bullets hissed over their heads. Now they raised themselves and continued to run towards the wagons, shrieking and brandishing their spears above their shields. But not all of them. Hurriedly ramming in another round, Fonthill had time to see three of the warriors slinking away from the charge, clearly declining to risk their lives in the last few yards of the dash to the wagons. The others, however, came on.

Again, at such short range it was impossible for anyone to miss, and Fonthill, firing from Jenkins's old wagon, felled one man, reloaded and killed another before he turned to his left, where the line was almost upon Alice's wagon. He brought down a third, who was attempting to reach up to Alice with his knobkerrie. But the boys in the wagons were now involved, and they stood manfully along the side boardings, thrusting and stabbing downwards. In his wagon, Simon joined them, swinging his rifle by the barrel as a club.

A thrown assegai thudded into the side of the wagon and he plucked it out and threw it back, swinging the gun again and smashing its heavy barrel on the head of a warrior who was attempting to climb on to a wheel. He thrust the muzzle into the face of a second, who fell back on to those behind, giving Simon time to look up. He could see the bush! Quickly – too quickly – he aimed and fired. Nothing! Before he could reload, however, there was an explosion from the other side of the compound. Turning, he saw a flame rise and then fall, before running along spluttering and dancing, virtually at ground level, as the fire took hold of the powder and then leaped into the dry brush all around. In seconds, the bush beyond the far side of the wagons was a wall of flame. It reached the edges of the vegetation but there, starved of fuel, it spluttered and died. Nevertheless, although it did not vault the barren trail, it continued to burn behind it, crackling and rising in a yellow wall, causing the attackers in front of it to run, screaming, away from the flames towards the northern part of the trail.

'Three five two,' shrieked Fonthill. 'Come over here and protect Alice. I'm going out to fire the trail. Cover me if you can.'

Without waiting for a reply, he rammed a round into the breech of his rifle and leapt down on the inside of the laager, pushing his way desperately between oxen and wagons until he reached the point nearest the end of the flame wall. He shot one attacker and then vaulted from the wagon and ran headlong through a narrow gap in the warriors until he reached the unfired end of the powder trail. There he turned, in time to swing his rifle at a large native, who took the blow on his forearm, causing him to stumble backwards. Fonthill was conscious that another attacker had been brought down by a bullet from the laager, and he crouched and fumbled for his matches, praying that one would strike first time. It spluttered into life and he just had time to roll away from an assegai thrust that plunged into the ground near his hip before the powder trail hissed and then broke into life. The fire immediately danced away until it broke into a wall of flame on reaching the vegetation, complemented by an explosion as the second bottle was reached. The laager was now in the centre of a fire storm.

Fonthill threw himself forward, away from the fire, and lay prostrate. He, however, was no longer of interest to the warriors nearest to him. The effect of the blaze and the explosion on them and the remaining attackers had been immediate. Those who had reached the wagons turned and fled, rushing into the warriors behind, so that the ground between the flaming bush and the laager became a maelstrom of black figures, silhouetted against the yellow flames.

'Keep firing,' shouted Fonthill, now crouching and running back towards the wagons, but he could not be heard above the roar of the flames. It was a superfluous order in any case. The black figures starkly illuminated against the flames made perfect targets, and the firing continued from the wagons. The terrified attackers, not knowing which way to turn at first, had now found one escape route, however. The line of powder across the trail to the north had found no vegetation to feed on and had now spluttered to extinction, leaving a narrow gap between the fires. Through it ran what was left of the attackers, hurling away their weapons as they fled.

'Alice!' shouted Fonthill, hauling himself into her wagon.

'Yes, I'm all right.' She rose from behind the little barricade she had made, her face smudged black with cordite and her eyes looking at the flames in wonder. 'What on earth have you done?'

'Just a few fireworks. Thank God you're safe. Whoa!' The

last exclamation came as the oxen nudged at the wagon, causing it to shudder. 'Boys.' He gestured to the thorn-filled gaps, and at the black figures in the wagons, who were staring wide-eyed at the flames. He pointed to their two comrades who were mingling with the oxen, attempting to soothe them, and in dumb show indicated that they should join them. He bit his lip. If the beasts did stampede, then the wagons would be easily overturned.

He jumped down himself and joined the boys, who were all now thrusting their way between the horns, patting necks, talking quietly and gently calming the animals. The horses were wide-eyed, but Mzingeli and Jenkins made their way to the middle of the herd to quieten them too, and the compound was soon more tranquil, if still a little disturbed.

They were helped by the fact that the fire had run its course on both edges of the wide trail, where the vegetation ran out and offered it no fuel, so leaving the laager untouched. The flames still ran back a little into the bush, but there was no wind and it was clear that, amongst the stony outcrops, the fire was beginning slowly to burn itself out.

'Blimey,' said Jenkins. 'Just like bonfire night, bach. Bloody good idea.' He grinned broadly. 'I'm glad I thought of it.'

Fonthill turned to the tracker. 'Mzingeli, see if any of the boys have been hurt, and Jenkins and I will make sure that the varmints have actually gone. We must be careful.'

Treading carefully, their rifles at the ready, the two moved between the figures lying around the clearing. There were, in fact, no wounded, for the range had been too short to inflict light wounds and those seen moving on the ground earlier had obviously succumbed. Even Alice's hunting rifle seemed to have proved effective. They counted twenty-three corpses and then, horrifyingly, another three blackened figures where the flames had taken them in the bush. Nowhere was there evidence of a uniformed figure.

Fonthill climbed on to the north-facing wagon and levelled his field glasses up the trail. He could clearly see the last of the retreating warriors and . . . was that a litter being carried, bearing a figure in yellow? He refocused but the distance was too great.

'Only two boys hurt little bit by spears,' reported Mzingeli. 'But they happy with fight. They think they now great warriors and are excited about the oxen promised to them.'

'Well.' Fonthill. grinned 'That's one way of getting rid of the animals when we reach Bulawayo.'

'Will they try and 'ave another go when we cross into Mattabellyland?' asked Jenkins. 'Or even, look you, on the other side of those koppy things?'

Fonthill pursed his lips. 'I think we've hurt them badly enough. We must have killed almost half of them and I doubt de Sousa is paying 'em enough to persuade them to have another go at us. The fire, I think, would have really frightened them.'

Mzingeli nodded. 'They think you great witch doctors,' he intoned. 'Masters of fire. They don't attack again.'

'Good. Now . . .' Simon looked around. 'Where the hell is Alice?'

'She's scribblin' again,' said Jenkins. 'Would it be a letter to 'er mother, then, d'you think?'

Fonthill sighed. 'I doubt it, old chap. I rather feel she is recording for posterity what she will probably call the Battle of Tuli Gap. But whatever she names it, I'm damned glad it's over.'

He sank to the ground, all the fatigue and misery of warfare suddenly descending upon him and the adrenalin raised by the excitement of battle now drained away. He wiped his blackened face with what was left of his handkerchief.

For a moment the two men, one squatting on the ground, the other standing protectively over him, were silent. Then Fonthill looked up and grinned sadly. 'Come on,' he said. 'We'd better organise a burial party.'

Chapter 9

It was late afternoon before the debris of the battle had been cleared away, and reluctant as he was to remain in this blackened, benighted spot, Fonthill decided that it would be best to stay in laager overnight before moving on. He sent Mzingeli and Ntini out to scout the other side of the kopjes and further ahead to the far bank of the little Shashe to ensure that the Portuguese and his men had retreated fully. They returned to say that the tracks of the attackers had ended at the Shashe Drift and then reappeared on the other side, heading north. They were, it appeared, quite safe. For now.

While the burial parties worked, Alice attended to the minor cuts sustained by two of the boys and then stayed in her wagon, head down, writing on her pad. She broke off only to stride into the blackened bush to estimate distances, speaking to no one, her brow wrinkled in concentration. Only on Mzingeli's return, when Simon broke open the whisky to celebrate, albeit wearily, the victory, did she join the others.

Later, as the boys cooked, she settled by Fonthill's side. 'I have written my story,' she said, 'and I must send it back to the cable station. May I have Ntini set off to do this tomorrow?'

Simon shook his head. 'Sorry. That's just not possible. Once we are in Bulawayo, I have to deliver the goods to the king and then persuade him to allow Rhodes to send off his pioneer column. When, hopefully, he has agreed, Ntini can leave to send my telegram to Rhodes and he can carry your cable at the same time.'

'Hell, Simon, this is a *news* story, for goodness' sake! I must get if off *immediately*.'

'Oh come along, Alice! Who is going to scoop you out here? I agree that news travels amazingly fast across this emptiness, but none of your competitors will trust native rumours, and anyway, you will have the kind of details that no one else could possible garner. I'm sure you can afford to wait.'

'No I can't.' Her eyes were cold and hard. 'You can surely spare just one man for me.'

Fonthill sighed. 'I am afraid not. I am sorry, my dear. You must wait. This mission is more important than your story.'

Alice's eyes came alight. '*Your mission*.' The words were a sneer. 'Do you really consider that taking guns to a native chief is an honourable mission? We have seen today another example of the criminal brutality that exists everywhere out here. By bribing tribes with guns – bloody *guns*, for God's sake – do you really think that Rhodes is peacefully settling this territory?' She grabbed her husband's arm. 'Of course he's not. He is just stirring the pot. It's not *his* country to settle anyway. It belongs to Lobengula. Why can't he leave the man alone? You are not on a *mission*, Simon. You are just running guns, like any other disreputable smuggler, although you seem to manage to kill more people in the doing of it. Don't talk to me about your *mission*!'

Simon tried to reach for her hand, but she withdrew it. He frowned at her vehemence. Then his own temper rose. 'Dammit all, woman. Only a few minutes ago I was being kissed as a hero of the Empire. Now I am being condemned as a murdering gun-runner. I think you had better make up your mind.'

Their voices had risen, and Mzingeli and Jenkins, washing their cups from a water bag, looked up in surprise, while the boys bent their heads to their tasks in some embarrassment. A silence descended on the little camp.

Fonthill swallowed. 'It's silly to quarrel like this, Alice,' he said, his voice low. 'I had not realised that you felt like this about this journey, and I am sorry that you are upset.'

She looked at him stonily for a moment, and then her face softened and she leaned towards him and took his hand. 'We were all very nearly killed today, Simon,' she said, 'and I have to confess that I am still trembling. Writing my story made me realise how stupid – how pathetically stupid – all this killing is. We could have been speared to death, and more than twenty of these tribesmen were killed by us. And for what? A tribal home that is not ours nor that of Portugal. You know,' she gripped his hand tightly, 'this man Rhodes is nothing more than a rich adventurer who has now turned his hand to land-grabbing. He has become a despot whom I regard as being far worse than poor old Lobengula with his gout.'

Fonthill shook his head. 'No. I disagree. Rhodes may be a rich adventurer, but he is a man with a vision who is not after further pecuniary gain for himself. He has as much money as he wants.' He enfolded her hand in both of his. 'Alice, dear Alice, things are moving at a fast pace in this damned continent. Rhodes believes fervently that the Matabele – and particularly their subject tribes – would be far better off as part of the British Empire than under some somnolent European country represented here by that cruel bastard de Sousa. And that's really the choice, you know, with probably the Boers of the Transvaal thrown into the equation. Them or us. Slavery, or freedom under the British flag. Poor old Lobengula cannot stay sitting like a fly in aspic, guzzling champagne and brandy while the world moves on around him. I think he knows that too.'

Alice wrinkled her nose. 'Yes, but what if Rhodes has to kill the whole Matabele nation to give them this "freedom"? He's quite likely to do that, isn't he? He's a ruthless man. It's clear that Lamb, Wolseley and the British Government are worried about it too.'

'He has promised not to do that unless provoked, and I doubt if that will happen. But anyway, that's part of my job, don't forget. To stop the man going in with all guns blazing.'

'Hmm. So you won't object, then, if I take one of the boys and go back myself to cable my story?' She could not resist grinning.

'Yes I bloody well would. I can't spare another man, and most of all I can't spare you. Who is going to treat poor old Lobengula's gout? He may well treasure me as a dear and close friend of Queen Victoria, but he treasures his own personal witch doctor even more. If he finds that you are not part of the parcel I have brought, he's likely to slit my belly open and feed me to the crocodiles.' Her grin widened and he went on: 'And what about the bigger story about him conceding agreement for Rhodes to allow his column of pioneers in to start digging – or colonising – Mashonaland? If you are not with me, you will miss that, my love, won't you?'

She shook her head resignedly. 'Oh, very well. You win. I will wait until you have got your own story for Rhodes. But please, please, no more killing, darling. I have become so weary of it.'

'So have I.' They exchanged a kiss, and it seemed as if a collective sigh of relief ran through the whole camp.

They inspanned early the next morning, but, still cautious, Fonthill sent Mzingeli ahead to cross the river and ride ahead to the village of Makobistown, the 'gateway' to Matabeleland, where the task of the *inDuna* there was to report to Bulawayo the entry of strangers to the country from the south. On their first, unheralded visit, Fonthill and his party had crossed the border from the Transvaal over the Limpopo, much further to the east. Given the importance of his cargo, Fonthill instructed the tracker to request an escort from the border to the king's capital. This would remove once and for all the threat of another attack from Gouela.

In the event, the progress to Bulawayo was uneventful, in fact almost regal, for the border *inDuna* was quick to recognise the importance of the party and he provided fifty plumed Matabele warriors, in full regalia, to act as escort for the journey.

'Blimey,' observed Jenkins, 'now I know 'ow our Queen feels.' To emphasise the point, he bestowed a wave of the hand, a gracious nod of the head and a regal smile on the many villagers who turned out to watch the procession go by.

The biggest crowd of all, of course, was provided in Bulawayo itself, where it seemed that many hundreds of people swarmed out to accompany the party on the last mile or so of the entry into the capital. Here, the escort took its duty very seriously, using spear and shield to keep the crowds away from the wagons as the little procession approached the outlying thorn *zariba* that enclosed the town. Now, however, there was no praise-singing to precede the meeting with the king, for Lobengula was waiting for them outside his house, sitting under the shade of the great indaba tree, on an ox cart where, Fonthill was later told, he often preferred to sleep. Despite the heat, he was dressed in his European garb, complete with billycock hat, and carrying a short assegai. He descended with great care, for it was clear that his right foot was still swollen, and as his wooden throne was quickly brought from his house, he gestured with a broad grin and his spear for the visitors to sit on the goatskins laid before him.

No provision for interpretation had been made, so Fonthill nudged Mzingeli to translate as Lobengula began to speak.

'He say,' began the tracker, 'that his good friends are welcome once again to his kingdom. He does not care what they bring for it is their good company he wishes.'

Fonthill, Alice at his side, inclined his head. 'I too am delighted to see his majesty again and I thank him for his warm welcome.' He had agonised for days wondering how to address the fact that his cargo was not all that had been promised, and in the end he had decided simply to ignore the matter until it was raised. 'I bring warm greetings to the king from Mr Rhodes, who apologises for the fact that he could not come himself. This is because he is about to be made prime minister of the Cape Colony, and he was forced to remain in the great city of Cape Town to receive this honour.'

The king waved his assegai in acceptance. 'It is understandable,' translated Mzingeli, perspiration beginning to appear on his brow as he grappled with his unfamiliar and important task. Fonthill waited for Lobengula to make some reference to the cargo, but the king remained silent, beaming at Simon and his wife. It was obviously beneath his dignity to refer in public to the gold, guns and ammunition. Again Fonthill marvelled at the innate good manners of the man.

Simon cleared his throat, but Alice spoke first. 'How is his majesty's foot?' she enquired, with a sweet smile.

'Ah.' A comic expression of great suffering came over Lobengula's face. 'It is . . . what you say?' enquired Mzingeli desperately.

'Hurting?' offered Alice.

'Yes, hurting.'

'Is the king still drinking much champagne and brandy?'

A frown descended upon the royal countenance, to be replaced by a look of petulant annoyance that in turn gave way to another of his face-splitting grins. 'Less than before but still too much. Does the Nkosana doctor bring with her the painkiller?'

Alice inclined her head. 'As before, I can help a little, but the main cure will come from the king drinking less of the white man's alcohol and eating less red meat. It is, I fear, the only way.'

'Good. Then the Nkosana perhaps will visit later to put the little spear into bottom . . . ?'

'Of course.' The king's relief was clear.

Fonthill cleared his throat. 'We have brought with us, your majesty, the . . . er . . . goods that Mr Rhodes promised as his part of the treaty he signed with you—'

Lobengula interrupted the translation by waving his assegai across his face, as though brushing away impertinent flies. 'That is good but not of great importance. We can talk of this later. Now we have beer . . .'

''Ow very, very sensible,' breathed Jenkins.

'. . . and then, when you have rested from journey, you will eat with us.' He clapped his hands, and gourds of beer were brought by young Zulu girls, shepherded in by the great bulk of Nini, the king's sister, who beamed on them all. This time, Fonthill noted with approval, Mzingeli, Ntini and all the boys were served also.

Small talk ensued for a few minutes as the king enquired about their long journey. Simon had decided that he would make no reference to the two attacks on them by de Sousa – at least not in public – and conversation quickly petered out. Then the king waved his assegai again.

'You go to huts now,' he said. 'Then, at sunset, we eat. Good meat,' he caught Alice's eye and finished lamely, 'with many berries. Can Nkosana come early and cure foot?'

'I will come, of course.'

With that the meeting broke up and the party retreated to their wagons, where Ntini presided over the unloading of the personal possessions, which were taken to the huts that had housed them before. Fonthill was glad to see that the hole cut into the back of his hut had been carefully repaired.

'What about the gold an' stuff?' enquired Jenkins.

'Look.'

Silently, six of the king's men had appeared and were quietly offloading the cases. 'He can't get into them until I unlock them,' said Fonthill, 'but it's clear that he is not so uninterested in them as he made out. At least everything will be under guard overnight and we won't have to worry about them.' He turned to Alice. 'Shall I come with you into the treatment room?'

'No. Witch doctors don't like to be watched when they're casting their spells.'

'All right. But take Mzingeli with you.'

'Of course. I shall need him to translate anyway.'

Alice carefully unpacked her medicine bag and checked its contents. 'Right, Mzingeli. Let's go.'

This time, however, they were forced to wait outside the king's house by a very nervous servant as loud voices came from within. Mzingeli frowned. 'King angry with someone,'

178

he whispered. 'Man inside steal royal cattle, I think. Ah. Yes. Man is to have hand cut off and he thrown to crocodiles in river.'

'Oh my God.' Alice blanched. 'How disgusting. He can't do that.'

The tracker shrugged. 'It is the way here. He not always cheerful man. He very cruel.'

Alice took a deep breath. 'Then he can cure his own blasted gout.'

'No, no, Nkosana. Don't make him more angry. We all in his power here. He . . . er . . . value you. Perhaps if you make him angry, we all die.'

They were forced to remain silent, until a scream came from within. At that, Alice thrust her way past the servant and entered the smoke-filled interior. The sight that met their eyes was repellent. Lobengula had removed his European clothes and was standing, wearing just a loincloth. The black folds of his skin were glistening in the firelight and his eyes were aflame. Kneeling in front of him, writhing in agony, was a native, whose right hand had been hacked away by an axe. Blood was spurting from the stump.

As Alice watched, he was dragged to his feet by two men and hauled towards the door, presumably on his way to the river. She barred the way.

'Put that man down,' she cried, pointing to the ground. A silence fell on the room, broken only by the crackling of the fire. The two men stood, gripping the victim, who had now slumped into unconsciousness. Their jaws had dropped and their eyes, widened in surprise, were white spheres in the half-light. They turned in consternation, looking for direction from the king, but Lobengula stood immobile, frozen by surprise.

Alice turned. 'Mzingeli, bring my bag. Quickly now, or this man will bleed to death.'

The tracker shook his head. 'No, Nkosana. No interfere. They kill us.'

'Do as I say. Here, yes. Good, thank you. Now, hold the man's arm up. Quickly.' She unclipped her bag and fumbled inside. 'Higher than that. I don't want the bag filled with blood. That's better.'

Kneeling and working quickly, she produced a narrow strip of bandage, which she folded lengthways and wrapped around the stricken man's arm above the elbow, knotting it loosely. Then she looked around, plucked a knife from the girdle of one of the two executioners, thrust its handle into a fold of the bandage and twisted it to act as a tourniquet. 'Hold this, Mzingeli,' she said. 'Keep it tight until the bleeding stops, then, when it does stop, loosen it slightly, and tighten it again. Now . . .'

Alice rummaged in her bag once again and produced a large pad of cotton wool, which she screwed tightly, wrapped in gauze and drenched in antiseptic from a bottle. Perspiration was now pouring from her brow. Wiping it away with the back of her hand, she pressed the pad on to the bloody stump and looked around in some desperation. Her eye fell on the nearest of the executioners.

'You,' she cried. 'Yes, dammit, you. Come here.'

Uncomprehending and fearful, the man remained unmoving. Alice reached across and pulled him towards her roughly by his forearm. 'Here. Hold this. *This*, you bloody fool. Look.' She gently pressed her hand on to the pad. 'Hold it like this. Yes, well done, you great barbarian. Hold it still while I bandage.'

Kneeling awkwardly, Alice wound a bandage around the

thief's forearm and then crossed it several times over the pad to hold it in place on the stump, before doubling it back to the forearm, cutting it off with her scissors, slicing the cotton into two strips and firmly knotting the two together to hold the bandage in place. She looked up and blew out her cheeks. 'Keep the tourniquet tight for the moment,' she ordered the tracker.

Then she caught the eye of the king.

There was no sign now of the grinning, genial monarch. Lobengula's face was contorted with rage. The King of the Matabele had never in all his life had his way thwarted when ordering an execution – and certainly not by a woman, whatever her colour. He opened his mouth to speak – or scream – but Alice interrupted him.

'Your majesty,' she said in a loud but precise tone that seemed to cut through the hot, smoky atmosphere like a jet of cold water, 'this man has suffered enough for his crime.' She turned to the kneeling Mzingeli. 'Go on. Interpret.'

The tracker did so, in a low, hesitant voice. 'I have tried to staunch the bleeding,' Alice continued, 'but I am not sure I have succeeded. The man may well die during the night. So it will certainly not be necessary to feed him to the crocodiles. If you are a wise and tolerant ruler, as I am sure you are, the compassionate thing to do would be to leave him to die in his bed, with his family at his side. By severing his hand, you have already punished him for his crime. I am sure you agree.' She summoned up a smile.

It was clear, however, that the king did not agree. He gave a shouted order and the victim, now regaining consciousness, was roughly seized again by his captors, so that Mzingeli was forced to remove the knife from the tourniquet loop.

Alice took a deep breath. 'Ah, I see that your majesty has

lost respect for my healing powers. In that case, of course, I can no longer treat your painful foot. I wish you good evening.'

As Mzingeli translated, Alice bent down and slowly began repacking her medical bag. Then she stood, and with a deferential nod, turned and began making her way to the door.

A shout from the king halted her. 'Why you interfere with our customs and judgement?' he demanded. 'Do I do this with Queen Victoria in your country?'

There was a logic to the question that confounded Alice for a moment. 'Ah, but Queen Victoria would never give two punishments to one man for the same crime,' she said. 'The loss of the hand would be considered sufficient in any civilised country.' The criticism implied by the use of the word 'civilised' put her on even more dangerous ground, she realised, but she was determined to hold her position.

Mzingeli translated, though unhappily. 'Careful, Nkosana, please,' he pleaded. But the king was speaking again. This time he was addressing the *inDunas*, wives and others crowded into the room. The tracker continued: 'He say your words have wisdom and ask why no adviser said same to him in past. He say he cannot do all thinking himself. *InDunas* should advise like you. You clever woman. You heal and you speak well. Man shall go to his family.'

Alice felt relief flood over her. 'The king is gracious, wise and compassionate,' she said. 'If he will allow me to finish my work with this man, I will attend to his majesty's foot.'

Lobengula nodded, a touch petulantly, and Alice knelt again at the thief's side. The stump was still bleeding, of course, but less so. She applied a second pad, bound it more tightly, and retied the tourniquet, less tightly. Then she selected a white cotton sling from her bag and arranged it around the man's neck, so that the arm was held pointing upwards, close to the chest. Finally she nodded. 'Take him,' she said.

The king gestured with his assegai, and while the mutilated man was helped to his feet and escorted from the room, Lobengula lowered himself on to his couch. Alice asked for water to wash, and a bowl was brought. Then she inspected the royal foot. It was swollen, of course, and still discoloured, but not as enlarged as when last she had seen it. Perhaps the king was, indeed, reducing his indulgences. Certainly the pile of bottles had disappeared.

Alice returned to her bag. In Cape Town she had resorted to a pharmacy, and now she laid out on the beaten earth the fruits of her visit: a box of Blair's Gout Pills, 'The Great English Remedy', and a bottle of Clarke's World Famed Blood Mixture. She had been assured by a doctor she had consulted in the Cape that these, coupled with a restrained and balanced diet, would reduce the symptoms of the affliction and indeed help to remove it altogether. She was anxious to lessen the king's reliance on her injections of morphine, for she wished to keep the drug for more serious emergencies.

She doled out a week's supply of the pills and explained that one should be taken every day with water, supplemented by a teaspoonful of the Blood Mixture. Then she injected the king, as before, with morphine, this time reducing the dose.

Immediately the king's good humour was restored, although it was unclear whether this was because the drugs took immediate effect – which was unlikely – or because he had managed, narrowly, to keep face over the sentencing of the thief. The great beam came back.

'How long you stay this time?' he asked.

'I am not sure,' replied Alice, thinking quickly. 'I know that my husband is anxious to seek the king's agreement to a question he will put to your majesty, but certainly we are not anxious to leave Bulawayo. In due course, however, I understand that we intend to explore to the east, towards the Indian Ocean coast.'

'Oh! Very difficult country that way. Very dangerous. Why you go?'

'Er . . . I understand that Mr Rhodes is anxious to find a route to the coast, either by river or by land.'

'Why he want that?'

'Your majesty must ask my husband. I do not know.'

'Ah. Rhodes always want something.'

'Um . . . yes.' She smiled, packed her bag, bowed and left, Mzingeli in tow.

The two walked together in silence back to the huts until, nearly there, Mzingeli spoke. 'You very brave woman,' he said. 'Very fine.'

Alice gave the tracker a sad smile. 'Thank you. The trouble is that I very much doubt whether it was worthwhile, for I am sure that the man will die, probably of shock or blood poisoning. Still, better he dies in bed than being dragged under by some foul-smelling crocodile.' And she gave an involuntary shudder.

Alice decided not to tell Simon of her intervention, and they prepared for their dinner with the king in companionable silence – broken, inevitably, by the arrival of Jenkins, who still perforce shared their hut.

'Been to Mr Fairbairn's,' confided the Welshman, 'just to see if 'e'd 'eard anythin' about the Portuguese bloke, look you.' The strong smell of whisky he exuded gave the lie to that, but apart from exchanging glances, neither Simon nor Alice decided to issue a rebuke.

'And what did he say?' asked Fonthill.

Jenkins gave a chortle. 'I got Gouela all right. In the shoulder. 'E's walkin' about with 'is arm in a sling. An 'untin' accident, 'e's tellin' everybody.'

Simon nodded. 'Well,' he reflected, squatting on a stool and pulling his head through his best shirt, 'if there was any doubt about who was behind that attack, that settles it.'

'Do you intend to tell the king?' asked Alice.

'I think not. However . . .'

'Yes?'

Fonthill grinned. 'If Lobengula does make a fuss about being short-changed with the number of guns I have brought, I would be sorely tempted to say that old Gouela took half of them when he attacked us.'

'Oh, I don't think . . .'

'No, neither do I. It would be wrong to lie about it, and anyway, I could never prove it. So I will just keep quiet and see how things develop.'

Alice sat for a moment in silence, and then decided it would be wise to tell Simon about her intervention after the mutilation, and of her brief conversation with the king following her treatment of his foot. Jenkins and her husband listened with rapt attention as she unfolded her brief tale, and at its end, Fonthill shook his head slowly.

'My dear Alice,' he said. 'I don't know what to say . . .'

'I do,' said Jenkins. 'It was a very brave thing to do. I wouldn't 'ave pushed my nose in there, with the old bastard in 'is 'and-choppin' mood. You did very well, Miss Alice, if I may say so. But blimey. It just shows what these people are capable of, isn't it?'

Fonthill stood and wrapped his arms around his wife. 'Yes, it does. So don't do anything like that again, my love. Will you promise?'

She pushed him away. 'Certainly not. I had him over a barrel and he knew it. I wouldn't have treated him if he had let the poor wretch be taken to the river. And that was that. I would do it again if necessary.'

Fonthill raised his eyebrows to Jenkins, shrugged his shoulders and resumed dressing. 'What did he say when you mentioned the exploration trip to the east?'

'He wanted to know why Rhodes wanted you to go, but I told him he had better ask you.' She grinned, her grey eyes sparkling in the gloom. 'I thought I had got into enough trouble for one day.'

'Ah.' Fonthill gave a histrionic sigh. 'Acknowledgement at last! But thank you for telling me. I had better think of a good reason.'

As the sun dipped away and the brief African twilight began to disappear, revealing the first spray of stars in the blue-black sky, the three walked together down to the king's hut. The heat had gone, taking the flies with it, and the evening was soft and delightful. After careful thought, Alice had decided to wear her only dress, having smoothed out the wrinkles with a sprinkling of water and the application of her hand. A touch of femininity, she had reasoned, would not be out of place after her show of masculine determination earlier.

Fonthill regarded her with approval as they strolled together, arm in arm. Alice had tied back her hair with her favourite apple-green silk scarf – a treasure of much importance in her tiny wardrobe – and donned open-toed sandals. A touch of face powder and a little rouge had smoothed her sunburned cheeks, and her eyes were sparkling.

'How nice to go to an elegant dinner in the tropics,' she said. 'I wonder if the old boy will serve us champagne.'

'Hmm. Equally, he might decide to cut our hands off. Which reminds me.' He turned to Jenkins, walking amiably by their side. 'I know you've had a touch of whisky, 352,' he said, 'so do please behave yourself tonight. If somebody stamps on your foot, take it as a compliment. Don't punch him on the jaw, there's a good fellow. The family has been in enough trouble for one day.'

'I shall be 'ave with great property ... propoty ... prop ...'

'Propriety?'

'That's the word, Miss Alice. On the tip of me tongue. Not a finger out of place, see. Oh, incidentally, old Fairbairn 'as been invited.'

Fonthill's eyebrows rose. 'Ah, so it's a kind of diplomatic party all round, probably to celebrate the fact that Lobengula's got his guns and gold.' A second thought struck him. 'I wonder if de Sousa will be invited. We shall see.'

They entered the large hut to find that, thankfully, the fire had been allowed to die down, even though the evening had become cooler with the descent of the sun. Benches of differing heights and provenance had been arranged in a great circle around the fire, with Lobengula's old wooden throne arranged on one side of the circle, facing the door. The king had not yet made his appearance, but all of the senior *inDunas* were there, including the man who had led them to the king on their first entrance to the country and who had been saved from punishment by Fonthill on their arrival at Bulawayo. He came forward with a grin, and made a great show of shaking hands, European style, with Simon, Alice and Jenkins, as though they were old friends. Fonthill took this as a good sign.

Nini, too, came bustling over, an ironmongery of copper charms and medallions cascading over her huge bosoms. 'How is you?' she enquired.

'We is . . . ah . . . we are very well, thank you, Princess,' said Simon, bowing over her hand.

The king's sister made an impatient gesture, and beer was immediately produced for all three. Receiving his, Jenkins gave an extravagant bow and immediately caught the attention of Nini. 'You not married?' enquired the princess.

'Ooh, yes,' the Welshman hurriedly replied. 'I 'ave three wives back 'ome.'

Nini immediately whirled round to Fonthill. 'He say you only allowed one wife at a time.'

Jenkins thought quickly. 'Ah well, you see, your majesty, two of 'em are dead an' buried, like. I've got one that is very much alive, look you. An' that's all I'm allowed, see. Great pity it is.'

The princess looked puzzled, but let it pass. Now she put her face close to Jenkins's and examined his great moustache, taking its end between plump finger and thumb and rubbing the hairs vigorously. 'Why you grow this?' she asked.

'Er . . . to make me look pretty, see.'

At this, Nini threw back her head and roared with laughter, giving a lead to all of the wives and girl servers in the hut, who laughed along dutifully, although they could not have understood for a moment the meaning of the joke. Fairbairn now joined the party, bringing with him his distinctive aura of tobacco smoke and whisky, and he immediately engaged the princess in fluent Zulu, which relieved Jenkins of his duties as purveyor of pre-dinner small talk.

The Welshman caught a stir in the far corner of the room – was there another entrance? – and he immediately turned to Fonthill. ''E's 'ere, bach sir.' He jerked his head.

Simon followed the direction of the nod and caught a glimpse of the familiar yellow uniform. De Sousa was talking to a couple of *inDunas*, standing firmly and with his right hand nonchalantly tucked into his unbuttoned jacket, Napoleon style. No sling was evident. Fonthill grinned. 'He's not prepared to show us that he's been wounded,' he said. Well, well, well. I must go across and pay my respects and . . . ah . . . offer him the hand of friendship.'

He strode across and interrupted the conversation. 'Ah, Mr de Sousa,' he said, 'how good to see you again. I hope you are well.' He extended his hand, but the Portuguese ignored it.

'Perfectly well, thank you.'

'Good. I had heard that you had suffered an injury while . . . ah . . . out hunting.'

'It was nothing. Just a slight mishap. The beast I was hunting, however, was wounded.' He gave a faint smile, revealing a gold tooth. 'He will die the next time. I always get the animal I am pursuing. Always.'

'Quite so. Sentiments I echo. I am the same.' And with exaggerated jocularity, he slapped de Sousa on the shoulder – the injured shoulder, of course – causing the Portuguese to wince and turn away in half-disguised agony. 'Oh goodness,' exclaimed Fonthill. 'Was that your bad shoulder? I am so sorry.'

Further exchanges, however, were prevented by the arrival of the king, who entered accompanied by his chief wife, a lady of proportions very similar to those of Nini but who carried herself with far less confidence than the princess. The king was dressed in his best European apparel, the billycock hat tilted at an audacious angle and his round face wreathed in a grin that indicated, perhaps, that Alice's new pills and potions, together with the morphine, were promising a pain-free evening.

Lobengula raised his fly whisk, which for social events seemed to have replaced his short assegai, and acknowledged his guests by pointing it to them all as he turned. Then he shouted an order, and everyone scuttled to take their places on the benches as more beer on wooden trays was brought in by the young girls. Significant gaps were left on either side of Lobengula's chair, and the *inDuna* who had greeted Fonthill on arrival now hurried over to indicate that Alice should sit on the king's right, with Fairbairn, rather surprisingly, at her side, and Simon, flanked by Jenkins, next to the trader. Disconcertingly, de Sousa was placed on the king's left, with the chief wife on his other side.

Alice leaned across to the Scotsman. 'We seem to be honoured, Mr Fairbairn,' she said.

The trader gave a wry smile. 'Oh, you may be, ma'am, but I'm just here to interpret, y'see.'

Alice gave him her best smile. 'Well I am jolly glad that you are here, whatever your role.'

The king clapped his hands, and immediately great wooden platters were borne in containing mounds of beef, which steamed as they were placed on rough stools in front of all the guests. Alice sighed, as she could see no sign of vegetables or bread, but could not resist a smile when piles of berries were placed ostentatiously in front of herself and the king. Lobengula caught her eye and winked. She was, it seemed, forgiven for her intrusion of a few hours ago – at least for the moment.

The monarch leaned forward and grabbed a choice piece of

meat, and fastidiously picking off the gristle, which he threw over his shoulder, he handed it to Alice. She nodded her acceptance and took it. It was the signal for everyone on the benches to bend to the task of selecting beef from the platters and begin wolfing down the prime cuts. Immediately a hum of conversation rose, and Alice could not but smile at the resemblance to a sophisticated dinner party in London, where the guests would wait for the host to begin before raising knife and fork and embarking on the tedious business of engaging in conversation with the person to left or right. The setting, though, could not have been more different. She looked around her with interest. The fire in the middle of the hut had been built up again, alas, and the flames cast a flickering glow across the half-naked figures that constituted most of the ring, their black skin glistening and the firelight reflected in the copper accoutrements of the women. White teeth and protuberant eyeballs shone in the half-light, and the murmur of conversation was low and guttural. There was no glitter of silver, no sparkle of diamonds, and the hum of voices certainly did not tinkle.

She could not resist grinning at the king. He leaned forward and spoke, his black eyes gleaming. 'The king says, eat your berries,' translated Fairbairn. 'Now what's that about?'

Alice nodded. 'A private joke,' she said. 'Tell me, Mr Fairbairn, why is that man,' she gave an almost imperceptible nod of the head, 'sitting next to the king?'

'Aye, the snake man. Well, Lobengula seems to like him, or to respect him at least. He knows that the Portuguese to the east have vast territories and wants to keep in with them. Gouela appears to have quite a personal bodyguard living here in the capital, and the king believes that the man is well regarded in Lisbon, which he ain't, ma'am, he's only an agent.

But I shouldn't worry too much about all that. Lobengula has sat him there just to balance things a bit with your husband – to let him know that even though he has brought a box or two of lollipops from Kimberley, it doesn't mean that Rhodes can just walk into the place.'

'Ah, so you know about the cargo we have brought.'

Fairbairn nodded his head as he munched. 'Oh yes. Everybody does.'

Simon leaned across his wife to address the trader. 'Would you ask the king if I can call and see him tomorrow, please? I have some keys I must hand over to him and other things to discuss.'

The king nodded equably. 'Come before sun is highest.'

The evening meandered its way to a conclusion, with the pyramids of beef disappearing under the attacks from the ravenous guests. Nothing more was served – it seemed that the berries were only a gesture towards Alice – except flagon after flagon of beer. Fonthill was glad that Jenkins was sitting beside him, and the Welshman behaved impeccably, even talking endlessly to the friendly *inDuna* on his right, who had not the slightest idea what was being said, but kept nodding amiably.

'Well,' asked Alice, as the three wandered back to their hut, 'what was all that about?'

'Fairbairn seemed to think,' said Fonthill, 'that although the king pretends to be uninterested in the guns, ammunition and gold, he is pleased that Rhodes has kept his side of the bargain. He says that the Portuguese talk and promise a lot, but nothing happens. Now the British have shown that they keep their word . . .'

'Even though we've only brought five hundred rifles?'

'Well, he doesn't know that yet, and, anyway, that's still a hell of a lot of firearms. He could frighten even the Boers with them.'

'And the British, eh?' Jenkins chimed in.

'No. We are not looking for confrontation.'

Alice gave a cynical smile. 'We will just have to wait and see about that, my dear.'

The next morning Fonthill removed a parchment document from its oilskin covering and spread it out on his sleeping mat. He had had it prepared in Cape Town and it looked impressive enough, with Cecil John Rhodes's signature at the bottom, beside the chartered company's crest, and leaving space for Lobengula's mark and his great elephant seal.

'What's it say?' asked Jenkins.

'Oh, the content is simple enough. It states that the king has given permission for surveyors and engineers from the company to enter the king's domain and to build a road through Mashonaland to the north and prospect for minerals there.'

Alice sniffed. 'Does it say anything about settling the land?'

'No. That is not the purpose of the expedition.'

'I don't believe that. Anyway, I thought Lobengula had already signed a similar document.'

'Yes, but the point of this is that now that the king has received his guns and cash, he will permit the column to enter his land *now*. There was only a rather vague reference to the future in the original treaty. Rhodes wants it all watertight before he invokes the great expense of getting his column together and moving north.'

'Well, good luck.'

Fonthill took the precaution of asking Fairbairn to accompany him this time to act as interpreter, instead of

Mzingeli. It would be sensible, he reasoned, to have another European present as witness.

The king welcomed them both with the inevitable beer, and accepted imperturbably the keys that Fonthill presented to him. He continued to give the impression that the cargo was of no importance to him. Then, with great care, Simon began the task of gaining the king's acceptance of the need for a column to enter his country imminently to begin the road-building work.

'Why we need this road?' asked the king.

'Because, your majesty, it is impossible to bring in the equipment needed to mine without having a road through to the north. There is a well-defined trail through Bechuanaland to your border, as you know, but not through Matabeleland.'

'Humph. How many men come?'

'I do not know, but it is likely to be several hundred.'

'Sounds like an impi.'

'No, sir. They will be pioneers, not soldiers.'

'I give permission already for Rhodes to mine. Why I have to sign new paper?'

'This will be more specific, giving him permission to enter your country very soon – as soon as he can form his column, that is.'

'My *inDunas* don't like me signing all this paper.'

'It is merely confirming your word, your majesty. It is normal in dealings between European countries. There is nothing sinister in it.'

Lobengula looked around anxiously, as though looking for some escape. But there was no one else present. Eventually he clapped his hands to summon one of his wives and then gave orders to have his seal prepared. His face, however, remained heavy.

'I sign,' he said, 'because I trust you. You are English gentleman and know the Queen of England. I take your word I am not giving away my country.'

Fonthill writhed internally. He could not take responsibility for something over which he had no control. Yet he could not be seen to dissemble. That would throw even more doubt into Lobengula's mind. He cleared his throat. 'Your majesty, there is nothing in this paper that gives away your country, I promise. You are only allowing these people in to build a road to the north and then start mining.'

The king grunted but still looked unhappy. A silence fell on the room, which was broken by an *inDuna* bringing in a blob of still smoking wax, together with the great seal, fashioned from ivory. A quill and a small pot of ink was also produced.

Lobengula ignored them for a moment, and then directed his gaze at Fonthill. He did not speak, but looking into the man's black eyes, Simon could see a bewilderment, an uncertainty – even a touch of fear – that plucked at his own heart. It was like confronting a caged animal, a beast that had great power and was used to striking fear into everyone with whom it came into contact, but which realised that it was now confronted by something intangibly more powerful. Lobengula had the innate intelligence that sent warning signals to his brain, yet he did not know how to evade this all-pervading pressure. His look now to Fonthill was almost an appeal. Then he shook his head and very slowly reached for the pen.

'Just there, sir,' said Fonthill, pointing to the space left for the king's mark. He felt like a crooked solicitor, forging a will.

Lobengula scratched his mark and then, sighing, reached for the wax. He scooped a little out with a broad finger, spread it on the paper alongside his cross, and then firmly impressed his seal on to the still warm wax, with a finality that seemed to express relief. The deed was done.

'Thank you, sir,' said Simon, sharing the relief. 'I will see that this is taken directly to Cape Town. He looked up at the king. 'As this is an important document and,' he coughed, 'I believe there are people near here who would wish to see that it is not delivered, may I ask your majesty if he would provide a guard to see that, at least, it gets to the border safely?'

The king waved a hand airily. 'You shall have fifty warriors,' he said. 'They shall leave tomorrow.'

Fonthill inclined his head. 'The king is most kind.'

Lobengula nodded. 'I am told you want to go to the east. Why?'

'Ah yes, sir. Mr Rhodes is anxious that once the road to the north is established, some way is found to make a passage to the Indian Ocean, so that a supply route is set up and it will be easier to trade with Matabeleland and Mashonaland by sea from the south. He has asked me to explore to examine the possibilities. I intend to begin this journey as soon as I am equipped, with, I hope, the help of Mr Fairbairn here.'

'You go so quick?'

'I fear so, sir.'

'You take your wife with you? It is dangerous country that way.'

Fonthill gave a rueful smile. 'As I think you . . . er . . . know, sir, she is a strong woman. She insists on accompanying me, and I must confess, I will find her support and company on this difficult expedition of great value.'

'Umph. Matabele men don't take women with them when they go to war.'

'Well, I am not exactly going to war. I hope that I shall not encounter violence where I go.'

A grin came over the king's face. 'You will. The tribes that way are fighting people, not ...' his lip curled, 'like the Bechuanas the other way.'

There seemed little more to be said, so Fonthill inclined his head. Then he rose. 'If the king will excuse me, there is much to be done.'

Lobengula dismissed them both with a wave of his hand, and they left him disconsolately picking shreds of wax from the bottom of his ivory seal.

Once outside, Fonthill let out a sigh of relief. He rolled the parchment up and tied it firmly with a red ribbon. 'I'm glad that's over,' he confided to Fairbairn. 'I was never sure that he would sign it.'

'Come back to the shop and have a dram,' said the Scotsman. 'In celebration if you like – and you'd better tell me about this expedition of yours and how I can help.'

'Thank you, I could do with a whisky. Yes, I shall need your help with provisions, and rather more than that, I fear.'

The two trudged up the hill towards the trading post. 'It sounds as though you will have to go through de Sousa's province,' said Fairbairn. 'You will walk into trouble there.'

'Not if I can avoid his land, or if I can leave him behind here. Slip away before he knows about my departure. I intend to travel light and fast, if I can.'

'Huh, that depends on the terrain. There is some pretty thick bush that way – and Gouela is not the only one you have to worry about. This is slavers' country.'

'What, this far south? I thought they did not come further down than the Sudan.'

'Good lord, no. The Arabs are all over central Africa, including the Congo. They stop short at Mashonaland, though. The Matabele would be too much of a handful for them. But they are a fierce lot. They employ mercenary tribesmen who can fight, and they have their raiding down to a fine art. It doesn't do to tangle with them. They raid down to the east here, next to Portuguese East Africa and Matabeleland, although there is no precise border – just a jumble of small tribes – ideal hunting ground for them, of course.'

They reached the store and ducked under the low lintel of its doorway. 'Here, sit down,' said Fairbairn. 'I'll bring us a wee dram – on me. Take a look at this.'

Fonthill sank into a cane armchair that creaked with his weight and picked up the old map that Fairbairn flung at him. He spread it out on his lap. It showed the east coast of southern Africa, accurately, as far as he could see, with the formidable block of Portuguese East Africa dominating the coastline north to south for about a thousand miles. No getting round that. The blue line of the Zambezi snaked its way down from the north, eventually curving to debouch into the Indian Ocean. But it was far too far to the north, perhaps some four hundred miles away from Bulawayo, to offer the convenience of a riverside road. And what good would a steamboat be for Lobengula at that distance? Fonthill had brought with him from the Cape a couple of maps that charted expertly the Indian Ocean coast but did little to help inland. Now this map shared the same fault. It too showed no distinct frontiers between Matabeleland/Mashonaland and its northern neighbour, a kind of no-man's-land round Lake Nyasa, nor to the west towards Portuguese Angola or the east and the huge Portuguese possessions along the coast. What was more disturbing, however, was that the map was virtually blank between Bulawayo and the nearest point to the Portuguese eastern territory: just a reference to 'swamp' and the brown shading of a mountain range. It was, without a doubt, a wilderness.

'Have you been out this way?' he enquired of Fairbairn.

'No fear,' said the Scotsman. 'No real reason to go, and wouldn't want to anyway. Not much more than tsetse fly, swamp, spears and slavers. I wouldn't recommend it to anyone.'

'Where is Gouela's territory exactly?'

'Exactly, I don't know. But I think you can expect it to be pretty much due east of here. Just in the Portuguese eastern territory, of course. Border country. The dagoes claim all the land west of there to be under their control, or "protection", of course. The British Government disputes this. But neither side seems really anxious to do much about it, though de Sousa huffs and puffs here.'

At that point a Matabele crept deferentially into the shop and bent to whisper in Fairbairn's ear.

The Scotsman nodded and looked up. 'You should know this,' he said to Fonthill. 'I've just heard that de Sousa decamped before daylight this morning. Gone, with his little army. The word is that he has returned to his territory. Just the way you are planning to go, I'm afraid, old chap.'

Chapter 10

Fonthill returned to his hut, the map and his signed agreement with Lobengula under his arm but his brain a-jumble with conflicting thoughts. He had to go east to explore the possibilities of finding a route to the sea, but that way would lead him right into Gouela's arms. To detour would obviously be sensible, but he had no idea of the precise location of de Sousa's province, the better to avoid it. Before leaving the Cape, Rhodes had told him that he intended the road to continue the well-established trail through Bechuanaland, then, after crossing to the border, to skirt well to the east of Bulawayo – 'to keep out of trouble with the old boy' – and then curl north and east into Mashonaland proper. But where exactly? First, however, there was the task of getting the new agreement back to Rhodes and Alice's story back to the cable station.

Simon did his best to give answers to the many questions with which Alice plied him on his return, and was able at least to assure her that Ntini would be protected by an escort to the Transvaal border, beyond which the Portuguese would not dare to go, even if his leaving of the king's kraal did turn out to be a ruse.

Alice immediately set about writing a separate story –

to follow on from the battle at the border – confirming Lobengula's agreement to the entry of the road-builders, and Fonthill began to sort out his requirements for the exploration to the east. He wanted at least five of the ten Kaffir boys with them as bearers on the new journey. Would they agree to come, leaving behind their newly acquired oxen and accepting instead the promise of good cash payments at the end of the journey? He would certainly need Joshua, who had proved himself to be a good right-hand man to Mzingeli.

He asked Mzingeli to pick out the five who had fought the best at the Tuli kopjes and offer them £25 each to make the journey. The tracker advised mules, salted against the tsetse fly, as the best means of carrying their loads through the heavy bush, and undertook to see if there were any locally that could be bought to supplement his own animal. The wagons and the surplus oxen Fonthill decided to present as a gift to the king.

The tracker returned to say that he had been able to persuade only four of the Kaffirs to accompany them on the journey and had been forced to increase the payment offer to £30. Fonthill shrugged. There was no alternative and they would have to make do. The good news was that bright-eyed Joshua had been eager to come.

Alice completed her story early that afternoon, and Ntini was instructed to travel south with it together with the escort and the other boys, and then return to wait for them at Bulawayo.

Shortly after dawn, the fifty plumed and armed warriors reported for duty and they all set off: the oxen herded by the six boys, now returning home with the cattle as prizes, Ntini proudly astride his horse, carrying his precious documents –

the signed agreement, Fonthill's telegram to Rhodes and Alice's long message in cable form – strapped behind him, and his escort walking, assegais and shields in hand, on either side of him.

That evening Alice, accompanied by Mzingeli, called on the king to treat his painful foot. She found him relaxed and, as ever, delighted to see her.

'You should not go with husband on stupid journey,' he said. 'Stay here until he come back. You safe here. We all look after you. Good food, no work, except to treat foot. Plenty beer . . .' he giggled, 'and a little champagne if you like – too much bad for you, you know.'

She smiled. 'You are very kind, sir, but where my husband goes, I go.'

'You got no children? I have many – too many.'

'Yes, but you have sixty-three wives. No, we have no children. Our only child died in childbirth. I was lucky to survive but we lost our son.'

'Yes, but you still young. Don't you try no more? Is husband no good on sleeping mat?'

The question was put without embarrassment, although Mzingeli hesitated to find words to reduce its coarseness. Alice looked away for a moment but realised it would be ridiculous to take offence. This was not genteel Norfolk.

'He is splendid there as elsewhere, your majesty. It is just that we have not been blessed. So we accept it now.'

'Ah.' The first sign of empathy crossed the king's broad features. 'King is sorry. Now, stick little spear into bottom. Pain not so bad today.'

'Have you been taking the medicine and pills?'

'Yes. As you say.'

'Then I think that is helping you as much as the morphine. Now, please roll over.'

That evening after dinner, as the firelight flickered outside their hut, Fonthill called on Mzingeli and Joshua to join Alice, Jenkins and himself in a whisky – heavily laced with water for Joshua – and a briefing on the journey ahead. The tracker, who had returned with the good news that he had procured five good mules, interpreted in a low voice for Joshua.

Simon spread out Fairbairn's map. 'This is the best chart I've got,' he said, 'but as you can see, it doesn't tell us much.' He took out a small ruler. 'I estimate that it's about two hundred miles as the crow flies between here and the Portuguese border. Firstly, we are not crows, and secondly, I understand that it is very rough ground indeed – swamp, heavy bush and mountains, or at least very big and awkward hills. That is why we are not taking oxen or wagons. Count the distance, in fact, as the equivalent of four hundred miles on easy going.'

No one spoke, and in the near distance two dogs howled their frustration. Simon continued. 'However, I don't wish to go out on a route directly to the east. Again, there are two reasons for that. Firstly, old Gouela's territory lies that way, and although he would love to see us again, I wouldn't want to experience his welcome. The second reason is that the route to the ocean – if we find a way, that is – should link up with Rhodes's projected road coming up to Mashonaland from the south, and I think that that will terminate somewhere north or north-east of here.' He stabbed at the map with his ruler.

'So . . . ?' asked Jenkins.

'So, we set out from here in a north-easterly direction, before turning to the right and making for the Mozambique border. If we get that far, our journey in fact will be much longer than two hundred miles anyway.'

Alice frowned. 'Why don't we go further north and use the Zambezi as a river road, so to speak?'

'Because Rhodes knows about the Zambezi. He is not convinced that it is the best way to the east. There could well be problems with the Portuguese at its mouth, on their territory, and there are other, navigational problems about using it as the main entry into Matabeleland. No. Rhodes wants a road. A proper land road.'

'Blimey!' exclaimed Jenkins. ''E doesn't want us to build the bloody thing too, does 'e?'

Fonthill grinned. 'Well, if I had offered, no doubt he would have accepted the idea. But no. What he wants is to find a way that is roughly geographically suitable in the long term and politically acceptable in the short term.'

'I don't understand,' said Alice.

'He wants us to link up with the local tribes, once we are out of Lobengula's sphere of influence, and get them to sign treaties with his chartered company, which will offer them protection under the company's flag and be the first step in the road-building procedure.

'What Rhodes wants is a progression like the one he has achieved with Lobengula: a basic agreement, a payment of sorts and then a road-building programme that will lead inevitably to some sort of settlement – small at first but larger later. Maybe one that will not even take place properly until the twentieth century.'

A silence fell on the circle once more. It was broken by a question from Mzingeli. 'How long we away?'

Fonthill nodded at the question's relevance. 'I just don't know,' he said. 'Maybe six, maybe nine months. I can't be sure. It depends upon so many things, in particular the terrain and our welcome or otherwise from the tribes.'

Mzingeli translated quickly for Joshua.

'Is this all right for him?' asked Alice.

The tracker smiled his slow smile. 'He say he go where I go.'

'Oh, there's cosy then, isn't it,' said Jenkins. 'I'll come with you as well.'

'Now,' Fonthill pointed again at the map, 'it's a hell of a long way, but I have worked out what we need for provisions, and by the look of it, Fairbairn can provide virtually all we want, particularly native presents.' His face slipped into a frown. 'I am afraid that we must be prepared for anything, and the man has some old Sniders that should be all right for the boys to use if they have to, so I have bought them. Can you give them shooting lessons, 352?'

'Of course.'

The silence returned, to be broken, inevitably, by Jenkins. 'Do you think you could spare just a drop more?' he asked, holding out his empty mug. In fact, they all – except for Joshua – took one more drink before, deep in thought, they retired to sleep.

The next three days were spent in steady preparation for their journey. Thinking of the possible dangers, Fonthill ensured that every morning Jenkins took Joshua and the four Kaffir boys, together with their Sniders, away from the kraal to teach them target practice, speed reloading and rifle care. Their new skills could be vital in the weeks to come. As he watched, however, he became more concerned than ever about the perils that almost certainly lay ahead. So few riflemen against Gouela – and who else? He shrugged his shoulders. They were committed now and they must just prepare as best they could.

Alice continued her evening visits to the king. Concerned that rheumatism was affecting the royal joints, she added sweet spirits of nitre and quinine to Lobengula's daily dosage. She had also acquired a second patient. The cattle thief had made a good recovery and was now taking his place in looking after his family. Alice showed his wife how to change the dressing on his stump, left her a precious supply of bandage, padding and a little antiseptic, and recommended, through Mzingeli, that they leave Bulawayo to be away from the king.

On the eve of their own departure, she found Lobengula in a particularly melancholy mood as she completed his treatment.

'You don't go on this bad journey,' he said.

Alice, methodically packing away her bottles, shook her head and smiled. 'I must,' she said. 'I am not really a doctor, as you know, and I must accompany my husband.'

The king growled. 'I need you here. I am getting better. You help me. You stay. He not need you as I need you.'

'No, sir. I must go.'

'I pay you to stay. I give you cattle and little house. Wait here until Fonthill come back.'

Alice frowned. There was a note of angry anxiety in the king's tone, and a warning light flashed in her brain. She remembered only too clearly the blood gushing from the thief's forearm. The jocular, beaming monarch could change into a despot immediately he was crossed. She must be careful.

'Your majesty has sixty-three wives,' she said slowly, anxious that Mzingeli should translate every nuance. 'That means that you have much love and care. Because of our custom, my husband only has one wife. He needs me and I must be with him. Now, I do believe that your condition is improving and that your foot will recover if you take the medicine I leave with you and change your diet and drinking habits. The choice is yours.'

She allowed herself a smile after this homily. 'We expect to be away only about six months. Then I shall return to see how you have progressed. It will not seem long. But then, of course, I must return with my husband to our own homeland. The king will understand that, I know.'

But there was no answering smile from Lobengula. 'You go now,' he said shortly.

Bowing, Alice picked up her bag and left.

Outside, she mopped her brow. 'I think that the sooner we leave, the better,' she said to the tracker.

Mzingeli nodded. 'King is now ... what is word ... depending on you. That is bad. He has everything he want here. Now he want you.'

'Well he can't bloody well have me.' She tucked away a stray lock of blond hair. 'He is a petulant bully. He has to learn that he can't have everything he wants in this world. Good God – he's got sixty-three wives already. He mustn't be too greedy.' A sudden thought occurred to her. 'Mzingeli, I have never asked you. Do you have a wife or ... er ... perhaps more, at home?'

The tall man shook his head slowly. 'One wife,' he said, 'but she die ten years ago.'

'Oh, I am sorry. Children?'

'Two. They die also.'

'Oh dear.' She felt a warm surge of affection for this quiet, resourceful man with whom they had already shared moments of great danger. She touched his arm. 'I think I know how you must feel.' They walked in silence for a moment. Then, 'Come on. If we are leaving tomorrow, we still have much to do.'

The next morning, the expedition was ready to leave and Fonthill, Alice and Mzingeli called on the king early to bid him goodbye. They found him clothed only in his waist circle of monkey skins, sitting on his cart under the great tree and in a surprisingly avuncular mood. Bowing, Simon asked him if he would accept the wagons and the remaining oxen as a parting present.

'Good,' said Lobengula. 'I add to my herd. You come back soon and we drink beer together.'

'How is the foot this morning, your majesty?' enquired Alice.

The king gave an airy wave. 'Ah, foot is nothing. I can live with bad foot.'

Alice and Simon exchanged glances. 'Then,' said Simon, 'I will bid the king goodbye and thank him for his hospitality and many courtesies.'

'Good travel. Go well. My heart is white for you.'

The couple nodded their heads low at this traditional, warm farewell and left the king's dwelling – perhaps for the last time.

They set out as the sun crested the hill above the kraal, sending their shadows stretching along the ground to their left as they headed to the north-east. Fonthill had decided reluctantly that the rough nature of the terrain ahead precluded the use of horses, and he left them behind in the care of Fairbairn. He and Mzingeli now strode ahead in the lead, followed by Alice and then Jenkins. Behind them came the five mules, heavily laden with their provisions and kept moving by the urgings of Joshua and the four Kaffir boys.

It was a fine, bright morning, but Fonthill felt no elation. To Mashonaland – but then where? To slavers, swamps and, somewhere, the Portuguese, de Sousa? He gulped, but set his jaw and lengthened his stride.

Chapter 11

Initially, Fonthill set off aiming for the range of high hills that sat on the horizon to the north-east of Bulawayo. These formed the watershed for a fistful of rivers flowing north into the Zambezi and also south into the Limpopo, but they looked formidable so he tacked to the north to avoid them and skirted around until on their fifth day they approached a singular mountain called, by some lone Englishman years before, Mount Hampden. Here he set course due east, and then they felt that they were in Mashonaland proper.

Now the country was indeed magnificent: league after league of rolling plain, a grassy vista dotted with clumps of trees and bush, interspersed with the mighty baobab tree, whose pods, Alice had earlier established in Cape Town, contained liquid that was both thirst-quenching and fever-curing. The visibility was clear and the air was good, despite the heat.

The little party's demeanour had changed gradually as the journey had progressed. As Bulawayo, with its potential threat from de Sousa, the king and his impis, dropped well behind them and the country opened out, so their mood lightened. The few Mashonas they met were curious but diffident and clearly offered no threat. Game, if not exactly plentiful, was on offer and they feasted for two days on the meat from two impala that Jenkins shot.

They did not press hard, for in anticipation of hard times ahead, Fonthill was anxious to preserve their energies. So day followed pleasant day. 'If Rhodes wants to build his road this way,' Simon confided to his wife, 'then I can't see what there is to stop him. But more to the point, we could farm here, darling,' he added. 'Good soil, plenty of water from these little rivers and the grass looks sweet. What do you think?'

Alice tried to prevent a smile, but her husband's enthusiasm was infectious. 'Well,' she said, 'I have to agree that it all looks very fine, and the air is good, too. But settlements here would very much depend upon the king, surely. Building a road and making the odd excavation for gold or copper is one thing. Letting in people to farm is very much another.'

Fonthill reached across and seized his wife's hand. 'Oh don't be such a grouch, darling. Old Lobengula would certainly let *you* in. One wave of your hypodermic thing-ummyjig and thousands of acres would be ours. But one thing is certain. There is no one else here farming the land or making the most of it. It's just lying gloriously fallow.'

And indeed it was. The local Mashonas lived in small, isolated villages and the few cattle they seemed to possess grazed in enclosed paddocks close to their wickerwork houses. Only wild game roamed the open plateau.

'Lions,' said Mzingeli quietly. But no one heard him.

As they pressed on to the east, however, the terrain became less hospitable. The land was now an ochre red, and as they dropped down from the plateau, the going became less hard underfoot. They had to cross more spruits and, importantly, the bush became thicker. For the first time, they decided to set up some form of protection for their camps overnight.

Mzingeli explained that, in addition to lions, this could be buffalo and elephant country, and showed them how to make a scarum for the camp. This involved cutting large boughs or stakes and driving them into the ground on the windward side to form a semicircle capable of containing the whole party, mules and all. Then small bushes were cut and interwoven into the boughs, making a hedge some nine feet high, capable of withstanding a large shock, on three sides of the encampment. At the open end, wood was stacked and fires lit at night. They all slept out of doors, cutting grass to form a mattress with a blanket laid on top. Saddles or spare clothes were used as pillows.

Some four weeks after leaving Bulawayo, as they sat near their roaring fire, Fonthill consulted his compass and the map that Fairbairn had provided. 'I have no scale for this damned thing,' he confided to Alice, Jenkins and Mzingeli, 'but I reckon that we have left the Matabele kingdom now and are well out of Mashonaland. We should be somewhere in this area of small tribes and therefore not far from the border with Portuguese East Africa.'

'Strange that we have not seen any natives,' said Alice.

'They here,' murmured Mzingeli.

'What?' Jenkins looked perturbed. 'I 'aven't seen a damned thing.'

'No.' The tracker nodded to the bush pressing in on them all around. 'They watch us. I see. I think they frightened of us.'

'Why?'

'Perhaps they think we slavers.'

Fonthill frowned, mindful of Rhodes's injunction to befriend the tribes. 'Well I would like to make contact. Can you speak their language, do you think?'

'Not well, but I try if they come.'

'How can we make them come?'

The tracker shrugged his shoulders. If he had nothing to say, he rarely spoke.

'Right.' Fonthill stood. 'We will stay here all tomorrow. Tonight we will put a few of the trade goods just outside the opening. Let's see if that will induce them to come forward, although . . .' he looked around and wrinkled his nose, 'I don't think this is the best country for laying down a new road, I must say. But perhaps we can discover if the terrain is better elsewhere, if they will talk to us, that is.'

Before retiring to his blanket, Fonthill hung a few brightly coloured lengths of cotton fabric, two axes and some copper trinkets on the edge of their scarum.

The night was dark when something woke him. Immediately awake, he reached for his rifle and sat up. The fires at the edge of the scarum were still guttering and the low flame was reflected in the copper amulets hanging from the hedge. So they had not been taken. What, then, had woken him? He narrowed his eyes the better to see through the opening, and as he focused he made out several large grey shapes, as tall, it seemed, as the scarum, moving slowly, ponderously, past the opening.

'Elephant,' said Mzingeli from his blanket. 'Stay quiet. They don't harm us.'

By the morning, both the elephants and the trinkets had gone.

'Good,' said Fonthill. 'Joshua' – the boy had now picked up a serviceable knowledge of English – 'put some more of those things outside. Then we must just sit and wait.'

It was well past midday when Mzingeli nodded. 'They come now,' he said. 'Don't show rifles. They frightened if you do.'

Gradually, as they watched, three men emerged from the bush and stood tentatively just beyond the ashes of the fire, at the opening of the scarum. Very slowly, Mzingeli rose and ambled towards them, his arm lifted in greeting. He spoke a few words but there was no reply, so he squatted on the camp side of the ashes and silently regarded the natives. After a while, they lowered themselves to the ground and sat cross-legged.

'Is it goin' to be a card game, then?' enquired Jenkins quietly of Fonthill.

'Shush. Let's leave it to Mzingeli.'

Simon looked at the natives. They were of far less impressive stature than the Matabeles, and seemed unwarlike, in that they were not painted and carried no weapons. They were naked except for loincloths of some animal skin, and their hair was plastered down with red earth. The middle of the three now spoke hesitantly to Mzingeli. The tracker responded, picking his words as though only partly understanding the language. Then he stood nonchalantly, handed down the trinkets and gave them to the three.

As a result, the conversation improved considerably, although it was clear that Mzingeli did not speak the language fluently. The tracker stood, walked back into the compound and, turning, beckoned the men to follow him. Reluctantly they did so until they stood facing Fonthill and Jenkins. Simon immediately made a gesture towards the ground and the three, followed by Mzingeli, squatted before him.

'There's cosy now, isn't it?' said the Welshman, grinning.

Jenkins's ability, proven in so many different countries and continents, to break through all kinds of linguistic barriers worked again, and his grin was immediately returned by the visitors, who revealed great yellow tombstone-like teeth.

'Who are they?' enquired Fonthill of Mzingeli. 'Can you communicate?'

'Yes, but not fluent. They Manica people, ruled by king called Umtasa. Their land goes up to Portuguese land. But Portuguese claim their land too. They heard of English and are glad we not Portuguese.'

'Good. How far away is their king?'

The tracker directed the question to the man sitting in the middle of the trio, who seemed to be senior. He had taken the gifts to himself and now sat with the cloth draped over his shoulders and the copper artefacts hanging around his neck. He replied at some length.

'He say that Umtasa is at kraal, say a day's march to east. He can take us to his village nearby and then come with us to Umtasa.'

'Good. Thank you, Mzingeli. Have Joshua offer them some food and we will make ready to go. I think we will leave Joshua, Alice and the boys here – they should be all right within the scarum – and the three of us will go to the king's kraal. It will be quicker that way.'

'Thank you very much, but I am not going to be left behind.' Alice had quietly approached. 'Simon, will you stop treating me as some kind of fragile supernumerary who is to be perpetually excluded from the more exciting parts of this expedition. Really, I am tired of it, my dear.'

Fonthill sighed. 'Very well, Alice. We will leave Joshua in charge. We will be away overnight so we must go prepared. Quickly now. I would like to be there by nightfall.'

As soon as the visitors had eaten their rice and biltong, the party moved off, taking one mule, laden with presents, food and their bedding, with them. The bush was now very thick and the going soft underfoot, deteriorating now and then to semi-swamp. Mosquitoes were accompanying them step by sodden step, and Alice was glad that she had brought quinine with her. To them all the unspoken thought occurred: this is no place for road-building.

They reached the village after a four-hour trudge. It was a poor affair, just a few huts set in a small clearing by a stream, but so hidden by thorn bushes and low trees that even invaders knowing the territory would have difficulty in finding it. It was clear that the man leading the trio was the local headman, and Fonthill prevailed upon him that they should not pause at the village but press on towards the king's kraal. He was retrospectively anxious that their scarum, containing most of their possessions, had been left so lightly defended, and wished to return to it as soon as possible.

They passed several other villages on the way to the Manican capital. The people were shy but friendly, not at all militant and more pastoral than the Matabele. They possessed few cattle – indeed the land did not encourage grazing – but they grew maize and grain where they could. It was clear that if they decided to come this way, Rhodes's engineers would have no trouble with the natives. The terrain and climate, however, could be another matter. It was hot, and the dreaded tsetse flies seemed to be as numerous as the mosquitoes. Fonthill kept a concerned eye on the mule, but, having been treated with salt, it seemed to be impervious to the insects.

It was nearly nightfall before they came to King Umtasa's kraal. It was set in clear land on a slight rise that took it away from the swamp and the worst of the mosquitoes and tsetses. It was not as large as Bulawayo, but was similar in shape and style, with thorn bushes providing a series of enclosures that led to the king's own house, a circular construction of wickerwork and red clay only slightly larger than those that surrounded it. The usual chorus of barking dogs and excited children ushered them into the heart of the town. Unlike in Bulawayo, however, the adult Manicans hung back.

The headman prostrated himself before a large man who appeared from the house, and taking their cue, Simon and his entourage bowed their heads before the king. The man was dressed inconspicuously in a loincloth of some animal skin and little else, except for a necklace of animal's teeth – lion's? – around his throat. His skin was very, very black and glistened in the reflection of the flames that danced from several fires lit outside the entrance to his house. Unusually, he affected a short white beard that contrasted strangely with the tight black curls of his hair. His frown on first seeing the Europeans disappeared as the headman, still prostrate, spoke.

'He say we not Portuguese,' murmured Mzingeli. 'That good.'

The king grunted to the headman, who rose to his feet, and raised his forearm, the palm of his hand facing Fonthill, in greeting.

'Please tell him,' said Simon, 'that we bring greetings from the Queen of England and from her representative in Africa, Mr Cecil Rhodes.'

'Huh,' grunted Alice. 'That's a bit much.'

Ignoring her, Fonthill continued. 'We come to offer a treaty of friendship between the British and the Manican people. We would like to present some small gifts as a token of our goodwill. Jenkins, please . . .'

The Welshman turned back to the mule, whose load he had begun unfastening on their way through the township. From the packs he produced lengths of cloth, several knives and axes, more of the copper decorations, two small hand mirrors, and – to gasps from the spectators who had now gathered near – two Snider rifles. He laid the gifts at the king's feet, gave a cheery nod and said, 'Merry Christmas, your worship.'

The king immediately picked up a rifle, weighed it in his hand, sighted along the barrel and spoke to Mzingeli.

'He say good, but no good without bullets.'

''E's no fool,' breathed Jenkins, who turned back to the packs and produced three small boxes of cartridges and laid them on the ground with the other gifts.

The king nodded and spoke again, flashing a sly glance at Alice. 'He say we are welcome. We come a long way, so stay with him to recover from journey. Lady particularly welcome. He not seen white lady before. Eat with him tonight. Take beer now.'

A signal was given, mats were brought for them to sit on, and after a slight delay, the inevitable gourds of beer were produced by smiling women. Fonthill noticed that the gifts were left lying on the ground, as though they were of no importance, although everyone was eyeing them. He liked that. It showed good manners.

They were given one hut for them all to share, and then joined the king and some of his *inDunas* – no wives – at a meal around the fires. Seated on logs, they ate meat that had a strangely fishy taste and which was served with mealies. On asking, Simon was told that it was crocodile. He decided to keep the news from Jenkins, who was conversing merrily but one-sidedly with an *inDuna*. Jenkins did not like crocodiles.

Through Mzingeli, whose proficiency in the language seemed to have improved considerably, he asked the king about the nature of the terrain throughout his kingdom. Did the semi-swampland continue to the north and south?

The king shook his head. 'Better land to the north. Firmer. Take wagons easily. That is best way to Mashonaland. But further. He take you there tomorrow.'

'Thank you. We must return to our camp first, but with the king's permission, we will return immediately with our mules and people to look at that land.'

'King want to know why you interested.'

Fonthill cleared his throat and felt Alice's gaze on him. 'If the king is prepared to sign a treaty of friendship with the Queen's company in South Africa, then one day it could be that a road will be built – with his permission, of course – through his country to link Mashonaland with the Indian Ocean.'

'That Portuguese territory.'

'Yes. An agreement would also need to be reached between the Queen of England and the King of Portugal.'

'You know the Portuguese?'

'Er . . . yes. I have met one of their agents.'

'They say that they own my country. They do not. Would your Queen give me protection from Portuguese?'

'If you reject the Portuguese claim to your land and sign a treaty with the South African charter company, which has powers under the British Government, then this can be done.'

'Are you sure, Simon?' The question came very quietly from Alice, but he was forced to ignore it because the king was speaking.

'He say that he will sign it but he will need more guns.'

'I will pass on his request to Mr Rhodes in the Cape, who is the chief of the company.'

'Then he sign.'

'Good. I have a copy of the treaty back at my camp and I will bring it to him for his signature tomorrow.'

The evening ended early, for Simon was anxious to set off back to the camp at dawn the next day. Predictably, before turning in, Alice raised the question of the treaty.

'Have you really brought a proper document with you?'

'Yes, of course. In fact I brought three with me from Cape Town, duly signed by Rhodes. We didn't know the tribes then, of course, because we didn't know whom we would meet, but all I have to do is fill in their names and those of the kings and get them to sign.'

She screwed up her features. 'Gracious, this all sounds so . . . tawdry. And what on earth could Rhodes – let alone the British Government – do if the Portuguese came here and started to throw their weight around? Think of Gouela. A bit of paper isn't going to stop him.'

'One thing at a time, Alice. The process has to be started somewhere, and it starts with this bit of paper, as you call it. Once the charter company is established in Matabeleland – and that means the road – then Rhodes can extend his protection to outlying provinces like this.'

Alice sniffed but said nothing more.

The next morning they set off back to their scarum even before the king had risen, although the village headman and his two villagers kept their promise to accompany them. As always, the return journey seemed quicker than the outgoing one, and it felt like only a couple of hours before they reached, and passed through, the village, dropping off the natives there. In the early evening they caught sight of the tall tips of the scarum fence. Everything seemed quiet and peaceful as they approached. Perhaps too quiet.

'Joshua should have been keeping a lookout,' said Fonthill testily. Then he held up a hand to restrain the party. 'Wait,' he said.

From the fringe of the bush cover they studied the make-shift stockade. Nothing could be seen through the opening and no sound came from within it. Their mule brayed, but no answering call came from the animals that should have been inside. Fonthill withdrew his rifle from its saddle holster and slipped off the safety catch. He signed for the others to do the same. Then, cautiously, they began to advance, only to be halted by Mzingeli's hand on Simon's arm.

The tracker nodded to marks on the floor of the clearing. 'Big party been here,' he mouthed.

'Damn! Do you think there are any still inside?'

'Think no. They move out. See spoor.' He pointed to where the marks went off through the bush to the south. Now the trail was there for all to see: broken branches and scuffed earth, winding away.

'Inside, quickly,' cried Fonthill and they moved into the scarum, their rifles at the ready. It was, however, a ghost camp. There was little sign of a struggle, except that their packs had been slashed away from the mules and left, unopened, on the ground. Of Joshua, the boys and the mules there was no trace.

'They couldn't have deserted and gone back to Bulawayo, surely?' asked Alice.

'No.' Mzingeli pointed to the ground to their left, by the exit from the scarum. 'Look. Blood.'

The stains were splattered in a strange, uneven sequence that led off into the bush. Everyone looked at the tracker in horror. He glanced up, his face expressionless as usual. 'Slavers,' he said. 'They whip.'

'Oh dear God,' murmured Alice. 'The boys. They've taken the boys.'

'How long ago, Mzingeli?' asked Fonthill.

The tracker kneeled down and rubbed his finger in the

marks. Then he walked to the broken foliage and examined it, fingering the broken twigs and branches with his thumb. 'Maybe five hours ago. Maybe six.'

'Blimey.' Jenkins spat on to the ground. 'They'll be miles away by now.'

'Not necessarily.' Fonthill joined the tracker. 'How many were there, do you think, and could they move fast in this bush?'

Mzingeli squatted and examined the tracks carefully. Eventually he looked up. 'They have captured slaves with them, walking in chains like this.' He gestured with his fingers to show a single file. 'Gun has been fired here. See marks of powder. Old gun. Like Arabs use.' Simon's brain immediately conjured up the picture of an old musket or *jezhail* that he remembered the Pathans using in the North-West Frontier of India – and he winced as he recalled a butt smashing into his nose.

But Mzingeli was continuing. 'No one killed. See, here they kneel to have chains fitted. Blood only from whip marks. Whips used to make them move.'

'Yes, but how many?'

The tracker shrugged. 'Cannot say. Cannot tell difference between slaves and slavers. Say thirty or forty. But party on foot – no hoof marks except our mules at end of train. They many people for this bush and mules slow them. They don't move quick.'

Fonthill drew in his breath and looked around carefully. 'Strange, they have left our packs. Why?'

Mzingeli shrugged again. 'They don't want to carry. They would like to move quick, though they don't.' He looked up at Fonthill, his face showing concern for the first time. 'Good spoor,' he said. 'We follow, yes? Get our boys back?'

'Of course. But we must be careful. There are only four of us, and they are used to fighting.'

'So are we, bach sir.' Jenkins spoke quietly and looked around, his gaze lingering on Alice as he added, 'All of us.'

Alice smiled, although it did not hide her anxiety. 'Couldn't we get help from the village?' she asked.

'No.' Fonthill was emphatic. 'That would slow us down, and even if some of them came, they would be useless. They are not fighters.'

'No,' agreed Mzingeli. 'They all frightened of slavers.'

'Then we will go as quickly as we can,' said Simon. 'Alice, please check on our rations and see if we need to supplement them from those packs over there . . . and,' he forced a grin, 'before you plead to be left behind, let me tell you now that you are very much part of this party. We need someone who can shoot.'

'Yes,' grunted Jenkins, 'that will make two of us.'

'Don't be insubordinate. Check the ammunition, 352, and fill up the water bottles. Mzingeli, hide the packs. We leave in five minutes.'

They set off in less time than that, in single file, with Mzingeli treading softly some way ahead, followed by Fonthill, then Alice and Jenkins bringing up the rear. Surprisingly, they had found two of the boys' Sniders, buried under their blankets in a corner of the scarum. They took them, one each slung over the shoulders of Simon and Jenkins, to supplement their firepower.

As they walked, Fonthill's brain was busy. Once they caught up with the slavers, they would be heavily out-numbered. Mzingeli had estimated that as slaving parties went, this one was comparatively small, made up of perhaps only five Arabs, armed with their *jezhails*, plus maybe twenty warriors, carrying spears and whips. They were not accustomed to opposition, for they inspired terror from the natives wherever they went and deliberately did not plunder nations of warriors, like the Matabele. Nevertheless, they moved stealthily and fell upon a village before their presence was detected. They did not take all the villagers, for this would denude them of further pickings, only selecting the healthiest men and women. Joshua and the four boys, big and strong, would have been a welcome bonus. Fonthill's jaw tightened. A small party – but still big enough! How to tackle it?

The trail was, indeed, easy to follow. Even though the slaves were walking in single file, the column had pushed its way through the bush heedlessly, leaving broken stems and torn foliage. Footprints were easy to see, even in the fading light, and the mules, of course, had left their droppings.

'Don't they care about being followed?' Fonthill asked Mzingeli.

'They don't care. People don't follow them. Everyone afraid of slavers.'

'Good. We shall be the exception.'

The four were striding quickly, and they stopped only once, for just five minutes, to drink water and eat biltong and berries. Fonthill had not worked out his tactics, for they would depend upon the deposition of the slavers, but he was sure enough of his strategy. They would reach the slavers' camp before dawn and attack at once, using surprise and the cover of darkness to reduce their enemy's advantage in numbers.

Accordingly, after four hours, he sent Mzingeli much further ahead to ensure that they would not all blunder on the camp itself or a rearguard. The prizes at stake – and the danger involved – were too high to make a stupid mistake.

Slave traders struck terror into the hearts of those upon whom they preyed, not just because of the disgusting nature of their predations, but because they could fight. They could defend themselves. Care was needed.

The forest – for that was what the bush had become – was thick and the trail was becoming difficult to follow when Mzingeli could be seen approaching, running softly and weaving his way between the trees.

'They about five minutes' walk ahead,' he said. 'They make camp. Built fires.'

'Good. Take me there now. You two stay here. I won't be long.'

The slavers had made their bivouac for the night in a little clearing, near a stream, and Fonthill followed Mzingeli, treading softly as they approached the edge of the bushes and trees. The Arabs had made no attempt to build a scarum, and seemed confident that an irregular ring of fires, now burning low, would keep out predators. Two small 'Crusader' tents had been erected, presumably to give the Arabs comfortable night quarters, and two spearmen, huddled in blankets, had squatted at either side of the circle and appeared to be dozing. Inside it, the slaves lay in an irregular line.

It was they who caught the eye, presenting a sight of such misery that Simon felt a lump rise in his throat. There were perhaps thirty of them, men and women, linked together in single file by straight wooden yokes, the Y-shaped end of which encircled the throats and was closed at the back of the neck by chains. Their ankles were shackled, and links of chain attached them to the person behind. The chains and the yokes prevented them from finding comfortable postures for sleep, and they half sat, half sprawled. Bowls at their side, however, showed that at least they had been given food.

'Can you see our boys?' hissed Fonthill.

Mzingeli indicated with a nod of his head. There, at the end of the line, were Joshua and the four bearers, all stripped naked like the rest. Joshua's back carried four whip marks, from which the blood still oozed.

Suddenly, some of the women in the line began singing softly. It was a song the like of which Fonthill had never heard before. It was clearly a lament, a slow ululation that bespoke desperation and the realisation of a great, consuming sadness. Tears were in every syllable, and as others joined in, the melancholy rose and settled above the little clearing like a thundercloud.

Then an Arab, a trim figure with a pointed beard, emerged from one of the tents, shrugging on his white burnous. He barked a command, and from out of the shadows appeared a huge, very black man – probably a Nubian from the Sudan, speculated Fonthill – wielding a long whip of buffalo hide. Immediately the whip cracked and hissed through the air, singling out the women and lashing their backs and bowed heads. The song died and silence of a sort descended on the clearing. Fonthill winced. His mind flashed back for a moment to a whipping post in Omdurman and the beat of a drum.

'If we can't kill 'em all, I know which ones we *will* kill,' he whispered. 'Now, Mzingeli. Please go and bring the others up. No. Wait a second. Am I right that the wind is coming this way,' he gestured, 'from the north?'

The tracker twisted his face to catch the breeze, and then nodded. 'Not much, though.'

'Good. Go now.'

As the tracker glided away, Fonthill began to move with great care around the edge of the camp, to the south. One rash move now could lead to disaster and upset his plans. He found the spot he was looking for, fringed on the camp side with bushes and low trees, but behind this foliage was another small clearing, its edges strewn with dead wood and dry grass. He hurried back, treading carefully. All was quiet in the camp now that the women had been silenced. Only a distant growl and then a bark showed that they were not alone in the forest.

A rustle presaged the appearance of Jenkins, Alice and Mzingeli out of the darkness. They gathered around Fonthill.

'Right,' he whispered, 'the plan is simple. We will take up various vantage points around the camp under cover but close enough to open fire when I give the signal. Alice and I will stay here; 352, you will go directly opposite us on the other side; Mzingeli, you go down ahead there to the south. You will find a little clearing behind a fringe of bush. Once there, I want you to gather some brushwood – dry tinder wood, to make sure that it will burn. There is plenty about. I want it to be big enough to frighten the camp but not big enough to set the whole damned forest ablaze. The wind is coming from the north, so if the blaze does spread, it will go away from us and the camp. But I hope that in the panic, none of these bastards will realise that.' He pressed a box of matches into the tracker's hand.

'When do I light?'

'Once you are in position, give us a good ten minutes – 352 has the furthest to go – and then light it.'

'Then what do we do, bach sir?' Jenkins's eyes were glowing in the semi-darkness.

'Wait until I fire from this side. I will take out the two guards.' He turned to Alice. 'I am sorry, but this will be cold-blooded killing,' he said. 'We must take advantage of surprise. If we don't kill quickly, they could overwhelm us. But I shall quite understand if you do not wish to fire.'

Alice's face showed white. 'I will do whatever you want me to do,' she said. 'I quite understand the need. These men are depraved.'

'Very well. Now, 352, as our best shot, you will have the key role. Here, take one of the Sniders as well as your rifle. The blaze will raise the alarm, of course, and then my shots. There are Arabs sleeping in those tents there, I don't know how many. The openings are on your side. They will turn out, of course, when the alarm is given. Kill them – or as many as you can. Mzingeli, you shoot as many of the natives as possible, but of course avoid the slaves, as we will on this side.'

He looked at them in turn. 'I am banking on the fact that the fire will cause initial alarm; then, when the shooting sets in from different sections of the forest, panic should ensue. Key to this, of course, is the killing of the Arabs. I want the natives to be leaderless. I will try and pick off any that you miss . . .'

'I'll not miss, bach sir.'

'Of course you won't. If you are attacked, duck and run and try and make it back to Alice and me here. Understood? Any questions?'

Alice cleared her throat. 'Where are the mules?'

'Good point. I have to confess that I don't know. Did you see them, Mzingeli?'

'No.'

'I suppose they will be somewhere in the compound. If they get excited, they might break their tethers and run about; that should help us. Cause a bit of panic. Just be sure we don't kill any of them. We will need 'em. Anything else? Good. Now go to your posts, and good luck.'

Jenkins and the tracker slipped away. Fonthill looked at his wife anxiously. 'Would you rather use this Snider instead of your own rifle?'

'No thank you. I am happier with this. It may not kill but it will cause a nasty wound. The Snider is too heavy for me.'

'Very well. Alice, let me take the guards, then you shoot at the Kaffirs who are nearest as they rush out. Is that all right?'

She nodded. She seemed completely calm, yet Fonthill knew that within she would be apprehensive at the prospect of having to kill. Oh, she had shot men before, but not like this, in cold blood. Nevertheless, he wished he had her composure. He licked his lips. The waiting was the worst part. He raised his Martini-Henry and sighted it on the guard furthest away. Then he realised that the muzzle was beginning to sway and he lowered it. Mustn't get tired. He frowned and wished – not for the first time – that he was a better shot.

Then, at last, about a hundred and fifty yards away down the trail, a thin flicker of light appeared in the bush. It danced tantalisingly in the darkness for a moment and almost went out, then it took hold, and suddenly that area of the forest was illuminated as a sheet of flame licked upwards.

Fonthill waited for a moment, and then, slowly, he raised his rifle. 'Now,' he muttered, and squeezed the trigger. The bullet took the sleeping warrior fully in the chest, and he sighed and then toppled over. Quickly Simon jerked down the extractor handle behind the trigger guard, inserted another round into the breech and aimed again. Almost inevitably, he missed the second guard as the man rose to his feet quickly, too quickly.

'Damn!' he cursed under his breath. Then Alice's Westley Richards barked at his right elbow, and the man staggered and fell. 'Good girl,' said Fonthill as he inserted a third cartridge and fired it into the figure of the guard, who, wounded, was now trying to totter to his feet. The man went down again immediately.

The sleeping camp suddenly became a scene of hectic activity. The Kaffirs appeared as if from nowhere – in reality, from their sleeping mats on the far side of the camp – and stood waving their spears and pointing, first to the fire and then to where Fonthill and Alice were now shooting at them systematically. To their shouts were now added screams as two, three and then four of them fell to the ground, clutching at gunshot wounds that sent blood gushing from between their fingers. The confusion was heightened as Mzingeli's rifle opened fire from the south.

'Why doesn't Jenkins fire?' hissed Fonthill.

'He's probably waiting to get a shot at the Arabs but the Kaffirs are in the way,' muttered Alice as she methodically loaded and fired, loaded and fired.

This seemed to be proven as two of the white-robed Muslims now came running into view from the side of their tents, bent low and carrying their *jezhails*.

'They're coming towards us,' cried Alice.

'Pick 'em off before they get near enough to use their muskets.'

Fonthill pulled his trigger, but the bullet only spurted dust from in front of the feet of the nearest Arab, who immediately knelt, levelled his *jezhail* and fired. The ball took Alice in the thigh, and she gasped, dropped her rifle and fell to the ground, clutching at the wound. Simon, quickly reloading, had time only to glance down and then fire at the first slaver, who was almost upon him. The bullet took the man in the chest, and he sprawled forward on to his face, his momentum taking him skidding along the ground until he lay still.

Fonthill knelt down quickly at Alice's side. The action almost certainly saved his life, for a second musket ball sang over his head and buried itself into the trunk of the tree above him.

'Behind you,' hissed Alice, her face contorted with pain. Fonthill just had time to turn and avoid the butt of a musket as the second Arab swung it at his head. The momentum took the man around, and Simon clenched his right fist and hit him hard in the ribs, following it with a left hook to the face. But his half-kneeling posture meant that he could get no power into either blow, and the folds of the man's unravelled turban softened much of the impact of the punch to the head. He staggered back, regained his balance and swung the *jezhail* again. Fonthill ducked under it but caught his foot on a tree root and sprawled forward, rolling on to his side to avoid the butt of the musket, which thudded into the earth beside his temple. He grabbed the stock to help him regain his feet, and for a matter of seconds he and the Arab fought for possession of the gun. The Muslim was taller than Fonthill, but he was also older, and years of being indulged by slaves had done nothing to toughen his body, whereas the last few months of trekking had left Simon with not an ounce of superfluous fat on his frame. He pulled the Arab towards him, then hooked his leg around that of the other man and pushed hard. The Arab twisted and then sprawled backwards on to the ground. Fonthill picked up the musket and brought it down on the slaver's head. This time the unwound turban did nothing to protect him, and his skull cracked with a sickening sound.

'Simon . . .'

Fonthill whirled and threw the *jezhail* at a native who, spear upraised, came at him from out of the forest. Then in one quick movement he bent, picked up the Snider, cocked it and fired from the hip at the native, who collapsed with a bullet in his stomach. Gasping, he picked up his Martini-Henry and looked about him quickly before crawling to Alice's side.

'Where are you hit, my love?'

'In the leg.' Perspiration was pouring down her face as she held out her hand. 'Help me up. It's only a flesh wound, but the rest of them will be on us in a moment. I must be standing.'

'Yes, but can you?'

'I can. Let me lean on this tree. Reload, for goodness' sake, Simon. They know where we are.'

Fonthill picked up his rifle and thrust another round into the breech. He could now hear shots coming from both Mzingeli's and Jenkins's positions, and pandemonium seemed to reign within the slavers' camp. One Arab was standing within a circle of Kaffirs, attempting to direct operations – were there others? Had Jenkins got them? The man was pointing towards the positions of the three rifles, obviously attempting to divide his force into three to launch separate attacks on the source of the fire. But the Kaffirs were clearly reluctant to move. The blaze that Mzingeli had created had taken hold and seemed to be threatening the camp; the rifle fire from three different points was now bringing down a man with each shot; and panic, as Fonthill had hoped, was beginning to set in.

First one man, and then two and three began to slip away from the edge of the group surrounding the Arab, and suddenly the rest threw away their spears and ran to the only point of the compass, the south, that offered them escape. They ran as fast as their legs could take them and disappeared into the bush, leaving the slaver standing, waving a curved sword and cursing them. He stood, however, for only a few seconds more before Jenkins's shot shattered his head.

Fonthill looked anxiously towards where the slaves lay. It looked as though none had been hit in the affray, for they all had remained as close to the earth as possible as the gunfire sounded all around. They were now lifting their heads cautiously to look around, and Simon could see that Joshua, at the end of the line, was attempting to stand, although the wooden yoke, attached to the next man, still lying, was preventing him.

It seemed that all the slavers had fled, but then he saw the Nubian slave master. The man, distinguished by the long coiled whip hanging from his cummerbund, had emerged from the edge of one of the tents and was crawling towards the line of slaves. He had a knife in his hand.

Alice had seen him too. 'My God, Simon. He's going to kill the slaves!'

Fonthill raised his rifle to his shoulder and took careful aim. But the Martini-Henry, so terrible a man-stopper, was never happy at being fired consistently without being allowed to cool – as the defenders at Rorke's Drift had found – and now it jammed.

'Damn!' Simon threw the rifle to the ground and ran forward, crashing through the undergrowth and leaping over the embers of the perimeter fires. He was too late to save the first man in the slave line, who succumbed with a slashed throat, but he threw himself on to the assassin, landing on his back as he crouched, preparing to continue his grisly work. The man lurched forward, arms outstretched and spreadeagled across the second slave, who screamed in terror. Fonthill recovered quickly, and straddling the two, he slipped his arms under the slave master's shoulders and locked his hands together at the back of the neck in the classic half-nelson hold. The Nubian, big and strong, hunched his shoulders and flung Simon to and fro, but was unable to break the lock as Fonthill hung on like a terrier clinging to a fox.

Then the man went limp as Jenkins's rifle butt thudded into his head.

'Sorry, bach sir. Couldn't shoot the bugger because you was 'uggin' 'im so close. Didn't know you fancied 'im, like.'

'Thanks, 352,' Fonthill gasped, scrambling to his feet. 'Search him for a key to the chains and unlock these poor devils. I must get back to Alice.'

He found his wife now sitting at the base of the tree, her face completely white, hacking away the cloth of her breeches with a knife.

'Here, let me do that.' He took the knife from her and slit the seam of the breeches. She gave a little gasp and bit her lip. The musket ball had buried itself into her thigh, leaving a neat, plum-coloured hole from which blood was oozing.

'Lucky it wasn't a rifle cartridge,' said Fonthill. 'That would have gone through and done a lot of damage, but I think we shall be able to get it out without too much trouble.' He looked up, his eyes moist. 'You are a strong, brave girl.'

'No I'm not.' Alice's voice seemed to come from far away. 'I really want to have a good cry. At this moment, Norfolk seems a very nice place to be. I've had enough of bloody Africa . . .' Then she slumped forward.

As Simon knelt and gathered her in his arms, he became aware that Mzingeli was at his side. He stood, lifting Alice, and adjusted her tenderly to avoid putting pressure on the wound. 'Have they all gone, Mzingeli, do you think?'

The tracker nodded. 'We kill many. Only maybe nine or ten left and they run. They don't come back. All Arabs killed.'

'Good. Pick up the rifles and please go on and find somewhere where I can lay Alice and build up one of the fires. We shall need to get this musket ball out of her leg.'

Carrying Alice into the clearing, he found Jenkins unlocking the big padlock that secured all the chains at the head of the line. He acknowledged the cries that came from the slaves as, one by one, the chains were threaded through and they were freed. Fonthill exchanged grins with Joshua and the other boys at the end of the line, and then the women began to sing again. This time it was no lament.

Alice had regained consciousness as Simon lowered her on to a divan of sorts within one of the tents. He tipped water from his bag on to his handkerchief and wiped her brow, and then gave her some to drink. Although beads of perspiration were beginning to fringe her hairline, he wrapped a blanket around her. Delayed shock and perhaps fever, he knew, would be a danger now.

'Three five two,' he hailed through the tent opening. 'Did you get the rest of those Arabs?'

'Yes, bach sir. I couldn't get a bead on 'em to start with, because of the black fellers in between. Then I got the first one, you got two and I eventually put away the last. There was only four, see.'

'Good. Now stand guard just in case any of the other bastards try to come back. Oh – and get Joshua to see if he can find clothes for the slaves. There must be some somewhere, and they should have their dignity back.'

Mzingeli had now joined him. 'I've left my pack by the tree over there,' said Fonthill. 'Please fetch it.' He lowered his voice. 'Then I shall need your help in getting this musket ball out. I'm no doctor, blast it.'

The tracker nodded and ran off. Simon returned to his wife and knelt by her side. 'We will soon have this damned thing out,' he murmured. 'Did you bring your first-aid bits and pieces with you by any chance?'

She nodded. 'I thrust a small bundle into the top of your pack before we left,' she whispered, her eyes heavy. 'Not much. Just a bandage or two, a little morphine, some antiseptic. Had to leave my bag hidden where we camped. Too heavy . . .' Her voiced tailed away.

'Splendid. Hold on. Won't be long now.' But he did not share the confidence his voice expressed. He held his wife's hand tightly until Mzingeli returned carrying his pack. Fonthill foraged inside it and produced the little bundle, wrapped in oilskin, that Alice had prepared. He unrolled it and laid the contents carefully on a blanket at the side of the divan: three tightly rolled bandages, some lint and a cotton pad, a jar of antiseptic cream, a small bottle of painkilling pills – and a broken bottle of morphine, its precious liquid long since drained away.

Hurling the bottle away with a curse, he fumbled once more in the pack and produced a half-bottle of whisky, now containing only a little of the spirit. He beckoned Mzingeli outside. 'Let me see your knife,' he said. The tracker produced it. 'Good. Better than mine. Thinner and sharper. Now, go and put the blade into a fire until it glows completely red. Let it cool – but don't touch it or let the blade touch anything else. It's got to be completely clean. Then bring it back here.'

Fonthill re-entered the tent, his wife's anxious eyes following his every movement. He took the cork out of the whisky bottle, put his other hand behind Alice's head and lifted it up. 'Now,' he said, 'drink a little of this, my love, please.'

Her wide eyes on his, she took the bottle and swallowed, spluttered and handed it back. 'I hate whisky,' she coughed.

'I know, my darling, but you must finish the bottle. Come along now. Do what Dr Fonthill says, there's a good girl.' He gave a mirthless smile and handed her the bottle again. 'Do it in your own good time, but drink it all, please.'

Pulling a face, she raised the bottle to her lips again, and eventually drank all the amber liquid. Her head sank back on the sheet that Simon had folded for her as a pillow. 'Oh God,' she whispered, 'I feel awful.'

'Lie there for a moment, my darling. Sleep if you want to.'

He put down her hand and left the tent. All of the slaves were now unshackled and were standing or lying, rubbing their ankles and necks where the chains and yokes had chafed their skin. Jenkins, rifle cradled, was talking to Joshua, and Mzingeli was gingerly holding his knife blade in the flames of a rekindled fire.

'Ready yet?' called Fonthill.

The tracker held up his free hand to quell Simon's impatience, and Jenkins came hurrying over. 'I didn't realise she'd been 'it,' he said, his face showing lugubrious concern. ''Ow bad?'

'She has a musket ball in her thigh. I am going to try to dig it out as soon as Mzingeli gets that knife clean.' He pulled a face. 'I'm not looking forward to it.'

'Excuse me if I don't come in. I'll be sick if I do.'

'No. Stand guard and make sure that none of the Kaffirs return. Oh.' He nodded to the slave master. 'Tie him up. We have unfinished business with him for the morning.'

Jenkins gave a puzzled look, then nodded. 'Very good, bach sir.'

The tracker held the knife up into the night air to cool it. Behind him, the fire he had started in the bush began to flicker and die as it ran on to the stony ground of the clearing. He strode towards Fonthill and offered him the knife, handle first. 'Still bit warm,' he said.

'Yes. Perhaps better to wait a minute anyway. I've given her some whisky. It's the only anaesthetic I had. She's not used to it, so I hope it does the job.'

The tracker nodded sympathetically. Then they both re-entered the tent. Alice was lying back, half unconscious, her head rolling from side to side.

Simon licked his lips. 'Right. Might as well start. You hold her leg very tightly and make sure that it does not jerk. Press down. I expect it will start to bleed again when I fish for the bloody ball, so staunch the bleeding with this felt. I want to be able to see what I am doing.' He shook his head. 'Oh dear. My poor Alice.'

As Mzingeli crouched on one side, Fonthill settled on the other and began very slowly to peel back the skin surrounding the wound. 'Forceps is what we want,' he breathed, 'not this damned butcher's knife.'

At first Alice seemed to feel no pain, but then, as Simon began gently probing to locate the ball, she jerked and then moaned.

'All right, darling,' he mouthed, 'won't be long. Nearly there. Ah, found it!'

With as much care as he could muster, he pushed the tip of the knife around the side of the ball and then, very slowly, worked it underneath the lead. At this point, Alice opened her eyes and then screamed. 'Hold her,' breathed Fonthill, 'nearly there. Now . . .' He levered the ball upwards until, in a welter of blood, he could seize it with his thumb and forefinger and flick it away.

As he did so, Alice sat upright and, eyes staring, grabbed his shoulder. 'Brave girl, brave girl,' he soothed. 'It's out now. Clean as a whistle. Lie back, my darling.' He pushed her gently back on to the bed. 'Just got to clean it up now. Lie still, there's a good girl.'

He seized the whisky bottle and emptied the last drops of the liquor directly on to the wound, before pouring a little water around the edges and wiping them gently. Then he opened the antiseptic cream and – all the finer points of hygiene lost in his anxiety – scooped a little out with the tip of the knife and spread it on the cotton pad. Handing the knife to Mzingeli, he pressed the pad down firmly on the wound and began winding a bandage around it to keep it in place. As he finished with a knot, he realised that Alice was watching him.

'Oh my love,' he whispered, 'I am sorry to have hurt you.'

She shook her head slowly and summoned up the palest of smiles. 'Don't be silly. Couldn't have done better myself. Do you know, I might take to whisky.' Then she closed her eyes and her head sank back on to the folded sheet.

'Can we find another blanket?' Fonthill asked Mzingeli. 'Shock is a danger now. We must keep her warm.'

The tracker nodded and stole out of the tent, to be replaced by Jenkins. 'Oh blimey, bach.' The Welshman's face was as white as Alice's. 'I was outside listenin'. I couldn't 'ave done what you just did. Do you think she will be all right?'

Fonthill wiped the perspiration from his brow and shook his head. 'I don't know,' he said. He looked around. 'It was just so . . . so . . . bloody primitive. I only hope I did the right thing and that infection hasn't got into the wound.' He looked unspeaking into the Welshman's eyes for a moment. 'You know, 352, I don't know what I would do if I lost her. Bringing her out here, exposing her to all this violence . . . She fought as coolly as a Guardsman and certainly saved my life by shooting one of those spearmen. And now, if I've botched this up . . . Oh lord!' He put his hand over his eyes.

Jenkins patted his shoulder. 'You've done all you could,

bach,' he said. 'A bloody wonderful job, I'd say. Now it's up to the man upstairs, see. I think you need a rest. Just you lie down on that bed thing there. Go on now. You'll be near 'er if she wants anythin'. I'll watch over the camp.'

Reluctantly Fonthill nodded and sprawled on to the other divan. Then he rose, pulled the bed so that it was next to Alice's and lay down on it again, reaching across so that he could take her hand. He was already asleep when Mzingeli crept in with two blankets, one of which he added to Alice's covering; the other he laid across Simon, before tiptoeing out.

Chapter 12

When Fonthill awoke, sun was streaming in through the tent opening and the camp was clearly active, for he could hear the sound of mules braying, the clanging of cooking utensils and voices singing. He had cramp in his arm from where he lay awkwardly, still holding Alice's hand. He looked across sharply at her. She lay peacefully asleep, her breast rising rhythmically to her breathing, colour now back in her cheeks. He smiled in relief, gently disengaged his fingers from hers and threw back his blanket.

Outside, fires had been lit and the wooden neck yokes were proving to be excellent fuel underneath two cooking pots. Some of the women, now chastely wearing brief garments that seemed to have been roughly fashioned from the Arabs' white burnouses, were stirring the contents of the pots, and others were helping the men throw earth into pits that had been dug on the periphery of the camp. Away to his left, the mules grazed. It was a scene of pastoral activity.

'Ah, good mornin', bach sir.' Jenkins hove into view, chains wrapped around his shoulders and arms. 'You got a bit of sleep, then? 'Ow's Miss Alice? I looked in about an hour ago an' she was sleepin' like a baby.'

Fonthill yawned. 'Thank you, yes. She's still asleep, thank goodness. Are you going to start an ironmongery business?'

'Ah, this lot. Thought I'd throw 'em all in on top of the bodies I've 'ad the lads bury up there, see.' He gave a theatrical shudder. 'These irons – awful bloody things.'

'Good idea. How are the boys?'

'Joshua's back is still a bit sore but 'e's all right really – at least now. So are the others, although, as you know, we lost one of the slaves. I've 'ad 'im buried separately.' He sniffed and then grinned. 'Everybody's very relieved to be free again. We would 'ave the freedom of Africa if they could give it to us.'

Fonthill returned the grin. 'Where's Mzingeli?'

''E went out early and shot us a bit of meat, an' that's what's stewin' now. Now 'e's in the other tent, rubbin' some leaf stuff into Joshua's poor old back. It'll probably kill 'im.'

'Well I'm glad I'm not being asked to do it. I don't think I'm much of a doctor.'

'Don't say that. Miss Alice is goin' to be all right, look you. Right as rain, I tell you. You can see to my 'angovers any time.'

Fonthill yawned again and stretched. 'Well, she will need rest. I think we had better stay here for at least two days. Can Mzingeli feed us all with his rifle, do you think?'

Jenkins munched his moustache. 'Should think so. What are you goin' to do with this slave lot?'

'Give them the choice of coming back to the local village with us or making their own way back to where they were taken.'

'An' what about 'im?' Jenkins jerked his head to the side of the tent. Fonthill turned and saw the slave master lying on the ground, shackled in his own chains.

Fonthill's face seemed to be set in stone. 'Oh, *he* will be no problem,' he said.

'Yes, but what will we do with 'im?'

'We shall hang him.'

'What! Just like that?'

'Yes. The sooner the better.' Fonthill spoke slowly and decisively. 'The man is a slaver and a murderer. I saw him cut the throat of a defenceless slave. If any of the Arabs had survived, they would have met the same fate. Let us do it now, before Alice recovers. We will take him a little way into the bush, drape those bloody chains around him, string him up by his whip and leave him there. Anyone who comes this way – and it seems to be a slavers' route – will see him and know him for what he was. He will be a warning to others. Fetch Mzingeli and Joshua and we will do it now.'

Jenkins's eyes narrowed. 'Are you sure, bach sir? I mean, killin' a bloke in cold blood – even if 'e is evil – isn't like you, now is it? I mean, an officer an' a gentleman?'

'To hell with that.' Fonthill's expression had not changed. 'The British made slavery illegal eighty-three years ago. One day, perhaps sooner than we think, this territory will be under British rule, and I want these people here,' he gestured to the ex-slaves, 'to know that wherever we are, we will always strive to exterminate this filthy trade. It will be a lesson to them too. Come on. Let's get on with it.'

The Welshman, surprise still on his face, shrugged the chains to the ground and went to fetch Mzingeli and Joshua. Fonthill strode to the centre of the clearing, clapped his hands and waved everyone towards him. The singing stopped and he was soon surrounded. He waited until they were joined by the tracker and Joshua and then he asked Mzingeli to translate his intention.

The announcement, made hesitantly by the tracker, who seemed to share Jenkins's surprise at Fonthill's decision, was greeted by a low hiss and then, when the import of it sank in, by a fierce shout of approval. Immediately the men ran to the Nubian, picked him up, chains and all, on their shoulders and bore him out of the clearing.

Simon yelled to Jenkins, 'Stay with Alice!' and followed, with Mzingeli and a grinning Joshua. The execution was carried out with dispatch. A large baobab tree with a sturdy branch extending out some ten feet from the ground was found, and a man shinned up and secured the base of the slave master's whip to the branch. Within seconds the end of the whip was tied securely around the Nubian's neck and willing hands launched him to swing, weighed down by the chains that only hours before had marked their own captivity and passage into slavery.

Fonthill experienced a sudden, reactive surge of disgust as he saw the man's frozen expression of terror before the drop broke his neck. Then he turned on his heel and walked quickly back into the camp.

During the two days that they remained in the clearing, Fonthill and the others learned of how Joshua and the boys had been taken. They had stood guard in turns through the night, as Simon had instructed, but the guard had stood down with the dawn and they were all taking breakfast within the scarum when, without warning, the slavers had struck. The spearman had come running quickly into the camp, and it took only seconds to herd the five boys together within a ring of steel. The slave line had followed and they were immediately shackled and yoked. Only Joshua had tried to escape, and he had been flogged for his audacity. The slavers, it seemed, had come from the north, from a port called Bagamayo (meaning in Kiswahili 'lay down your heart'), and the slaves were destined to be exported from there. They had been captured from villages on the slavers' march to the south. Some had been in chains for two weeks. Listening to the story, Fonthill felt exonerated for hanging the slave master. Killing wasn't easy, but in some cases it was the only means of justice.

Alice continued to recover, and to Simon's huge relief, it became clear that his rough and ready surgery had proved effective and that no infection had entered the wound. Nevertheless, she still found it difficult to walk. The unpleasant associations of the clearing – the grave pit and the swinging, enchained body in the forest, although Alice knew nothing of the execution – began to press in on them all, however, and Fonthill decided that they should set off on the third day and make their way back to the scarum, where they had left their tents, supplies and, most importantly, Alice's medical bag. A litter was constructed for Alice from one of the divans, and they set off shortly after dawn.

It was an uneventful journey, made long by the necessity to put the litter down every hour to allow Alice some respite from the jarring, irregular movement she was forced to endure. They found their camp untouched, however, and were able to retrieve their possessions from where they had been hidden in the bush.

Once inside their tent, Simon examined Alice's wound. The antiseptic ointment seemed to have done its job well, for there was no sign of infection, but the hole made by the musket ball remained gaping and there was some suppuration. Fonthill caught Alice's eye.

'I'm afraid it needs stitching,' he said. 'Mustn't leave the hole like that in this climate.'

'Hmm.' Alice's face was white under her tan. 'Who is going to do that, then?'

'I . . . er . . . don't suppose that you . . . ?'

'No. I couldn't quite face that, and anyway, I am not as good a needlewoman as I claimed. I am afraid, my love, that it must be you. It isn't saying much, I fear, but you are far and away the best surgeon in our little group. You have already proved that.'

Fonthill gulped. 'Do we have a needle and some gut?'

'Yes. In my bag.'

'So I just . . . ?'

'Yes, dear.' She gave a wan smile. 'You just pierce the skin and draw the edges together. Neatly and tidily. While I scream.'

'Oh lord. Do you have any morphine in your bag?'

'Yes. And a syringe. Might as well get on with it, darling, while I have faith in you. I don't want people staring at a nasty hole in my leg while I bathe in the North Sea off the Norfolk coast, now do I? And if you do well, you can take on the task of mending your socks when we get home.'

Gloomily Fonthill opened up her precious medical bag, laid out a towel on a collapsible stool and placed upon it the necessary implements. He stuck his head out of the tent and called Joshua to bring soap and hot water and to summon Mzingeli.

'What's up?' enquired Jenkins.

Simon explained. 'Ah yes.' The Welshman's face looked drawn, then he nodded his head in appreciation of the task ahead. 'I'll just see to the lightin' of the fires for the night, then,' he said. 'Important, this fire-layin' business, see. Got to be done right. You won't need me in there.' And he strode away very quickly.

Alice, her jaw set squarely, supervised the injection of the morphine and then threaded the needle before lying back, waiting for the drug to take effect. 'Remember,' she said, her head on the pillow, 'you must make the edges of the flesh meet. No gaping gaps, please.' Then she nodded. 'I think the morphine has taken effect now. Stitch away.' And she took a deep breath and looked the other way.

Once again Mzingeli took on the task of holding down Alice's leg, and staunched the bleeding while Simon made the incisions. It took about fifteen minutes before he was able to draw the needle through for the last time, snip off the end of the gut and tie it in a knot to prevent it slipping back.

'There,' he said. 'Not a bad job.' He looked up at his wife, who had made no sound during the operation, but her face was wet with perspiration and blood was flowing from where she had bitten her lip. She was quite unconscious. It was clear that the anaesthetic, clumsily applied, had not been as effective as had been hoped. Cursing, Fonthill bandaged the wound, gently tucked Alice's leg beneath the blanket and, kneeling, began to wipe her brow with a cloth dipped in cold water.

Within a minute she had come round. She gazed at him dreamily. 'I don't suppose there is any whisky in the camp, is there?' she enquired.

'There is just one bottle left,' Simon breathed, 'and you can have all of its contents, my love. You have been a brave, brave girl.'

'Oh good.' And she went back to sleep.

Mzingeli allowed himself one of his rare smiles. 'Nkosana like a warrior,' he said.

They all stayed within the scarum for the next three days while Alice recovered, but the problem of what to do with the ex-slaves began to be pressing. They were becoming fractious, and yet were timorous of leaving the camp on their own. They still feared that the slavers, in some form or other, might return, although Mzingeli tried to assure them that this was most unlikely. The question was: where should they be taken? Most of them seemed to have come from outside the Manican territory. Could they find their own way back to their villages?

Fonthill called a meeting, and he, Jenkins, Mzingeli and Joshua, whose English had now improved to the point where he could understand most of what was said to him, sat around Alice's bed. It was Mzingeli who stated the obvious.

'We no nursemaids,' he grunted. 'Take them to nearest village. Then they decide what to do.'

Simon looked at his wife. 'I don't think you will be able to walk for a time,' he said. 'And I don't want to leave you here.'

Alice waved her hand. 'Don't worry about me. I want to start writing the story of the fight with the slavers anyway, and will need a bit of peace and quiet to concentrate. You must take Mzingeli with you to interpret and Jenkins to help you keep them all moving. I have a feeling that you will have to herd them like cattle, so you will also need some herdsmen.' She smiled. 'Just leave Joshua with me, with a couple of Martini-Henrys and that whisky you promised, and we will be as right as rain.'

'Well I don't know about that.' Fonthill looked at Jenkins, who shrugged his shoulders, and then Mzingeli, who gave an almost imperceptible nod of assent.

He sighed. 'All right. We will go tomorrow. If we make an early start, we should be back well before nightfall—'

Alice interrupted. 'No. It's pointless rushing. When you get to the village, you are virtually halfway to the king's kraal. Why don't you push on to see him and get him to sign your treaty? He will be so happy that you have sent the slavers packing that he will give you anything you want. Probably make you deputy king or Prince of Wales. Strike while the iron is hot. Joshua and I will be right as rain here for two days if you leave us food and drink. Eh, Joshua?'

The boy grinned, not quite comprehending the conversation but glad to be included, and nodded his head.

'Very well. But we won't be away longer than two days. Joshua, you keep a good watch and look after the Nkosana.'

Joshua's grin widened and he nodded again.

In truth, Fonthill was happy to accept Alice's suggestion. Her leg was healing well, but she would need to rest for at least another three days or so, and he did not relish the prospect of kicking his heels idly in the scarum for that time. He was anxious to pull King Umtasa into his bag, prospect a little to the north for firmer terrain for a road, and return to Bulawayo as quickly as possible before going south to meet Rhodes's column on the march. It would almost certainly be on its way now, and he was eager to march with it and look for possible farming land in Mashonaland. For Alice's safety he had no fear. The Manican people were not warlike and would cause her no harm, and Mzingeli had assured him that no slavers would come through this way now for a year or more after the rebuff the last party had received.

It was with a happy heart, then, that he, Jenkins, Mzingeli, the four boys and the chattering band of ex-slaves set off for the Manican village. Surprisingly, it seemed that two of the natives, a pair of brothers, were from the king's kraal and were anxious to return there. They had been taken when they had strayed too far to the west on a hunting expedition. Bringing them back safely would surely cement Fonthill's relationship with the king, and thus confirmed the good sense of pressing on to his kraal as soon as possible.

And so it proved. The majority of the ex-slaves were left at the village, and Fonthill, Jenkins, Mzingeli and the two

Manicans continued their journey, arriving at the kraal just before nightfall. They were met with cries of joy and dancing as the two brothers were welcomed back from the dead. Chattering children, singing adults and barking dogs formed an avenue through which they all marched to the king's hut. It was, Simon reflected, rather like the return of the prodigal son.

That evening they were once again the guests of King Umtasa at an outdoor feast. The king had insisted on interrogating the two brothers on their capture and learning how Fonthill and his party had rescued them. He nodded his head in particular approval at the hanging of the slave master. The man, it seemed, was known to the tribe, and although the king's own kraal was too large and well defended to be a target for their depredations, the slavers had raided other villages in Umtasa's territory and the big Nubian had earned a reputation for cruelty. It was good, said the king, that his new British protectors had already showed that they would and could keep their word.

Fonthill swallowed hard at this. It would be some time, he knew, before a British presence could be extended directly to the Manican people – and what about the Portuguese claim to their land? Through Mzingeli, he gently probed Umtasa on this. Was the king forced to pay allegiance to the European power?

The king shook his head. 'No. They want money. They come sometimes and want me pay taxes. I give little grain but nothing more. Their man comes with his men from the south. He used to take slaves and particularly women from my villages. But I say I complain to Mozambique so he don't no more.'

'What man was that?'

'His name de Sousa,' Mzingeli allowed himself a ghost of a smile as he translated, 'but everyone call him Gouela.'

Fonthill nodded. 'This man is known to me,' he explained. 'He is an agent for the Portuguese government in territories just over the border in Portuguese East Africa. But he has no claim on your country. He also makes claims on the land of the King of the Matabele, but King Lobengula does not accept them. You are right to reject him. He is no better than the Arab slavers who come from the north.'

The king listened impassively. 'Will your Rhodes protect me from him?'

'If your majesty will sign the treaty of friendship between your country and the charter company of Mr Rhodes, as has King Lobengula, then the company will be able to extend protection. Mr Rhodes has now begun building a road through Matabeleland and Mashonaland to the west that will bring him and his influence close to you. I must first return, of course, with the treaty signed by you.'

'And he will give me guns?'

'I shall relay your request to him.'

'This treaty don't take my country from me?'

'No. This is a treaty of friendship between your country and the British Government, as represented by the charter company. It will give the British the right to oppose the Portuguese claim to your land.

'Ah.' Umtasa pulled at his trim beard for a moment. Then he nodded his head. 'Your words are good. You fight slavers already and bring back two of my people. You show you can fight. You bring me treaty. I sign it now.'

Fonthill gave a quiet sight of relief. He was growing weary of the strain of picking his words carefully, and delicately balancing his answers. He was, he realised, tiptoeing between the truth and the near truth. It was a role he did not relish.

Jenkins, who had been listening, immediately rose and retrieved the carefully rolled piece of parchment from Simon's pack. He also brought a pen and a sealed bottle of ink. Umtasa called for a table to be provided, and then he spread out the document and, following Fonthill's pointed finger, laboriously made his cross. Simon scrawled his own name, on behalf of the charter company, and a frowning Jenkins, his tongue poking out from under his moustache, scratched his signature as a witness. Sprinkling a little sand on the signatures, Fonthill extended his hand, and he and Jenkins shook the king's hand as the last seal of goodwill.

The *inDunas* sitting around the fire, not quite under-standing what had just taken taken place but realising that it was a ceremony of some importance, set up a brief ululation in approval.

Jenkins carefully rolled up the document, put away the ink, pen and sand, wiped the back of his hand across his moustache and confided, 'Well, as we've just got married, so to speak, shall we 'ave another little drop of beer to celebrate, eh, your worship?' And he raised his empty cup in genial supplication.

The king grasped the meaning, nodded and ordered more beer, and the drinking continued until the fires were guttering low.

Fonthill rose the next morning with a throbbing head, although Jenkins and Mzingeli appeared to be completely unaffected by the night's carousing. During the evening, the king had repeated his claim that the country to the north offered more open and firm going, right through to the Portuguese border, but Simon resisted the temptation to detour on the way back to the scarum to see for himself. He was already feeling guilty about leaving Alice, and he decided that they would make all haste back to her and explore to the north-east as soon as she was able to walk.

They set off early, carrying with them a pair of medium-sized elephant's tusks that Umtasa had presented to Fonthill for freeing the slaves, and which the four boys carried slung between them.

It was, however, a long trek, and it was almost dark before they reached the scarum. The camp seemed quiet enough, with the mules grazing peacefully outside the stockade, and Fonthill raised a loud 'hello' as they approached. There was no reply, however, and Simon exchanged a puzzled glance with Jenkins. Then he broke into a run.

Alice's tent was empty, and there was no sign of Joshua either. Alice's travelling pack, her few clothes and her medical bag had gone, yet there was no evidence of a struggle. The two Martini-Henry rifles and her Westley Richards stood leaning in a corner of the tent. Alice and Joshua had disappeared without a trace.

Fonthill looked wide-eyed and despairingly at Jenkins and Mzingeli.

'P'raps they've just gone to pick berries or somethin',' offered Jenkins.

'Don't be bloody stupid, man. She can't walk.'

'Ah yes. Sorry, bach.'

In desperation, Fonthill looked around the interior of the tent once again. Something else was missing . . . Ah yes. 'The divan has gone!' he exclaimed. It was true. The bed from the Arabs' tent that had been converted into a rough litter to carry Alice had disappeared. So too had her blankets. 'Why the hell should she want to take her bed with her? Or, for that matter, who else would want to take it?'

Mzingeli had quietly walked outside. Now he re-entered the tent. 'Nkosana taken,' he said. 'Many men.'

Simon crashed his fist into an open palm. 'Oh my God! Who? Where?'

The tracker shrugged. 'Don't know. They go that way.' And he pointed to the west.

Chapter 13

Fonthill noted the direction of Mzingeli's pointed finger and ran outside the scarum and looked hard to the west. At first his unskilled eye could see little to help him. Then, on bending and examining the ground, he perceived the crushed grass and broken twigs that betrayed the passage of a considerable number of people. He turned to find Mzingeli and Jenkins at his elbow.

'Can you see anything that would tell us who they were,' he demanded of the tracker, 'and how long ago they struck?'

Mzingeli bent and put a long black finger into the disturbed grass. He wrinkled his nose. 'No, Nkosi. Not sure. But I think yesterday. And they don't wear shoes. Native men. Going fast. Look how . . . what is English? Yes, heel of foot don't show. Only ball. They running.'

Fonthill nodded, although he could detect nothing of the sort. 'Running? Why on earth should they do that?'

Jenkins sucked in his moustache. 'I suppose they'd be worryin' about us comin' after them, like.'

'Well they've got at least a day and a half's advantage on us anyway.' He bit the knuckles of his fist and tried to think rationally. He turned back to Mzingeli. 'Is there any sign of anyone being hurt?'

'No. No fight. No blood. Guns not moved. Bed gone. Blankets gone. They look after her. Take Joshua, too.'

'So they definitely wanted Alice,' mused Fonthill. 'They saw that, obviously, she couldn't walk, so they took her bed and probably carried her on that. Who would do that? Perhaps someone who wants to have a hold over us so has taken her as some sort of hostage. But who . . . ?' Then his eyes lit up. 'Of course, why didn't I think? De Sousa!'

He turned to the others, anguish showing in his face. 'This is virtually his territory anyway, and he has a score or two to settle with us. He obviously saw the scarum and swept in. It was just his luck to find us gone but Alice remaining. Oh why did I leave her?'

'Don't think about that, bach sir.' Jenkins was at his most pragmatic. 'Just think about gettin' 'er back, which we will, as surely as God made little apples. Now, look you, do we go after 'em right away, or wait until morning?'

Fonthill deflected the question to Mzingeli. 'Can you follow the spoor in the dark?'

'Perhaps, but can't go quick at night.'

'Very well.' Fonthill spoke quickly. 'Let us have something to eat and drink. We will have to leave the mules because they will slow us down, and we take only what we need: dried biltong, water bags; no tents, just blankets. Leave the ivory tusks. But we take Alice's Westley Richards and the other rifles. I want to be well armed and on the way before darkness falls.'

They all bustled about, unhobbling the mules, stuffing their packs with essentials, filling extra water bottles and then, squatting briefly, eating a quick supper. Fonthill was careful to ensure that the document he had signed with King Umtasa was safely stowed in his pack. They were still chewing when a crashing in the undergrowth made them grab their rifles and brought them to their feet.

From the direction in which they had come only a few minutes before, a figure emerged. He was a native, dressed only in loincloth and monkey-skin calf bands and carrying nothing except a water bag. Perspiration poured from his face and chest and he was gasping for breath. Fonthill raised his rifle but was restrained by Mzingeli.

'He from Umtasa kraal,' said the tracker, and he moved quickly towards the tribesman, who looked on the verge of exhaustion. Mzingeli seized the man's water bag to slake his thirst, but it was empty. Instead he raised his own bag to the runner's mouth and urged him to sit. They then engaged in conversation, conducted between the Manican's gasps.

'What does he say?' interrupted Fonthill.

Mzingeli lifted his hand for silence and continued to interrogate the runner. Eventually he rose. 'He come from King Umtasa,' he said. 'After we leave kraal, de Sousa arrive with men. He tell king that he heard we in area and want him to produce us for him to kill. King say we left day before. De Sousa go off to find us. This man sent by king to warn us. He been running all day.'

'Ah.' Fonthill clenched his fist. 'That settles it. The bastard arrived here before us and took . . . Wait.' He frowned. 'Ask him how long after we left the Portuguese set off.'

Mzingeli translated. 'He not sure but think about one hour. He run around Gouela and men and then come straight here. They not far behind him now.'

Fonthill's frown deepened. 'That means that de Sousa could not have got here before us and taken Alice. I just don't understand this, at all.'

'Well,' sniffed Jenkins. 'Do we wait 'ere an' give old

Saucepot another bloody nose, or do we bugger off after Miss Alice? Not much time to decide, bach sir.'

Fonthill raised his hand. 'Let me think. Now, if Gouela had been able to overtake us in some way, by design or accident, and taken Alice, then he would have waited here to surprise us. That means that he hasn't taken her and someone else has. Right. We go after Alice, and we start now before that greaser and his men arrive. Here.' He delved into his pack and pressed two golden sovereigns into the messenger's hand. 'Mzingeli, please give him our thanks and ask him to pass our gratitude on to the king. Give the man one of our spare water skins and tell him that if he can hide them from de Sousa, the mules are his. We leave now.'

Leaving the young man standing in the compound clutching his sovereigns, Fonthill and his party broke into a trot and set off into the bush, following a trail that was now only slightly discernible in the dusk. They alternately trotted and walked for about an hour, stringing out in single file with Mzingeli in the lead, followed by Simon, Jenkins and the four boys, before the tracker was forced to admit that he could not follow the spoor any longer in the growing darkness.

'Right,' grunted Fonthill, perspiration trickling down his face. 'We get off this track and bed down in the bush. No fire. No light. No talking . . .' He paused. 'Wait a minute, we are missing a boy.'

Indeed they were. Only three of the young men who had journeyed with them from Bulawayo had gathered around him. 'Mzingeli – find out what's happened.'

A quick conversation ensued between the tracker and the three boys. Then Mzingeli reported: 'Boy was last in line. Slow runner. Boy in front of him not realise he fall behind and disappear. Maybe he come soon.'

Fonthill shook his head. 'If you can't find the track in the dark, then this lad can't.' He sighed. 'All right. You and I had better go back and look for him. Jenkins, stay in charge here, and for goodness' sake don't let any of the boys stray.'

Jenkins pulled a face. 'Better I come with you, bach sir, with old Saucepot on our trail. Just in case you run into trouble.'

'No. You stay here with the boys. We don't want too many bodies wandering around in the bush in the dark. Keep a guard rota. We won't be long. I only hope we can retrace our steps.'

It was difficult, but they did so – at least for some forty minutes. Mzingeli was well in the lead and hardly visible in the darkness when a movement in the bush to his right caught Fonthill's eye. Something was swinging from a branch. Rifle at the ready, he took a couple of paces into the thicket before he stopped, his mouth opening in horror. Hanging from the branch by his neck was the young man who had fallen behind. Swinging at his side and equally dead was Umtasa's messenger. As Simon watched, the man's hand twitched and the two gold sovereigns slipped to the ground.

Fonthill was turning to shout to Mzingeli when something crashed on to his head and blackness descended.

Fonthill came round with excruciating pain consuming his mind and body. The throbbing in his head was as nothing compared to . . . what was it? He opened his eyes and realised that somebody, very close to him, was slowly cutting into the flesh of his chest with a knife. There was a strong smell of pomade, highly scented hair oil. He struggled but realised that his wrists were bound behind him and his ankles were similarly tied. The black eyes of de Sousa looked into his at a distance of some twelve inches, and then, realising that he had regained consciousness, the Portuguese held up a knife, from the end of which dripped blood.

'Ah, Mr Fonthill,' he said. 'I thought that a little surgery without the benefit of anaesthetic might bring you round. I was just carving my initials in your chest to while away the time until I could talk to you.'

Simon winced but refused to cry out. 'Where is my wife?' he demanded.

De Sousa indicated genuine puzzlement. 'Don't tell me you have lost her? Well I haven't got her, nor do I want her. But you, my dear friend, I do want. Oh yes. I want you. You have a debt to pay, do you remember?' And he dug the end of the knife into Fonthill's pectoral muscle, this time bringing a cry.

The Portuguese sat back. 'It's been quite a chase catching you, but I thought that getting the boy would bring you back. And here you are.'

Fonthill gritted his teeth at the pain from his chest. He realised that the shirt had been torn from his body and blood was dripping down on to his breeches from the cuts that had been made. He looked around. They were in a clearing of sorts and it was still dark. But fires had been lit, and some dozen large natives, some with spears at their sides, others with rifles, were lounging on the ground near the flames, devouring meat. There was no sign of Mzingeli.

'What the hell do you want with me?'

'What do I want?' Gouela revealed a gold tooth and, at very close observation, his pockmarked yellowish skin. 'Well, firstly I want to cause you pain. Then I want to kill you, rather slowly. But given my responsibilities for this area—'

'Neither you nor your government has any claim to this territory.'

The Portuguese ignored the interruption. 'Given my responsibilities for this area, I must make an example of you. I intend therefore to set off in the morning to take you back to Umtasa's kraal, and there, before his *inDunas* and his people, I shall roast you slowly over a very large fire, but not until you are dead. No. When we have turned this ridiculously white skin of yours into a fine piece of pork crackling, I shall hang you, Fonthill.'

Fonthill tried to summon up a dismissive grin. 'You won't do that. You know that I am a representative of Rhodes, and through him of the British Government. Your country and mine have a pact of non-aggression. The news would get back and you would have to answer to your government for my death.'

'No. I don't think so. This is a faraway, primitive country, Fonthill, and I have found that I can do more or less what I like here. I shall tell my friend King Lobengula that you tried to kill me and that I was forced to defend myself. But, of course, to Umtasa I shall demonstrate how the Portuguese crown treats those who attempt to persuade its subjects to defect to another colonial power. So you will roast for a while and then hang. Now,' he raised the knife again, 'where was I? Oh yes . . .'

The pain began again, and Fonthill clenched his jaw to prevent himself from screaming. Then came oblivion.

The fires were burning low and the darkness beyond the clearing seemed to have grown blacker when he regained consciousness. The pain was still burning his chest, but he forced himself to sit upright and look around. De Sousa seemed to have disappeared, but was probably sleeping in the small bivouac tent that had been erected in the centre of the clearing. Most of his men had wrapped themselves in blankets and were asleep, strewn around the ground. One guard, however, carrying a rifle of some make that Fonthill could not determine, was slowly, sleepily patrolling the perimeter of the camp, coming into and out of the light cast by the fires. Again Simon looked for Mzingeli, but there was no sign of the tracker.

Fonthill's mouth tasted as if it had been force-fed on ashes and it cried out for water, but he forced himself to check his bindings. They remained tight, and the effort nearly made him black out again, but he breathed deeply and sought to clear his head. He must consider his position rationally. The fact that Mzingeli had not been exhibited to him as a corpse surely meant that the tracker, with his innate sensibility in the bush, must have escaped, for there would be no particular kudos for de Sousa in taking him back to the king's kraal. He would be just another native to the Portuguese. Escaped, though, to do what? He pondered. Mzingeli, superb tracker and resourceful man though he was, was no soldier. If he had got away, then surely he would have made his way back to Jenkins.

Fonthill tried to roll over, and stifled a groan as the cuts burned into him and began to bleed again. Looking down at his blood-drenched torso, he rationalised that at least the wounds seemed to be only superficial, for if the knife had cut deeply, then surely he would have bled to death by now. He forced a grin. Small mercies!

Just then his hands, foraging around in the dust of the clearing, found a stone – a sharp-edged stone. He grasped it in his fingers and tried to force it backwards to saw the edge of the vine that bound him, but he could not reach. He looked around. A few feet away was a small grouping of stones.

Could he inch his way towards them and wedge the base of the sharp stone into the middle, firmly enough to use it as a saw? He jerked his knees upwards, and again the pain flooded through his body, but he gritted his teeth and persevered. Gradually, inch by agonising inch, he moved towards the stones. He swivelled his head. Was he being watched? No. He continued the movement, scraping his bottom along the ground. There! Now. He turned his back and thrust the base of the stone among the others. Yes – there was a hole. Would the base hold? Would it stay upright and firm enough to saw away? Somehow, clumsily, he inserted the bottom of the stone into the gap. Thank God, it stayed upright. He began sawing.

Almost immediately the stone toppled over. Damn! Fonthill fumbled again, this time managing to move one of the base stones a little to enable more of his cutting stone to wedge into the resulting gap. Yes, firmer this time. Much firmer!

He had been sawing away for perhaps three minutes with seemingly little effect, except to cause the blood to seep more strongly from the cuts in his chest, when a sound made his head jerk upright. It was a high-pitched scream, of a malevolence that Simon had never encountered in his life, and it seemed to emanate from the western side of the clearing. As he listened, it increased in intensity, and was joined by similar screams from the bush on the other three sides of the camp. The sleeping men in the centre of the clearing started awake and sat upright, their eyeballs showing white in the half-light, fear in their faces. The banshee cry was like that made by a handful of lost souls, bewailing their descent into hell, and Fonthill felt the hairs stand up at the base of his head. He saw a half-dressed Gouela scramble out of his tent and stand erect as his head swivelled round to detect the source of the sound.

The consternation caused by the wailing, however, was as nothing compared to the next development. As Fonthill watched in wonderment, two fires, some fifteen feet apart, sprang into life a little way back in the bush, on the western side. They were small, but the light they shed was effective enough to illuminate two grotesque figures, each hanging above one of the fires, swinging gently from branches some twelve feet above the ground. The heads of the figures were twisted to one side, but they were unmistakably the two boys who had been killed and strung up further back in the forest.

Fonthill's jaw gaped as the bodies swung like pendulums, first into view as they moved into the yellow firelight and then back again into the darkness. And the screaming continued, now ululating, but still seemingly having no source.

Now the noise was supplemented by a single, sharp cry that seemed to come from the solitary guard who had disappeared into the blackness of the forest. It was enough to send the Kaffirs rushing into a terrified group in the centre of the clearing, their mouths agape, their eyes like white marbles set into their dark faces. Their heads twisted, for they seemed not to know which way to run, because the banshees were all around them.

De Sousa snarled and shouted an order, but he was ignored, for the fear that gripped the men was greater than that they held for their master.

Then: 'Lie flat, bach.'

The words boomed from the western end of the clearing, from where the apparitions were still swinging, although the fires were now flickering low. Simon flung himself on to the dusty earth, just before a fusillade of shots came from scattered points on the perimeter of the bush. Much of the firing was inaccurate, either whining over the heads of the men bunched together in the centre of the camp or burying itself into the ground at their feet. But that which came from two separate places was deadly, and within seconds, five of the Kaffirs had staggered, doubled up and lay prostrate. Immediately, the rest turned and fled towards the east, the only point of the compass that did not seem to belch flame. They ran, throwing aside spears and rifles, their legs pumping as they weaved in and out of the trees and bushes until they had disappeared from sight.

De Sousa, however, turned towards where Fonthill lay and, crouching, ran towards him, knife in hand. A bullet took him in the upper arm, sending the knife spinning away and causing him to stagger and fall. He was struggling to rise when two of the fleeing Kaffirs, leaders of the group, or so it appeared from the traces of grey in their hair, doubled over to him, seized him under each armpit and dragged him away until he was able to regain his feet and stumble after the others, holding his arm.

For a moment, silence descended on the clearing, and then there was a whoop and Jenkins appeared, rifle in hand, and ran to where Fonthill lay.

He knelt at the side of the still pinioned man and reeled at the sight of the blood on Simon's chest. 'Good God, we didn't 'it you, did we? Our lads can't shoot for toffee.'

'No, and it's not as bad as it looks. Can you cut away this damned binding? The bastards may return when they get their nerve back.'

Jenkins produced a knife and sawed through the thick vine that bound his wrists and ankles. 'No, I don't think they'll be back. We've killed 'alf of them, look you, an' the others are frightened out of their nappies, see.' He helped Fonthill to stand. 'Bloody 'ell, man. What 'ave they done to you?'

Simon staggered for a moment and put a hand on Jenkins's shoulder. Then he summoned up a smile as the three boys, grinning and with their Martini-Henrys proudly shouldered, emerged from various sides of the clearing. 'Gouela cut me up a bit, but not deeply. My, 352! Your show scared the life out of me. Was it your idea?'

'As a matter of fact, it was, bach sir. Not bad, was it?' He gave a reciprocal grin to the boys. '*They* all enjoyed it, anyway, though I thought they'd shoot old Jelly and me before they 'it the black fellers. 'Ere, drink this.' He held a water bag to Fonthill's lips. 'Now lean on me and we'll get out of 'ere.'

'No. Wait a moment.' Fonthill nodded his head towards the two corpses, now clearly to be seen in the light of dawn, hanging inert, no longer swinging. 'They've served us well and we must not leave them there for the hyenas.' He looked over his shoulder to where de Sousa and the remnants of his band had disappeared, but there was no sign of them.

They were joined by Mzingeli, now wearing the half-smile that was as near as he ever came to showing pleasure.

Fonthill held out his hand. 'Thank you, Mzingeli. I didn't know you could sing so well. And you, lads.' He shook hands with them all before turning back to the tracker. He nodded his head in the direction taken by the Portuguese and his men. 'Do you think they will be back?'

'No. These men very soppos . . . what is English word?'

'Superstitious?'

'That is it. They think this bush haunted. They no come back.'

'Good. Then please ask the boys to take down our two old friends up there,' he nodded to the hanging corpses, 'and burn them. I'm afraid we have no time to bury them.

Jenkins and I will wait here with our rifles just in case those men return.'

'Yes, Nkosi.'

While they waited, Fonthill learned of how Mzingeli had melted into the bush when Simon was attacked, and of how he had followed the two men who had taken him back to the Portuguese camp, which had been set up about half an hour's march from the scarum. Then he had returned to an anxious Jenkins and together they had plotted the attack.

'It was old Jelly who really gave me the idea,' said Jenkins. 'He told me that these Kaffir blokes don't like being in the bush at night on their own – not just because of the animals, but because of the spirits of people killed in the place, y'see. I felt that an outright attack would 'ave been a bit chancy because only two of us could shoot – as you saw. I did think of your fire trick, but knowin' me, I would get it wrong and 'ave us all burned to death.'

Simon gave a weary smile. 'I have to say that the shooting was a bit haphazard, but that was the boys, I guess.'

'Ah yes. Sorry about that – an' I was worried that we might 'it you an' that's why I shouted. Mind you,' he sniffed, 'my shootin' wasn't the best it's ever been. I managed to pot quite a few of the black fellers, see, but I missed old Saucepot again, dammit. Only got 'im in the arm, so that's two lives 'e owes me. I'll get 'im next time, though.'

'No. I think he's reserved for me.' Fonthill looked up as smoke once again drifted down across the clearing. 'Right. It looks as though the lads have done that job. Let us go. We must find Alice.'

Jenkins laid a hand on his arm. ''Ere, 'alf a mo. What if old Yellow Pants 'as taken 'er?'

'I've thought of that. If he had got her, he would surely

have exhibited her to me in delight. And if he had . . .' he gulped, 'already killed her, he wouldn't have taken her bed. Above all that, as I've said before, there is no way he could have overtaken us in the bush and arrived at the scarum before us. If he had, he would have waited and ambushed us on arrival. No.' He shook his head wearily. 'Someone else has taken her. But they have left a good spoor and we must get on our way and catch them.'

Jenkins sniffed. 'That's all very well, but you've been carved about a bit and 'ad a fair old bump on the 'ead, an' with respect, bach sir, I don't see you doin' much forced marchin' for long, see.'

'Nonsense. I can march. Come on.'

But Jenkins was right. They made what progress they could through the bush, yet everyone was tired, and when eventually Fonthill collapsed, there was almost an air of relief. They carried him into a glade and made him as comfortable as possible, and took turns to stand guard through the day. The next morning, Simon was clearly delirious and moving into a fever. Mzingeli carefully examined the cuts on his chest and declared that there would be no marching that day. Instead, he dug into the earth until he found what he wanted, some strange-looking, bulbous roots. He made a small fire, carefully disseminating the smoke, and boiled the roots in the only kettle they had. Then he mashed them into a paste with a rifle butt, spread them on to a couple of leaves from a baobab tree and tied them to his patient's chest. Lastly, he took a couple of baobab buds, crushed them and forced Fonthill to drink the resulting liquid.

The next morning, Simon awoke clear-eyed and with no sign of fever. 'You're a bloody marvel,' said Jenkins, and patted the tracker on the back. Mzingeli just shrugged.

During this enforced stop, Jenkins had posted guards on a rota back in the bush the way they had come, but there was no sign of pursuit. It looked indeed as though the Portuguese and his men had been forced to flee and lick their wounds. So they set off again, this time at a slightly reduced pace to allow Fonthill time to recover fully.

However, they were soon confronted with what seemed a virtually impossible hurdle. The trail, so clearly marked and which they had been following so assiduously, now suddenly branched into three. 'Clever bastards,' cried Fonthill. 'Mzingeli, can you tell which one would have been carrying the litter?'

The tracker frowned. While the rest of the party waited impatiently, he carefully and slowly walked down each of the three spoors a little way, sometimes bending to inspect a piece of grass or the edge of a footprint in a patch of dust. Then he returned.

'Cannot tell,' he said. 'I go a longer way now down each spoor. This will take time. You wait.'

Fonthill shouted a curse. 'We are already behind by about four bloody days,' he cried. Then he regained his composure. 'Yes, of course, Mzingeli. Do what you can and take your time. We will wait here.'

But the tracker returned within ten minutes, holding out his hand and indulging in his joyful half-smile. 'Nkosana leave these,' he said. 'Very clever lady.' And he handed three gout pills to Simon.

'What . . . ?' Fonthill examined the little white capsules. 'Gout pills. What the hell could they . . . Ah!' He slapped his thigh with delight. 'Of course. Why didn't I think of this before? It's old Lobengula! He's sent half a bloody impi or whatever to take her back to Bulawayo to treat his damned gout. It all fits – not caring about the rifles, the tents or the mules, but taking her bed and Joshua to look after her. The old devil!'

Jenkins nodded. 'His worship might have left us a note or somethin'. It would 'ave saved us a lot of worry an' trouble, wouldn't it?'

Fonthill's relief was etched into his face. 'Well, Alice left us a note of sorts. It means that she's being looked after and she will be safe with his men, even with Gouela on the rampage.'

'Do we take it a bit easier, then?' asked Jenkins. 'Now that we know which way we're goin', like.'

'No. We carry on following the trail. I want to catch them up. And when we get to Bulawayo, the king is going to get a piece of my mind and . . .' He broke off as a disturbing thought struck him and he turned to Mzingeli. 'Could somebody just have taken her bag and the pills simply dropped out, do you think?'

The tracker shook his head. 'Don't think so. Pills not in little pile. Dropped regular. A trail to show us way. Clever lady. Perhaps she do this earlier but we missed in dark.'

'Yes. Bless her. Now, you found the pills on this trail?' He pointed.

Mzingeli nodded his head. Fonthill produced his compass, squinted at it and consulted the much-folded map from his pack. 'Yes, it is to the north-west, roughly in the direction where Bulawayo lies.' He nodded his head, relief etched into his face. 'That settles it. They are taking her back to the king.'

'So we don't need to rush about like blue-arsed flies tryin' to catch up, then?' Jenkins's question was more of a plea for mercy.

'Oh yes we do.' The frown had returned to Fonthill's face. 'Knowing Alice, she might very well tell the king to go to hell, and he could lose his temper and . . . and . . . anything might happen. I want to catch them up, if we can, before they reach Bulawayo.'

'But think about it, bach sir. They've got about five days' start on us, you said so yourself. We'll never catch them.'

'We might. If they've taken Alice's bed, then she'll be on it and they'll have to carry her and it. Whether she's able to or not, she will not leave that bed. She'll do everything she can to delay them. We should be able to move faster. Come on. Up, everybody. Take the north-west spoor.'

So they pressed on, no longer attempting to increase their pace by breaking into jog trots from time to time, for Fonthill, at least, could not sustain that effort. But they made good time, particularly once they had broken out of the bush country into the more open high veldt of what was now clearly Mashonaland. Here the signs of the passage of the Matabele party were less distinct, but Fonthill had set a compass course for them, removing the necessity to rely on Mzingeli's tracking skills, and he estimated that they were covering perhaps twenty miles a day. They must, he argued, be closing the gap. The pace could not be maintained, however, not least because Simon had by no means completely recovered from his treatment at the hands of de Sousa, and they were forced to take longer spells of rest at midday.

Fonthill was also showing the signs of the deprivations of the last two months. The years of peaceful farming in Norfolk had added flesh to what had always been a rather sparse frame, but all that had disappeared shortly after their arrival in Africa, and the recent fighting and forced marching had now left him gaunt and as taut as a bowstring. The threat of losing Alice had weighed heavily on his imagination and his conscience, and he was now hollow-eyed and drawn – a driven man, pushing himself and his party to the limits.

Nevertheless, they were now nearing the end of their stocks of biltong, and most of one day had perforce to be devoted to allowing Mzingeli to stalk and kill an impala. It gave them not only fresh meat and the chance to replenish their biltong, but also a blessed day's rest. The enforced break impelled Fonthill to consider his position vis-à-vis Lobengula and Cecil John Rhodes. He did so even while realising that his mind was perhaps not in its most balanced state to rationalise and draw conclusions. But his chest still hurt like hell and the muscles of his legs told him that there was now a limit to how fast and how far he could walk in a day.

So, sitting and chewing on the last of the biltong, he resolved that if the king had harmed Alice in any way, then he would kill the man. Life would not be worth living without his wife, and his act would show to the world that even the most powerful despot in Africa could not behave like a barbarian without attracting the consequences. If, however, he found Alice alive and unharmed, then he would have no more of this surrogate adventuring for Cecil John Rhodes. This strange millionaire would have to do his own exploring in future. Alice had never wished to come on this journey, and now she was being forced to suffer because of her husband's own arrogance and selfishness. No, he resolved, she would do whatever she wished now, and he would meekly follow her desires, even if it meant going back to sowing more wheat in flat bloody Norfolk!

The next day, their stomachs full and hopes renewed by the promise of another day of blue sky and scurrying snowball puffs of cloud, they set off as soon as the sun appeared over the hills behind them. It was towards the end of the day when they glimpsed a party of warriors trotting across the plain towards them.

Fonthill ordered a halt and they formed a square, their rifles at the ready. 'Who are they, do you think, Mzingeli? They don't look like Mashonas.'

The tracker shielded his eyes from the sun. 'They black blades,' he said. 'Matabele. They coming straight for us.'

Chapter 14

It was Fairbairn who told Alice that her husband had been found and was at that moment approaching the king's kraal. She immediately hurried to wash her face and comb her hair, then ran – for her leg had now completely healed – to meet Simon. She saw the party walking slowly down the hill, past the first thorn hedge, still accompanied by the platoon of warriors, who were anxious to reap the approval of the king for so successfully accomplishing their mission, but also by the usual cacophony of dogs and children barking and singing.

Alice strode forward to meet them and opened her arms in greeting. She could not help but release a sob, for Fonthill, Jenkins and Mzingeli now resembled scarecrows, their clothes torn, their bodies thin and, in the case of Simon and 352, wearing unkempt beards. Their eyes, however, were bright, and Simon, holding her close, whispered, 'Are you all right? They've not hurt you?'

'No, of course not. Now you are back I am perfectly fine.'

She made them all break away from their escort and walked them to her hut, where Joshua – and Ntini also – greeted them with a warmth that only diminished when they realised that just three of the boys, their friends and contemporaries, had returned. Alice made the two build a fire and she busied herself with boiling water so that they could all wash, including the boys. Then she made tea and they sat around the fire drinking it while she and Fonthill exchanged their stories.

Simon and his party had only been gone an hour, she explained, when about sixty warriors had descended on the camp. They had been led by an *inDuna* and at first she had been terrified, helpless and crippled as she was, because they were painted as for war and carried assegais. Joshua had whispered that they were Matabele, and when she shouted – through the boy – that her husband and his party would be back within minutes, their purpose became clear. They had gently pushed her back on to the bed, put blankets over her, bundled a change of clothes into her pack, picked up the bed and her medicine bag and jogged away into the bush, Joshua being forced to trot with them.

She was clearly being kidnapped, for there had been no attempt to take her rifle or other items that would have been attractive to natives. But the medicine bag had been a priority, and it was now being carried with care by a warrior just ahead of her litter. Her attempts to put a foot to the ground had been firmly resisted, but no extreme force had been used and it was evident that she was not to be harmed.

It did not take long for her to speculate that she was being taken to Bulawayo so that she could continue her treatment of the king's foot. She had been sure that Mzingeli could follow the signs that so large a party would make through the bush, but she had been able to take a few of the gout pills from her bag and drop them to indicate where they would be heading. She had saved her last three pills, and it was well that she had done so, for she had used them to indicate which of the three trails she had taken when the party split up.

Simon nodded. 'Clever girl,' he said. 'This finally confirmed to us where you were heading and who had taken you. We felt much better after that. But you must have been in great pain being jolted about on that litter.'

'It was not as bad as all that. They were very gentle with me, and later, I was able to wash and change the dressing.'

'What happened when you reached Bulawayo, and why did the king send a party to look for us? If he wanted me back here, he could simply have waited for our return.'

Alice grinned. 'I refused to see the old rascal. I was not going to let him think that he could just send his warriors and drag me back here. So when he summoned me, I told him to go to hell.'

Jenkins nodded his head approvingly. 'Good for you, Miss Alice.'

Alice's smile had disappeared, however. 'Yes, well, he sent his sister to fetch me, but I insisted on talking to Fairbairn first. It was he who told me that Rhodes had sent a huge column that had already crossed into Matabeleland, that the king was in great pain and that his relationship with the white men had worsened.' She pulled a face. 'I realised that it would do no one any good for me to continue playing the Great White Lady, so I struck a bargain with his majesty.'

Fonthill frowned. 'What sort of bargain, for goodness' sake?'

'Oh, don't worry. Your position has not been compromised and I haven't sold bloody Rhodes short. I said that I would treat his foot if he would send a party out to find you and bring you back here. Eventually,' her smile returned, 'after we had exchanged a few choice words through Fairbairn, he agreed. And here you all are at last, my darlings, though you look as though you could do with a good bath and a hot meal – which shall be forthcoming, I promise.'

Simon took her hand. 'And your leg . . . ?'

'It has healed perfectly well. Now, when you have eaten, I think you should go and see the king.' Her expression was now very serious. 'And I should be very careful about what you say to him, my dear.'

'To echo you, to hell with him.'

'Yes, well, you won't find him very contrite, I fear. He is not a happy monarch. Rhodes's column of pioneers has crossed over the Shashe into Matabeleland at Tuli and is building a fort there.'

'Rhodes has moved remarkably fast.'

'Yes, and I understand from Fairbairn that it's quite a crowd. The king thinks he is about to be invaded. This is a dangerous time, Simon.'

Fonthill lowered his brows over the edge of his cup. 'But he signed the agreement. He knew that a column would be coming sooner or later to build the road.'

Alice smiled wanly. 'Yes, but it's very much sooner rather than later, and it sounds as though it's a virtual army. Fairbairn tells me that there are some two hundred prospectors, a hundred and fifty native labourers and, would you believe it, five hundred "police" – they're really soldiers – together with the usual paraphernalia of about one hundred and twenty wagons and two thousand oxen. They have even brought along a giant naval searchlight, which they shine into the bush at night to deter attack. Fairbairn is drafting a letter of protest from the king.'

Fonthill nodded and then looked at her sharply. 'That still doesn't excuse the bloody man from abducting my wife.'

Alice reached across and gripped his knee. 'I think, darling, that you must be very careful how you handle Lobengula. He has not harmed me and he did agree to send men to find you. To repeat, my love, these are dangerous times. In fairness to the man, remember that he has about twenty thousand warriors who are just dying to wash their spears in British blood. He is trying to restrain them.'

Jenkins, who had been listening, pulled at his moustache. 'Sounds a bit to me like Zululand all over again, isn't it?'

Fonthill nodded. 'Hmm. I think we have all done our bit for Rhodes now. You, my love, have had a bullet in your thigh, I have had my chest used as a carving block by this Portuguese madman and we have all tramped more miles than I would have wished over this bit of Africa. I have no intention of doing any further exploration to the east. I think we now make our way back down to the Cape, don't you agree?'

''Ear, 'ear,' growled Jenkins.

There was, however, an awkward silence from Alice, who looked away with an air of embarrassment.

'What?' Fonthill frowned in puzzlement. 'You never wanted to come on this expedition in the first place. Whatever is the matter?'

Alice gave him a weak smile. 'You will see that Ntini is back,' she said. 'He arrived just a few days ago. He came with this cable for me. I think you had better read it.'

Simon took the cable form. It was from the editor of the *Morning Post* in London, and it read:

SPLENDID COPY STOP UNDERSTAND PIONEER COLUMN HEADING NORTHWARDS STOP TROUBLE EXPECTED FROM LOBENGULA STOP OPPOSITION PAPERS WITH COLUMN STOP CAN YOU JOIN IT SOONEST AND REPORT TROUBLE AND PROGRESS STOP CONGRATULATIONS STOP LIKE OLD TIMES STOP CORNFORD

Fonthill looked up in astonishment. 'You don't mean that you are going to join the column, surely?'

At this point, Jenkins rose and ostentatiously walked to where his pack lay. There he began unpacking it. Alice followed him with her eyes before replying.

'I must, Simon.' She spoke softly and slowly. 'When I agreed to accompany you on this expedition, I did so on the understanding that I would report it for the *Morning Post*. You know that. I made a commitment to Cornford.'

'Yes, but this thing could develop now into a full-scale war, another Isandlwana for all I know. You can't be involved in that, my darling. It would be far too dangerous.'

She blew out her cheeks. 'Well, my love, let's see.' She began counting on her fingers. 'So far on this trip I have been involved in a close-up encounter with lions; two attacks by Portuguese mercenaries; a fight with slavers; and I have been abducted. Now, a bit of old-fashioned campaigning with a British invading force – for that's what it sounds like – should really represent only a touch of light relief, don't you think?'

Fonthill's face was thunderous. 'Don't be flippant, Alice. We agreed that you would report for the *Morning Post* only on our expedition, not some bloody invasion of the whole territory.'

'Yes, but . . .' Alice now gave her husband her sweetest smile, 'did you not wish to see for yourself this wonderful farming country in Mashonaland that the prospecting column will discover? And didn't Mr Rhodes offer to give you some of this prime land – even though it wasn't his to give? Don't you think you should look at it?'

'Oh come along, Alice. You know that I never wished you to become involved with the column. I really thought that your journalistic days were over – with the exception, that is, of reporting on our particular expedition.' He held up the cable. 'Cornford speaks about "the opposition" accompanying the column. This means that you will be in it again up to your neck, trying to get scoops and all the rest of it. I know what you are like. You will be sticking your neck out, taking risks to get exclusives and so on. You will be well and truly back in the profession. And I shall lose you, I know it.' He floundered for a moment, lost for further words. 'Dammit all, it's not right, you know.'

Alice's face lost its expression of sweet cynicism and she reached out and took his hand. 'My darling, you will *never* lose me, you know that.' She paused for a moment and then spoke softly again. 'When I look at you, my love, I see a nose broken by a musket barrel in Afghanistan, a back terribly scarred by a Dervish whip in the Sudan, and now a chest cut horribly by a Portuguese knife. You have sustained all of this in the service of the Empire, although you haven't served formally in the army for years. Yet I do not begrudge you your adventuring, although I worry about you terribly. But I must have a life too, you know. It would perhaps be different if we had a child, but . . .' her voice faltered for a moment, 'we do not, so one half of us can't be off adventuring for the Queen and the other sitting at home knitting. Well, not this half anyway.'

Fonthill gripped her hand tightly in return.

'You see,' she continued, 'I have made a commitment to Cornford and he was kind enough to take me on. Now I don't anticipate for one moment returning to the *Morning Post* as a full-time correspondent, even if they would have me. But to be *here*, on the spot, so to speak, of this remarkable expansion of the Empire – even if I don't approve of it, perhaps particularly *because* I don't approve of it – and not write about it would be a terrible waste of the talent I know I have. I must report on what happens to this column and see it through. Then I can stop. Do you see?'

Simon sighed. 'Very well. I shall come with you, of course. But I must give 352 and Mzingeli the chance to opt out, if they wish.'

'Of course.'

Wearily, Fonthill stood and called Jenkins and Mzingeli over. They sat around Alice while Simon explained the situation. 'So,' he concluded, 'we cannot ask you to accompany us – nor the boys, of course – and I can understand why you in particular, Mzingeli, would want to return to the Transvaal. It is up to you.'

'Well.' Jenkins looked affronted. 'I go where you go, you know that, bach sir. But if you don't want . . .'

'Don't be silly. Of course we both want you. Please come with us. There will be plenty to do. What about you, Mzingeli? I would continue to pay you, of course, but we shall quite understand if you have had enough of danger and fighting.'

The tracker gave an almost imperceptible nod of the head. 'I come,' he said. 'You want Ntini and Joshua?'

'Oh yes please,' interjected Alice. 'I would like them to come and run my cables back for me.'

'Yes. Then they come.'

Simon gave a weary grin and rose to his feet. 'It seems,' he said, 'as though Fonthill's private army stays in being, then. Thank you both. Well done. Now, I suppose I ought to go and see the bloody king.'

'Not before you have shaved,' said Alice. 'And you, 352. You look like a pair of pirates. But you, Mzingeli, have managed to preserve your essential elegance and dignity. I am proud of you.'

She received the tracker's slightly embarrassed half-smile in return.

Later, Fonthill and Mzingeli walked down the hill to the king's house. Simon's anger at Lobengula's abduction of Alice had abated somewhat, not least because he had sensed a change in mood by the Matabele towards him and his party. The men who had met him out on the high veldt had been surly and had not engaged in conversation with Mzingeli, merely stating that they had come to fetch the white man back to his wife. In Bulawayo, there was now an undoubted air of hostility. Warriors were sitting outside their huts, ostentatiously sharpening their assegais and bending new hides around the framework of their shields. If Simon caught their eye, he received a scowl. It was not a good time to attempt to rebuke a king whose people were itching to go to war, to wash their spears in the blood of white men.

He found Lobengula standing, for once, and talking to his *inDunas*. The king whirled round and indicated that Fonthill and Mzingeli should sit, and then walked slowly to his couch.

Simon inclined his head. 'Tell the king,' he said to Mzingeli, 'that I hope I find him in good health and that his foot is causing him no pain.'

Lobengula ignored the pleasantries. 'I take back your wife because my foot bad,' he said, through the tracker. 'If you there when my men found her, they would explain that we borrow her. But you gone. We not harm her. Treat her well. And then send my people to tell you we have her safe here and bring you back.'

'I have to say, your majesty, that in my country it is a criminal offence to abduct someone's wife.'

At this, Lobengula stood and advanced on the seated pair, so that he loomed over them, his face like thunder. 'You not in your country,' he shouted, 'you in mine. I do what I want here. But I no harm your wife. I ask her to do service for me. If white men respect king, she should do that service.'

Fonthill kept his voice level and looked the king in the eye. 'You will know that my wife is not a doctor, and that in England, as in Matabeleland, her duty is to her husband. But she believes in trying to reduce pain with the drugs at her disposal. How is your foot now?'

The directness of the question and the refusal of Fonthill to be bullied slightly disconcerted Lobengula. He raised his eyebrows and then lifted his right foot and replaced it again. 'Foot better,' he said. 'King is grateful to Nkosana. What you do now?'

'Er . . . I understand that the prospectors that your majesty has kindly allowed to enter your country have arrived on the southern border. We intend to join them.'

'Ah!' The king pointed his assegai blade towards Fonthill. 'I agreed for men to come and make road and dig. Now I have foreign impi at my border. Guns and big witchcraft light. It is too much. There is a wall around the word of a chief. But white men always lie.' There was a murmur of approval from the inDunas.

'Well . . .' Fonthill began, hesitantly. But the king was speaking again, quickly and with vehemence.

'Look,' he said, putting aside his spear and using his hands to illustrate his words. 'England is like chameleon stalking a fly. Chameleon changes colour to go into background. It rocks to and fro on feet,' he cupped his hand, palm down, and imitated the actions, 'and advances so nobody notices. Then flashes out tongue and eats fly.' The fingers of his hand leapt forward. The king's eyes stared into Simon's. 'I am fly. England is chameleon.'

As if exhausted, Lobengula sank down on to his couch. 'When you go?' he asked.

'As soon as we are able to buy provisions for the journey.'

'Good. You take letter for me to chief of this impi, man called Jameson. I know him. Like you, I thought him friend. At one time.' The last three words were heavily emphasised, and Mzingeli translated them faithfully.

Fonthill chose to ignore the innuendo. 'Of course,' he said. 'I will take the letter.'

The king spoke to one of his *inDunas*, and an unsealed envelope was produced containing the letter. It was addressed, Simon noticed, to Dr L. S. Jameson. The king rose, indicating that the audience was over, and Fonthill and Mzingeli also stood, then bowed and left the hut.

Outside, Fonthill wiped his brow. 'Phew. That was not easy. Do you think they will go to war, Mzingeli?'

The tracker shrugged his shoulders. 'People and *inDunas* want to,' he said. 'But king knows power of white man and he afraid to throw assegai. He know you beat Zulu. Pot is boiling and he wants to keep lid on it. But maybe he don't.'

Back in their own hut, Alice and Jenkins had prepared a meal. Before eating, the four of them drank a little beer and

Simon recounted what had happened at his meeting. As the envelope was not sealed, he took out its contents and read it. It was written in English, in a hand accustomed to writing bills, and Fonthill recognised the long loops and crossed Ts of Fairbairn. Its message was a simple repetition of the king's complaints already expressed to Simon, but it ended on a note of diplomatic insolence that he could not resist reading out: 'Has the king killed any white men that an impi is on the border,' it ran, 'or have the white men lost something they are looking for?'

Alice slapped her thigh in delight. 'Good for him,' she said. 'The old devil has guts and also a good sense of humour. I can't help liking him, you know.'

'So it seems.' Fonthill sniffed. 'But you seem to have forgotten that he lops off his subject's hands and noses at the pop of a champagne cork. Speaking for myself, I shall be glad to get out of his kraal now. I must say I worry for Fairbairn if trouble breaks out.'

'Well,' said Jenkins, 'I'd wager that that old Jock can look after 'imself. 'E's well in with the king. Where else would the old boy get his grog, eh?'

Alice nodded. 'Quite. But Simon, I think you would be wise to go and see Fairbairn. He has his own source of contact with Rhodes, it seems, and he is well informed about the column and the politics involved there. I gather it is a bit of a witch's brew.'

'Good idea. He might be able to help me get this agreement document with King Umtasa safely back to Kimberley. You will need Ntini and perhaps Joshua for your dispatches. And we must get our horses back from him anyway. I will go after dinner.'

The smell of stale tobacco and personal functions met

Fonthill as he walked through the trader's door (did his shop never close?). Fairbairn, his pipe in mouth, came from behind his counter and extended his hand.

'Welcome back,' he said. 'I've heard you had a few knocks down in that swamp country, but at least you didn't get the fever.' He gestured to a rickety cane chair and picked up a whisky bottle. 'Rest your weary body. Care to join me in a wee dram?'

'Ah, that would be very kind of you. Thank you very much.'

'It'll only cost you two shillings.'

'What? Oh . . . er . . . yes, of course.'

Fairbairn poured out two minuscule measures and set them down on a dusty table before pulling up another chair. 'You'll have heard that the column has arrived, down in Tuli?'

'Yes, so I understand. We shall be setting off to join them once we've settled things up here. We will need some supplies from you and, of course, our horses.'

'That will be no problem. Cheers. Here's to the Queen, the poor lassie.'

'Er . . . yes. The Queen.' Fonthill tasted the whisky, coughed and replaced the glass. 'Lobengula has asked me to take the letter you presumably wrote for him to a Dr Jameson. Who is he?'

'Aye, I wrote it. I usually write the king's letters now. He knows what he wants to say, so I just put it into English. Jameson, you say? Ah, quite a character. He's become virtually Rhodes's right-hand man – outside business, that is. He was the first doctor to set up practice in Kimberley, and Rhodes took a shine to him. He's a little Scotsman and as tough as nails. Great horseman and traveller and even better talker; he's been up here several times and the king likes him. Makes him laugh. Now he seems to handle all the dirty work that Rhodes can't do himself.'

'These five hundred "police", or whatever they are – where do they come from and what's their purpose?'

'Well, Cecil John's original idea was that the settlers would be able to protect themselves. They would be stiffened, so to speak, with a few regular officers, and Frank Johnson, who has organised the column and is in charge of the workmen and settlers, himself has the rank of major. Rhodes would provide weapons and ammunition. There would be no line of communication stretching back because these chaps would be self-sufficient, able to look after themselves along the way and in Mashonaland. You get the drift?'

Fonthill nodded.

Fairbairn grinned. 'Well, the powers that be in Whitehall didn't like the sound of a bunch of amateur soldiers heading into a country bristling with natives just itching to get their assegais into their bellies, and they insisted that Rhodes should organise proper protection for the column, otherwise they'd cancel his charter. So Rhodes gave in. He's now got these police – so called so as not to upset his majesty here – with the column, armed to the teeth and under the command of a regular soldier from the Inniskilling Dragoons, a Colonel Pennefather. And they've got to leave a chain of forts behind them.'

'Good lord, said Fonthill. 'So who is in command of the whole column, then?'

'Ah, that's just the point. It was obvious that there would be trouble if the major who had organised the whole thing was out-ranked by a colonel. So Rhodes has sent his very canny Scots doctor along, with no obvious rank or position but with his power of attorney.' Fairbairn giggled into his pipe stem. 'That means that nobody can do anything without Jameson's approval, because he's the moneybags. Rhodes's company, of course, is paying for everything, so Jameson is in effective control.'

Fonthill frowned. 'It sounds a ridiculous situation to me. Very complicated and tortuous.'

Fairbairn leaned forward and slapped Fonthill on the knee. 'Ah, you know what Rhodes is like. Everything is done on the run, on the back of an envelope sort of thing. But it seems to work in the end. And that's true of this expedition. They've all worked harmoniously together through Bechuanaland, so I hear, and built a damned good road.'

'Yes, but the difficult bit is about to start. What happens if Lobengula attacks? You know his people are looking for a fight.'

'Aye, you're right there.' The Scotsman looked rueful for the first time. 'But Rhodes certainly doesn't want a fight. That's why the route for the road has been taken so far away from Bulawayo. The colonel will be looking to gain a medal or two by taking on the Matabele, but the civilians are in charge of the column, and Jameson and Johnson will be out to avoid bloodshed.' Then his face lit up. 'And it's my view that dear old Lobengula wouldn't want to unleash his warriors. He just wants a quiet life.'

Fonthill nodded. 'I hope you are right. But tell me, Mr Fairbairn, I believe you have a fairly regular means of communication with Rhodes.'

'Yes, I do. I've got a reliable set of laddies who can travel safely up and down to Kimberley. In fact, your wife has used me to get one of her stories back down to the cable station. There'll be a charge, o' course.'

'Of course. Let me know what it is. There is an important document that I wish to send back to Rhodes. I will bring it tomorrow. Now, can we talk about provisions for our trip to the Tuli . . .'

They set off two days later. There was no opportunity to say goodbye to the king, for he had left Bulawayo to visit one of his villages to the north. However, it seemed that he had had a pang of conscience about his abduction of Alice, for he gave Fonthill a farewell gift of a wagon and six oxen to carry them on their journey. His contrition might also have extended to the letter of complaint addressed to Jameson, for he asked Simon to tell the doctor that he would be dispatching one hundred and fifty native labourers to expand the work force of the column – 'Although,' said Fairbairn, who had passed on the message, 'whether he actually does so is entirely another matter, o' course.'

The party consisted of Simon, Alice, Jenkins, Mzingeli, Ntini and Joshua. The three boy bearers who had come with them on the long journey from Kimberley, out east to the forest and wetlands of Manica and back again to Bulawayo had been released, with a handful of gold sovereigns and a Snider rifle each.

The journey was uneventful and even enjoyable, for the weather was pleasant, the trail well defined and for once they all felt free from danger or the need to hurry. Alice's wound had long since healed, leaving hardly a trace of a scar, which produced much ribaldry between them about Simon's prowess with needle and thread. Good food and the healing powers of Mzingeli's herbs had hastened Fonthill's recovery from the effects of de Sousa's knife-work, and all in all, the party was in good spirits as the oxen plodded over the low veldt towards the Sashe river. Simon had dispatched his document signed by King Umtasa back to Rhodes with a letter explaining all that had happened in that region and telling the millionaire that he was about to join the column of pioneers. His disillusionment with Rhodes's expansionist ambitions and Alice's return to hard-nosed journalism had diminished with the promise of exploring the fine farming land of Mashonaland.

The further they rode south, the more they realised that this mopane woodland, which stretched throughout southern Matabeleland to the Macaloutsi and Shashe rivers at the border, was ideal country for an ambush. Although it was the height of the winter dry season and the thorn trees had lost their foliage and their bark had turned black, presenting a kind of charred, dead forest appearance, visibility was remarkably restricted. A man standing amidst it could only see for about one hundred yards. The impression of crossing burned-out country after a fire was heightened by the sun beating down day after day from a clear sky as the temperature soared, and heat seemed to bounce back from the dry soil, turning their nostrils into hot, acrid channels.

'If the Mattabellies want to come at this column thing,' sniffed Jenkins, 'this is the place for it. The blokes cuttin' trees and all wouldn't see a thing until the black fellers were on 'em, see.'

His view was more than confirmed when, at last, the party mounted a hill and saw below them the column at work. A party of pioneers – all white men – led the way, cutting down trees to the stumps with their axes, while a second group used horses and mules to pull the trunks away. Out ahead and on either side ranged horsemen, presumably of the 'police', acting as scouts to warn of potential attack. But as Fonthill watched from his high vantage point, he saw that some of these outriders were clearly lost, for they were slowly making their way in circles, often blundering back into the tree-cutters before turning and venturing back into the bush again. Behind the pioneers snaked a long column of wagons and oxen, stretching back for at least two miles. Halfway along the line, Simon picked out a large, low-slung trailer, carrying the searchlight, with its own steam engine, dynamo and battery. He shook his head. It was clear that it would take at least two hours for this clumsy line to form into a laager if it was attacked.

'God, they're vulnerable,' he muttered. 'If the Matabele attacked now, it would be a massacre.'

Jenkins cocked a quizzical eye. 'Best to tell 'em, then?'

Fonthill frowned. 'I don't want to get off on the wrong foot with this Jameson, or with the other two so-called commanders. But you are right. They can't go on like this.'

The little party allowed their horses and oxen to pick their own way down the side of the hill until they drew level with the first of the wood-clearers. Dr Jameson, Fonthill was told, was back in the leading wagon, and there they found him, sitting on the driver's seat, scribbling on a pad. Simon looked at him keenly. He was a little man, dressed for the trek in rough boots, old trousers and a flannel shirt, opened almost to the waist in the heat. His bush hat had been thrown aside to reveal a balding head and a moustached face that showed character: a fine forehead, full lips, a firm chin and eyes that were as bright as a monkey's.

Diffidently Fonthill introduced himself, with apologies for his intrusion. Immediately the doctor's face lit up and he took in the members of the party in one swift, appraising glance:

Simon, slim and weathered, with experience lining his face; Alice, her features tanned by the sun and dust-covered, but presenting a refreshingly feminine figure in her jodhpurs, cotton shirt and soft blue neckerchief; Jenkins with his immense moustache, width of shoulder and black button eyes; and Mzingeli, as dignified as a native chief with his erect posture and white hair, but holding back discreetly.

'My word, Fonthill,' said Jameson, jumping upright and reaching across to pump Simon's hand. 'I was hoping that we would meet up.' He spoke with only the softest of Edinburgh accents. 'I've heard so much about you and,' he gave a small bow to Alice, 'your wife and the rest of your party. Rhodes told me all about you, and I've been reading with fascination your pieces in the *Morning Post*, Mrs Fonthill. Och, what a time you seem to have had of it.'

Alice summoned up her sweetest smile, and relieved by the warmth of their welcome, Fonthill introduced her formally and then Jenkins and Mzingeli.

'Right,' said Jameson. 'Hitch your horses to the end of my wagon and pull yours in behind it, if you can get in. We only progress, of course, by fits and starts as the way is cleared up front, but we are still travelling at the rate of about ten miles a day, which I think is pretty good given the workload and this heat. Then you must all come and have a cup of tea with me and meet Johnson and Pennefather, my . . . er . . . colleagues.'

Fonthill was pleased that the invitation clearly included Mzingeli. It looked as though Jameson was one of the new breed of colonists who were relaxed about relationships between black and white – and that was a relief. Within minutes they were all sitting at the side of the column drinking tea from primitive and distinctly pioneering tin mugs. Johnson and Pennefather, it seemed, had ridden on ahead with the scouts in the van.

'Congratulations on your good work with Lobengula,' said Jameson. 'I can well imagine that getting him to agree to our entry was not easy. How is the old boy's gout?'

Fonthill gestured for Alice to speak. 'Oh, I'm only a first-aid practitioner,' she said quickly. 'I have been plying him with morphine injections and anti-gout pills. They seem to have begun to work, but the real problem is his drinking, his diet and his lack of exercise.'

'Oh aye.' The doctor nodded. 'I did exactly the same when I was up there and came to the same conclusion.' He turned back to Simon. 'But how did you get on out in the east? Last I heard formally was that you were setting out, and then of course I read Mrs Fonthill's account of the attack on the slavers. Marvellous stuff.'

Simon inclined his head, then related to Jameson his securing of a 'first stage' treaty with King Umtasa. He decided to omit the story of Lobengula's abduction of Alice, but described in full the clash with de Sousa and the man's claims to territorial suzerainty over Umtasa's kingdom, and also his persistence in cultivating Lobengula.

'The problem,' concluded Fonthill, 'is that whatever he has signed, the king is very uneasy about the size of the column here and particularly the police you have with you. I think he is coming to the conclusion that this is a virtual invasion of his country. Here, I have a letter for you from him.'

Jameson read it impassively, until giving a wry smile at the concluding questions. 'Aye,' he said, tapping the envelope against his moustache. 'I understand his worries and I can well imagine the pressures he's been under from all those supplicants at his court. What's more, I know that his *inDunas* think he's giving away too much and all his warriors want a fight. But, you know,' and he shrugged his shoulders, 'this is not the eighteen sixties. We're nearing the twentieth century now and the old boy has to move with the times. Civilisation will come to Matabeleland whether he likes it or not. And he has signed those treaties with us. We have the right to make our road and dig for minerals in Mashonaland.'

Alice leaned forward. 'But do you have the right to settle his land?' she enquired.

'Oh.' Jameson waved the envelope dismissively. 'That will come inevitably. Matabeleland will become a British protectorate sooner or later, just like Bechuanaland.'

Alice gave the little man the full benefit of her smile. 'Yes, but your treaties with the king acknowledge his ownership of both Matabeleland and Mashonaland. You cannot just ride roughshod over him and colonise the place, now can you?'

Jameson frowned, and seemed to recall the fact that Alice was not just Fonthill's wife but also a journalist for one of Britain's most influential newspapers. He was seeking a reply when Simon, uneasy about the direction the conversation had taken, intervened.

'When we left Bulawayo,' he said, 'the atmosphere was very uncomfortable. The warriors seemed to be preparing for war: there was much spear-sharpening and new shield construction, and the women were making sandals for their men, always a bad sign. And, of course, Lobengula has the five hundred rifles and the ammunition that I took to him, although I must say I have seen no sign of them practising with the guns. But do you expect to be attacked?'

'It is certainly a possibility. So, in the end, I am glad that we have the soldiers with us, although,' he gave a wry smile,

'Rhodes didn't want 'em. Soldiers, he said, always end up looking for a fight. But we do take good precautions. We laager every night, set off firecrackers at intervals in the bush through the hours of darkness, and we have this damned great searchlight, which,' his smile broadened into a grin, 'I borrowed from the British navy at Simonstown. We use it through the night, sweeping the bush. So far, it has frightened to death every Kaffir we've met.'

Fonthill acknowledged the ploy with a smile. 'The trouble, though,' he said, 'is that you are in ideal terrain for ambush – and you are likely to remain in it for another hundred miles or so. Your line stretches back for two miles. By the look of it, your scouts out in the bush wander a bit – and I don't blame them for it, because you can't really see your hand in front of your face out there – so you will get precious little warning of an attack. Like the Zulus, the Matabele like to attack at dawn. You would never have time to pull the wagons into a laager.'

Silence fell on the little gathering. It was broken eventually by Jenkins, who munched his moustache and nodded. 'The captain's right, sir,' he said. ''E knows about these things, see.'

Jameson glanced at them both. 'Look,' he said eventually. 'I'm really just a general practitioner from Edinburgh, so I wouldn't dream for a minute of arguing with two distinguished ex-soldiers who I know have fought at Isandlwana, Kabul, Kandahar, Majuba, El Kebir and Khartoum. What you say sounds sensible to me, but I shall have to put it to Pennefather. He should be back soon. Now, tell me what your plans are. I do hope you are joining us.'

Fonthill explained that Alice had been instructed by her editor to join the press contingent on the column (it turned out to be small – five only, all men, of course) and that they would indeed like to stay until some sort of settlement had been established at the end of the trek. He added that Rhodes had promised him land in the new territory and he wanted to see it for himself.

'Then you're most welcome. We can certainly use your knowledge of the country and your military expertise.'

At that point two men on horseback joined them. The first, a lithe figure, deeply tanned and dressed like a Boer, was introduced as Frank Johnson. Fonthill was surprised at how young he looked (he later learned that he was only twenty-four) for a man who had such a record. He had, of course, hunted and prospected through the country since his teens and he had the skill to put together the logistics of this remarkable operation, which was, so far, working well. The second man was easily recognisable as Colonel Pennefather, in that, despite the heat, he was wearing the uniform of a colonel in the Inniskilling Dragoons. A tall man, with a white moustache, he regarded Fonthill steadily.

'Heard about you,' he said abruptly. 'Who were you with?'

'Originally the 24th of Foot, Colonel, and then the Queen's Own Corps of Guides on the North-West Frontier.'

'Must say, you look damned young to have a CB.'

'Oh, that came up with the rations after the Sudan,' said Simon airily. 'The DCM of Jenkins here was far more important.'

Jenkins stood immediately and shook the hands of both men, bestowing on them his great moustache-bending smile. Johnson took this act of equality with equanimity, but Pennefather's jaw dropped momentarily, although he gave Jenkins's hand a firm enough grip.

'Er . . . Fonthill here has a point about our defences,' said Jameson.

'Ah.' Simon tried to look uninvolved. 'It was just something that occurred to Jenkins and me as we breasted that hill up there. It's probably not quite got home to you because you've not had the benefit of our vantage point. If you have a minute, perhaps I could show you.'

'Certainly,' said Pennefather, with a quickness that surprised Fonthill. 'I would be glad to have your view. Let's go now.'

At the top of the hill, Simon swept his hand back along the wagon line, the end of which was out of sight to the west. 'It's a single line, of course . . .' he said.

'And stretching about two miles,' Jenkins pointed out helpfully.

'. . . and I don't see how you could laager it in time if the Matabele attack.'

'Probably won't be necessary.' The colonel pulled on his moustache. 'We've got ample firepower, you know. Five hundred rifles should be able to stop any kaffirs coming at us, I'd say.'

Fonthill stifled a sigh. 'With respect, Colonel, Pulleine had one and a half thousand seasoned professional infantrymen at his disposal at Isandlwana – *and* he was on a plain and could see the Zulus coming at him for at least a mile. Yet he and his men were still massacred. Lobengula has about twenty thousand warriors, all descended from the Zulus. In this bush they could be on and through you in two minutes.'

Pennefather scowled and Simon took a deep breath, prepared to continue the argument. The old soldier, however, stiffened in the saddle, turned to Jameson and said, 'He's right. We *are* vulnerable.'

Jameson lifted his eyebrows and addressed Simon. 'What do you propose we should do?'

297

'If the colonel agrees, I would suggest that you change the method of advance. Instead of having your wagons in single file, you should have them in two parallel lines. This will reduce the length of the column and enable you to close the two lines at front and back in the event of an attack by just drawing over the leading and rear wagons. This could be done quickly, and although it would be a hell of a long laager, it *would* provide cover for the men to fall back into. And I believe you should have the scouts riding much further out from the wagons. The officers in charge don't seem to have sight of the column because of the thickness of the bush and are getting lost as a result. They should be given compasses so that they can plot their courses and range wider. This should give you more time to laager if there is an attack. And don't forget that like the Zulus, the Matabeles like to attack at dawn, so the pickets should be out during the night in extended order.' Fonthill paused, suddenly realising that he was sounding like a senior officer talking to three juniors. 'I . . . er . . . hope that this is helpful.'

Jameson, Johnson and Pennefather exchanged glances. Johnson spoke for the first time. 'This would halve your rate of progress, Doctor, and consequently cost more money,' he said. 'Can we afford it?'

The diminutive doctor looked across at Pennefather. 'Colonel?'

'It's a good idea,' said the tall man. 'But it will cost you.'

'We'll do it,' said Jameson. 'Johnson, you arrange it with the wagon master, and Colonel, I will leave the matter of the scouts to you, of course. Thank you, Fonthill and . . . er . . . Jenkins. Now, let's get back.'

When they returned, they found that Alice had gone to find

her fellow journalists and Mzingeli was erecting a tent for Simon and Alice, Jenkins having already elected to sleep in the wagon with the tracker.

'I don't mind tellin' you, bach sir,' said Jenkins, 'that I'm glad they've accepted what you suggested, like. I'd 'ave felt very, very exposed, see, sleeping in this long thin line with blokes out in the bush gettin' lost. Even I could see that this was barmy.'

Fonthill shrugged. 'Well, I must say, Pennefather took it well. I have a feeling that he hasn't seen much active service, so I hope these police chaps know what they're about.'

The night was not exactly passed tranquilly, for little landmines of gelignite, spread all around the laager and fired from the searchlight's battery, exploded throughout the dark hours. The searchlight itself stabbed the bush like some ghostly probing finger. Fonthill wondered if the column had the facilities to continue this nightly practice throughout the rest of the long trek, but had to confess that he could well understand these defences working against the superstitious Matabele.

The next morning, he found that the 'police' were, in fact, actual policemen, in that they were composed of five troops of the British South Africa Police and three troops of Bechuanaland Police, more militia cavalrymen than gendarmerie, but experienced horsemen who were used to putting down isolated instances of skirmishes with natives in the bush. He also learned that Pennefather had served in the Zulu and Boer campaigns. The puzzle of why the pioneers themselves were doing the labouring – an unheard-of thing in Africa, where black labour was plentiful and cheap – was explained when he was told that the original one hundred and fifty black labourers had been lent by King Khama in

Bechuanaland, but had been withdrawn once they had left their own country.

Fonthill realised that he had not passed on Lobengula's verbal promise to provide his own detachment of workers for the column, but when he confided this to Jameson, the doctor nodded and seemed unimpressed. 'I'll believe that when I see 'em,' he said. Simon's lingering doubts about discipline within the column, however, were dissipated to some extent early that morning when the pioneers assembled to begin their labours at the head of the line.

Setting off on their duties, they looked more like elite cavalry than labourers. They wore brown corduroy uniforms, yellow leather leggings and bush hats and had waterproof coats strapped behind their saddles. They carried Martini-Henry rifles in gun buckets, Webley revolvers in holsters at their waists and long-handled axes slung across their saddles. Fonthill could see that they were mounted on fine, well-salted horses and he could not help speculating how much this had all cost Rhodes. Later he learned that they were earning seven shillings and sixpence a day, with the policemen receiving five shillings, and that they had been promised a grant of five thousand acres of land each and the right to peg fifteen mining claims. He decided that he would not offer these details to Alice. She would only point out that the land was not Rhodes's to give. Once at the head of the column, the men stripped off and worked with a will, although their weapons were at their sides and their mounts tethered nearby, ready for them to join the police in defending the column at the sound of a bugle. The thud of axes cutting into wood and trees falling was soon to become a constant companion to Fonthill as the days passed.

He rode to meet Jameson, who was already out and about.

'I have written back to the king,' said the doctor. 'Tried to reassure him by saying that we have no militaristic ambitions at all and that the police are with us purely for protection, as insisted on by London. All of which is true, of course, although I don't suppose he will believe me.'

Fonthill nodded. 'Thank you. By the way, I would like us to be useful to you,' he said, 'but I don't think we would be much good wielding axes. What if my chaps and I scout ahead every day and even do a little shooting for the pot?'

'Excellent idea,' said the doctor. He reached out and caught Simon's arm. 'Look here,' he said. 'I am most grateful to you for your suggestions yesterday.' He nodded to where the wagons had been lined up in two rows. 'It's no good me saving Rhodes and the company money if we all end up disembowelled. And I was delighted to see the way Pennefather accepted you. It's a relief to me to have you on board, I must say.'

Fonthill smiled. 'Delighted to be of service.' He looked around at the busy scene. It still looked vulnerable. 'Tell me, Jameson. You know Lobengula. Do you think he will attack?'

Jameson frowned and lowered his voice. 'To be honest, my dear fellow, I don't see how he can resist doing so. As you know, we've deliberately mapped our route to keep as much distance between him and us as possible, but I know we offer such a juicy target that, considering how his warriors are jumping up and down and anxious to go to war, I don't see how we are going to get away without blood being shed.'

Smiling his thanks, Fonthill pulled at his bridle and rode away. Unbidden, terrible memories of Isandlwana and Rorke's Drift flooded into his mind as he made his way back towards the column. He saw again the Zulu warriors – 'Here they come, as thick as ants and as black as hell!' a terrified sentry had shouted – streaming across towards the red-coated defenders; he smelled the cordite and the blue smoke of battle; and he heard once more the screams of the wounded and the dying. Was it going to happen again – and this time with Alice amongst it all? He shook his head. He could not envisage how this attenuated and vulnerable column could escape the sort of massacre he had seen in Zululand eleven years ago. Surely it could not survive?

Chapter 15

Three months later, Simon, Alice, Jenkins, Mzingeli, Ntini and Joshua stood amongst cheering pioneers in the shade of jacaranda trees as the Union Jack was hauled up a very crooked pole and fluttered at the foot of Mount Hampden. The end of the trek had provided a rather embarrasing anti-climax, in that, having reached the high kopje, outspanned and declared the terminus Fort Salisbury, in honour of the Prime Minister of Britain, Johnson, as nominal leader, had sent a scout to the top of the kopje who had then seen the *real* Mount Hampden ten miles to the west. The ceremony had to be repeated at the new site, but this time the embryonic township was firmly declared to be the capital of their new country, which was then and there formally annexed in the name of Queen Victoria.

'Why don't they call it Fort Rhodes and have done with it?' whispered Alice.

'Probably will within a week,' grunted Simon. He was almost right, for it took only a few days before it had become common practice to call the new territory 'Rhodesia'.

The journey from the border to their destination, some two hundred miles to the north-east of Bulawayo, had not been without incident, for it had been a gruelling task to cut a road through the wooded territory of the south and then up over the mountain ridge that ushered them into Mashonaland. But despite all the threats and alarms along the way, Lobengula had not attacked. When the column reached the Lundi river, he had sent a message saying, 'Go back at once and take your young men,' but nothing ensued. Every night the searchlight had probed the bush, and every morning, from three a.m. until dawn, the column stood to, waiting for the attack that never came.

'Why didn't he come, eh, Fonthill?' asked Colonel Pennefather just after Mount Hampden had been reached. 'He could have taken us at any time, you and I know that. Why didn't he do it?'

Simon shrugged. 'I presume because he just didn't want to. For all his faults, Lobengula is a shrewd man. His spies were observing us all the time as we plodded and cut our way through the timber country in the low veldt in the south, and he knew that a couple of impis could have overwhelmed us at any time. Yet he also knew that a terrible retribution would come afterwards, which would mean the loss of his country. He remembered that eleven years ago, Ulundi followed Isandlwana. He doesn't want to take on the British Empire.'

'Hmm. Suppose you are right. Pity, in a way. I wouldn't have minded a bit of a scrap, don't you know.'

Along the route, Jameson had dutifully followed the instructions from Whitehall that the column should leave a string of forts behind it, with small garrisons, to protect the lines of communications to the south. The last one had been called Fort Charter, and the one preceding it, Fort Victoria, had been sited just after Providential Pass, the 1,500-foot-high passage through the escarpment that marked the entry into Mashonaland. From this vantage point, the pioneers had looked down across the rolling, lush plains of what was, literally, their promised land. Here, the high veldt offered long grass and distant views, merging into mauve hills on the far horizons. This was what they had been straining to reach as they chopped and sawed their way through the humid bush of the low veldt. Here, stretching before them, were the farmlands and rich mineral sites that would make all their labour worthwhile.

After the pioneers had finally been dismissed as semi-soldiers under the flagstaff at Salisbury, it was not at first the threat of war that caused them problems as they spread out across the thinly populated land of the new Rhodesia, looking to stake their claims. The Matabele was not the enemy as they ranged through the high veldt, anxious to stake and then register their precious acres. Fonthill, together with his little party, was among them. And he, like the others – prospective farmers and miners alike – suffered as nature turned on them all, as though she had decided that if Lobengula would not protect his own, she would.

The worst storms that the region had seen in many years swept across the high veldt in late 1890 and the early months of 1891, turning dried-up dongas into swollen rivers and washing away the early diggings that the miners had begun. After the rains came mosquitoes and the blackwater fever, and rough burial grounds sprang up, almost outnumbering the wooden shacks that formed the early townships.

Fonthill, with Alice, Jenkins and Mzingeli – plus Ntini and Joshua, who had agreed to stay and help establish the farm – suffered less than some of the others, in that Simon had staked his claim in the north of the territory, far away from the diggings in the foothills of the mountains of the south, which had been so badly affected. They rode out the storms in the little huts the men had built. The members of the press contingent had returned home, of course, after Mount Hampden had been reached, and Alice had contentedly stepped down from her assignment with the *Morning Post*, clutching to her the congratulations from her editor on the quality of her reporting and a request that she should contribute the occasional colour piece about life on the high veldt in the new country. She retained her indignation that Rhodes had succeeded in riding roughshod over Lobengula and had, as she had predicted, settled land that was not his. Within a year, some fifteen hundred settlers had followed the pioneers and were living in the old Mashonaland. But there was nothing, it seemed, that Alice or the king could do about it. She had long since acquiesced in Simon's determination to twin their land in Norfolk with a farm in the new territory, and they had all decided to grit their teeth and ride out the frightful weather to establish their holding, although it meant living the rough life of pioneers for a couple of years.

Fonthill had always known that it was Lobengula's practice to send out raiding parties among the Mashonas to keep them in line – to maintain his sovereignty over them, at least, if not on the ground they trod. He also knew that Jameson, who had been appointed by Rhodes administrator of the new territory, had attempted to keep the king sweet by giving him the ownership of a gold reef and even equipping the mine with a steam engine, with the king's initials picked out on the green paint of its boiler. It was Jameson who told Simon of the first dark shoots of unrest.

'The trouble is,' he confided, 'the Mashonas are perfectly happy to have white people living among them and don't see why they should pay tribute to old Lobengula any more. This has gone to the head of a Mashona chief called Lomagundi, who has refused to pay his dues to the old tyrant in Bulawayo. I am trying to soothe things down a bit and I don't think it will get out of hand.'

A Matabele troop was sent and Lomagundi was killed. Jameson protested, but Lobengula was evasive in his reply. Soon the incidents began to mount. Another Mashona chief cut five hundred yards of Rhodes's newly laid telegraph wire and was promptly fined by Jameson and ordered to pay the fine in cattle. He did so – but with Lobengula's cattle, which had been sent to graze on the chief's green land as part of his tribute. The king promptly sent his warriors, and this chief, too, paid the price for attempting to shield behind the white settlers. Once again Jameson's protest was met by the bland and not altogether illogical answer that while all the white men must abide by the laws of Mr Rhodes's company, the natives of Mashonaland and Matabeleland remained subject to the king's laws. Nothing in any of the treaties that had been agreed between him and Rhodes, Lobengula pointed out, negated that fact.

'I don't like any of this,' said Alice. 'The fundamentally immoral nature of Rhodes's position here is being exposed all the time. Things are building up. Rhodes must not push Lobengula too far. If he does, the lid really will come off the pot.'

There had been so many false alarms, however, both on the long journey to the north and in the petty skirmishes since the farmers and miners had become tentatively established, that few of the white folk in the tiny townships or out on the veldt believed that the explosion would come. For the Fonthills, the news was brought by a Kaffir on horseback, who arrived at their remote holding with a message from Jameson. It was terse and to the point:

Big trouble with Matabele around Fort Victoria. Can you come right away?

Simon had come to respect the little Scotsman, and such a request could not be resisted. With Jenkins and Mzingeli, therefore, he prepared to ride south. His intention was that Alice would stay with the two boys and look after the cattle. Inevitably, though, she insisted on joining them. Whatever the rights and wrongs of the 'big trouble', this would be too good a story to resist, and the arrival of the telegraph at Victoria meant that she could cable a dispatch to the *Morning Post* immediately. Simon's protests were easily overridden, and the four arrived to find that the situation around the little town had become critical.

They rode through country just outside Victoria that was littered with the corpses of killed and mutilated Mashonas. The Matabele impi had taken this opportunity to wash their spears, and it seemed that few had been spared, including natives working on the new farms, some of whom had been pursued into the farmhouses and butchered under the horrified eyes of the settlers.

Fonthill found Jameson in a determined but unfazed mood.

'Glad you could come with your private army, old chap,' he said, rising from the chair in a little hut near the ramparts where he had set up his headquarters. He bowed gallantly to Alice.

'How did it start?' asked Fonthill.

'Usual thing. The local Mashona chief here refused to bend the knee to Lobengula. In his time-honoured fashion, the king sent two and a half thousand warriors to carry out what he felt was some well-deserved disembowelling. This time, though, the chief lived close to the town. The arrival of an impi in full war regalia was frightening enough to our folk here, but then the Matabele proceeded to kill *all* of the Mashonas in the area, including, as you have seen, many who worked for the white men. Settlers from around have flocked into the town behind our rather flimsy walls and the war drums are beating.'

Alice looked up from her notebook. 'Have any white people been killed?'

'Not yet, although cattle have been stolen.' Jameson removed his spectacles and vigorously polished the lenses with his handkerchief. '*I* certainly don't want war and I am sure that Lobengula doesn't either. If we do have a little skirmish here, then I think the king might even be glad that we have relieved a bit of the pressure on him by thrashing some of his young warriors.'

'Depends upon whether his foot is achin' or not, I should think,' murmured Jenkins, but no one seemed to hear him.

'The trouble is,' continued Jameson, 'the settlers here have put up with a lot over the last few days. This impi is composed of very arrogant young bloods who undoubtedly have behaved extremely badly. I am afraid that, uncharacteristically, so has Lobengula.' The administrator leaned forward. 'He has sent a most brusque letter to the magistrate here, demanding that the Mashonas who are sheltering within the walls of the fort should be handed over to Manyao, the *inDuna* who is leading the impi. He has offered one insolent concession: he says that they will not be killed near the river, where they might pollute the water, but would be finished off in the bush.'

Fonthill frowned. 'It sounds as though things have gone too far.'

'Yes. The other complicating factor is that the settlers here, having been frightened out of their lives, are just itching for a fight, and are talking about dealing with the Matabele "now and for ever". So I've got two lots of hotheads on my hands, so to speak. Even so, I think I can handle it.' He sat back in his chair, his bald pate gleaming.

'What do you propose to do?' asked Fonthill.

'I have rushed a very polite but firm letter by special messenger over to Lobengula in Bulawayo, asking him to withdraw his impi at once. In the meantime, however, I have summoned Manyao to a meeting on the banks of the River Tokwe. As you know, I have always believed that talking is better than fighting. I think I can calm everyone down.'

Alice looked up from her pad, her face flushed. 'I do hope so,' she said. 'Lobengula has been pushed pretty far already in my view. I don't think anyone back home – and particularly in the government – wants another native war. It's Lord Salisbury in Number Ten now, you know. Not Disraeli.'

'Aye, I understand that. But if the members of the House of Commons could see the bodies that you saw when you rode in, then perhaps they might have a different view of things. But as I say, I am going to try and cool things down. You're welcome to come to the meeting.'

The following morning, Jameson took his kitchen chair down to the banks of the river and sat with his back to the fort, with a handful of settlers and Captain Lendy, the officer in charge of the modest detachment of soldiers based at Victoria. Fonthill, Alice, Jenkins and Mzingeli joined them.

As Fonthill arrived, he drew in his breath at the Matabele ranged opposite the little doctor, a small group of *inDunas* at their head. He had never before seen so many of Lobengula's men arrayed for battle. One hundred and fifty of the two and a half thousand massed on the other side of the river formed a semicircle in front of Jameson. They were splendid specimens. Tall and muscular, and naked except for their loincloths and monkey tails at calf and biceps, they wore warpaint on their faces and chests and their black skin glistened in the morning sunlight. Plumes nodded from their heads, and most carried assegais and shields, though some were proudly nursing new rifles. They were restive and their postures exuded hostility, most of the warriors jigging up and down. It was as if their killing spree had released a long-pent-up savagery within them.

'Blimey,' murmured Jenkins. 'I don't like the look of that lot. 'Ow many men 'ave we got to fight 'em, if it comes to it?'

Fonthill spoke softly so that Alice could not hear. 'About forty or so soldiers, I think, with probably the same number of settlers who can handle weapons. Not exactly an army. Let's hope that Jameson can talk them out of more killing.'

The doctors raised his hand for silence. For a moment all that could be heard was the buzzing of the thousands of flies that had decided to attend the conference, probably still gorged from feasting on the bodies that surrounded the fort. Then Jameson began to speak. He did so observing the etiquette that members of the Zulu race espoused at meetings of this sort: welcoming Manyao and his *inDunas* with compliments but suggesting that they had gone too far by indulging in the mass slaughter in the country that he, Jameson, now controlled.

Manyao was an elderly man, with the *isiCoco* ring of the *inDuna* woven into his grey hair, and he spoke with equal politeness and dignity. Through his interpreter he pointed out that the original treaty with Rhodes had acknowledged that Lobengula was king not only of Matabeleland but also of Mashonaland, and that the only powers given to the white men had been to dig for minerals, not to erect forts or settle the land. For more than a century the Matabele had collected tribute from the Mashona, and the law decreed that default was punishable by death. The action taken had been within the law and following precedent. No white people had been hurt.

Alice put her pencil in her mouth and tugged at her husband's sleeve. 'I don't approve of the killings,' she whispered in his ear, 'but if this was a court of law, old Manyao would have won the verdict hands down.'

The *inDuna* finished speaking, and it was clear that, for once, Jameson had no reply. The silence hung on the air like a blanket of embarrassment as the doctor sought unchar-acteristically for words. Then one of the minor *inDunas*, named Umgandaan, stepped forward. He was much younger than Manyao, tall and well muscled, a warrior in his prime. But while Manyao had been rational and elegant, Umgandaan was truculent and loud. His king, he said, was paramount in his own country, and he had been sent to perform the king's will. No white man would stop him.

His aggression produced a murmur of dissatisfaction from the small group of settlers behind Jameson's chair and gave the doctor his prompt. He cut the young man short and ordered Manyao to withdraw all of his impi across the river before sundown, or his white soldiers would drive them across.

'With what?' asked Jenkins sotto voce. 'Three blokes on 'orseback?'

The meeting broke up in surly disarray. Jameson picked up his chair and strode towards Fonthill, who blew out his cheeks in consternation. He remembered hearing that the doctor had earned a reputation in Kimberley as a hard-nosed poker player. 'You're taking a big risk, aren't you, Jameson? What will you do if they call your bluff? We're outnumbered by about fifty to one. And they've got rifles.'

The little man seemed completely unfazed. 'They'll go,' he said. 'I know these people. They think they're Zulus but they're not really. They will move back by tonight, you'll see.'

But they did not.

Looking down from the flimsy mud ramparts of the fort as the sun sank towards the horizon, Jameson, with Lendy and Fonthill, realised that the Matabele impi remained firmly encamped on the Victoria side of the river. Many of those who had remained on the far side for the morning's meeting had obviously crossed during the day and were now either sitting cross-legged on the bank or milling about, quite unperturbed, under the walls of the township. Fonthill noted, however, that all carried their weapons. In the distance, he saw that another kraal had been set on fire and more of the company's cattle were being rounded up.

'Well, I was wrong,' admitted Jameson.

'What are you going to do?' asked Fonthill.

The little Scotsman looked up sharply. 'Do? Why, disperse them, of course. Send 'em back across the river. Off you go, Lendy. How many men do you need?'

The captain looked down on the milling throng below. 'Well, it would be unwise to take all of my troop,' he said. 'Should keep some in reserve back here. I'll take forty. That should do it.'

Fonthill gulped. Forty against two and a half thousand! 'Jenkins and I will come with you,' he said.

'Rather you didn't, Fonthill,' said Jameson. 'I would be grateful if you two stayed back here with me and organised the manning of the walls. Haven't got too many chaps, you see, who know what they're doing in these matters.'

The doctor still seemed quite unconcerned. Simon's brain, unbidden, recalled the words to him of the British commander at Isandlwana when warned that twenty thousand Zulus were about to descend on him: 'I hope Johnny Zulu does attack. I'll give him a bloody nose . . .'

Captain Lendy strode away and Fonthill heard him giving orders to his little troop below. Simon exchanged glances with Jenkins. 'Right,' he said. 'We have little time. Come with me. We'll run through the streets calling for every fit man to bring his rifle and gather in the square below. Quickly now.'

The two ran down and took to the streets. Within the eight-foot-high mud walls – not high enough, thought Fonthill – the township was more of a hamlet, with insubstantial wooden huts radiating out from the square behind the wooden doors guarding the only entrance, and forming only four streets. It took barely five minutes, given that many men were already on the ramparts, for the main population of the town to gather around them. Fonthill counted: some seventy men, old and young, but all of them carrying rifles, some more than one. Almost as many women and children had accompanied them. To one side stood the ten troopers that Lendy had left behind.

Fonthill looked over his shoulder. Lendy and his men had not saddled up yet. 'Right,' he shouted to his little group. 'Ladies, go and fetch whatever spare ammunition you have. Bring it back as quickly as you can, then take the children and lock yourselves and them in the houses.'

'I'm not doin' that,' one amply proportioned woman called from the back. 'I'm stayin' with my man. And the little 'uns will do the same.' A chorus of approval rang out from the rest of the women.

Simon glimpsed Alice arriving and joining the crowd at the

back. He sighed. 'Very well, but please don't get in the way. We may have some hard fighting to do. Now.' He gestured with his hand to segregate about twenty men. 'You men stand over here with Sergeant-Major Jenkins. You will be in reserve and when I call will double to whatever part of the wall looks under pressure. The rest of you, space yourselves around the ramparts – but don't fire until I give the order. Troopers, come with me. I will spread you out among the civilians,' he lowered his voice, 'to give a bit of stiffening if it is needed. Right, go to your positions. Quickly now.'

He realised that Alice was at his side. Her eyes were pained. 'I have just used the telegraph to send my story,' she said. 'Oh, I do so wish it hadn't come to this.'

'So do I, darling.' Fonthill pulled her to him briefly. 'Look. I really can't see forty men dispelling two thousand. Where do you want to be?'

She looked up at him unflinchingly. 'With you, of course. I shall go and get my rifle.' And she turned on her heel and strode off.

'Strong lady, the Nkosana.' Mzingeli was at his shoulder, carrying his rifle.

'Are you going to fight, old chap?'

'Of course. Matabele long time enemy. They kill my people. Now I kill them. I stay with you.'

Fonthill nodded and looked across at Jenkins. 'You understand, 352? Hold your men back until I shout and tell you where to go on the wall.'

'Very good, bach sir.'

'Good. Come on, Mzingeli. Let's see what's happening on the other side.'

They scrambled up on to the ramparts. The natives below seemed to have sensed that battle was imminent, for those of them who had been seated had now risen and all were flourishing their spears at the men on the walls. To Fonthill, they seemed to stretch almost as far as the river and they presented a frightening sight, their plumes nodding as they danced and chanted and their painted faces contorted with derision.

He gulped. 'Throwing forty horsemen out into that lot is going to be suicide.' He spoke to himself.

Slowly the big wooden gates to the fort creaked open and Lendy and his men, their bush hats buttoned up to one side and the butts of their carbines resting on their thighs, trotted out in excellent order in two columns. Immediately the cries of the Matabele rose in a crescendo, but they did not attack. Instead they fell back a little, as though surprised at the audacity of the little group of horsemen who had come out calmly to face them.

Fonthill realised that the gates had been left gaping open. 'Close those bloody gates,' he called down. He was, of course, cutting off whatever chance of retreat Lendy's men might have, but he could not risk allowing the Matabele to cut through the horsemen and run on unimpeded into the heart of the settlement.

The troop split and wheeled to right and left, so that each man had a clear view of the enemy. Then Lendy shouted: 'Select your target. Take aim. Even-numbered troopers, FIRE!' Twenty rifles cracked as one and the same number of natives, standing at point-blank range, crumpled and fell. Lendy's voice, clipped and clear, rose up again to Fonthill. 'Reload. Odd numbers, FIRE! Reload. Even numbers, FIRE! Reload.'

Among the first to fall was Umgandaan, who ran forward brandishing his spear. Perhaps it was his loss or the steadiness of the volleys, but immediately the mass of warriors broke and ran as fast as they could back to the dubious safety of the river. Only a handful of young, brave men followed Umgandaan's example and ran towards the troopers, only to die in their turn. From a phalanx of threatening warriors, the Matabele had splintered within seconds to become hundreds of frightened individuals, turning their backs on the enemy and running away from the guns. It was a complete rout.

'Fire at will,' screamed Lendy. Then, 'Canter, follow them up. Fire as you go.'

A single shot rang out from the wall of the fort. 'No firing from the walls,' shouted Fonthill. He realised that the men on the ramparts, only a few of whom could be called good shots, were more likely to hit the troopers than the tribesmen. Even now, as the soldiers urged their horses forward, they were in great danger, for if the Matabele rallied and counter-attacked, they could surround the troopers and engulf them before the horsemen could reload. Then the fort would be virtually at their mercy, for the mud walls could be easily scaled.

But the warriors continued their headlong race towards the river, spreading out in a black mass, their truculence, like their pride, melting away as their strong legs took them from the fearful firepower of the forty white men on horses.

'Oh, thank God. Lendy is bringing them back.' Alice was at Simon's side, her rifle held listlessly at her side and tears pouring down her cheeks as her gaze took in the figures sprawled on the ground below. At least fifty of the tribesmen lay dead. All forty of the troopers, however, were trotting their horses back, their bush hats thrown back, their faces beaming with triumph. In the distance, a host of black figures could be seen wading and swimming across the river.

'It's the most amazing turnaround,' gasped Fonthill. 'Forty routing two and a half thousand. God, Lendy and his men were brave to ride out there. I am not sure I would have done it.'

'What's 'appenin' outside, then?' Jenkins called up from the square. ''Ave we won the war? Can we come up and 'ave a look?'

'Yes. Let all of them come up. The Matabele have fled.'

'Blimey. An' I didn't fire a bleedin' shot. Amazin'.'

Fonthill dropped down to order the opening of the gates and was met there by a sombre-faced Jameson. Simon shook his hand and congratulated him.

'Humph,' grunted the doctor. 'It's Lendy we must congratulate. It was the surprise, you know. The Matabele just didn't think *we* would attack *them*. They thought we would stay holed up behind these walls. Then the old fears about our guns stirred up among them when the shooting started and they just took to their heels.' He took off his hat and wiped the sweat off his pate with his handkerchief. 'Trouble is, Fonthill, I'm sure that this is not the last of it. I can't really see Lobengula accepting this. I shall have to tell Rhodes to prepare for war now. Dammit, it's going to cost the company a packet.'

He hurried forward to meet Lendy, while the settlers raised a cheer to welcome back the troopers as they rode through the gates. Fonthill and Jenkins joined in the applause, but Alice and Mzingeli watched silently.

'So Rhodes is going to have his war, then,' murmured Alice.

Fonthill sighed. 'It looks like it.' His face was sombre. 'I suppose it was inevitable, once Lobengula's men began all this killing.'

'No,' she said coldly. 'It was inevitable once Rhodes sent in his damned column to invade the king's country. And I shall say so in my dispatch.' She turned away, her face tear-stained but determined, and strode off to the telegraph station.

Just before dusk descended, Jameson had Lendy send out patrols to see if the Matabele were forming up again, but the horsemen returned to report that the shattered impi had remained broken and was limping back, in small groups, towards Bulawayo. It looked as if the danger to Fort Victoria was over – at least for the time being. The doctor, however, was convinced that the Matabele threat was not ended. He confided to Fonthill that Rhodes had been advised by military men in Cape Town that a force of at least seven thousand well-equipped troops would be needed to subjugate the Matabele nation if things got out of hand.

'The company can't afford that,' he said. 'Rhodes is very strapped for cash as it is. I've got to get a second opinion – one that knows these Kaffirs better than the colonels and generals in the Cape. I'm going to talk to the Boers.'

There were a handful of Dutchmen from the Transvaal who had moved north into Mashonaland and taken shelter in the fort. Most of them had had brushes of one sort of another with the Matabele in the past, and Jameson set about getting their advice. The next morning he took tea with Fonthill, Alice and Jenkins and told them the result of his soundings.

'These chaps say that seven thousand is ridiculous,' he said. 'They believe that a force of between eight hundred and a thousand men, well mounted and armed, will do the job.'

'Sounds light to me,' said Fonthill. 'They would need Maxims and cannon if they're going to take on all of Lobengula's impis. Where are those going to come from?'

Jameson sipped his tea and gave a rueful smile. 'That's the point. Rhodes abhors the thought of what he calls the Imperials – that's the redcoats in the Cape, with the Colonial

Office behind 'em – getting involved. As it is, we've now got a high commissioner appointed by the government in Salisbury to oversee the colony. But of course, he's got no money. It's the company that will have to raise the force and pay for it.'

He fished in his pocket. 'I cabled Rhodes late last night to put the situation to him. Here's his reply.' He handed the cable to Fonthill, who read it aloud.

'"Read Luke XIV: 31." Is that all? What does it mean?'

Jameson produced a battered pocket Bible. He read, '"Or what king, going down to make war against another king, sitteth not down first, and consulteth whether he be able with ten thousand men to meet him that cometh against him with twenty thousand."'

Fonthill frowned. 'I suppose he means that you've got to think carefully about expenditure.'

'Exactly. But Rhodes is down there and I am very much here. I have told him that I can do the job with a thousand men but they must be well armed and he will just have to find the money.'

Alice put down her cup in exasperation. 'Surely this war is not inevitable. You have always said, Doctor, that neither Rhodes nor Lobengula wants to fight. Can't you make a last appeal to the king? I am sure he would listen.'

'Hmm.' Jameson smoothed his moustache. 'It's not quite as simple as that, Mrs Fonthill. Y'see, time is not on our side. In a few weeks the rains will start, and mounted troops – our main weapon – will be immobilised. The settlers will be cut off from the south and the Matabele, in their own good time, could swoop down on the settlements and destroy them piecemeal. We would not be able to move our men about to protect them. Plus I've got idiots among the settlers who want to form their own militia and set off now to burn Bulawayo.

To go off at half-cock would be equally disadvantageous.'

He smiled. 'So, I really have to strike while the iron is more or less hot. Having said that, the High Commissioner is making one last appeal to Lobengula from the British Government to restrain his troops. But I think things have gone too far for that, and I can't afford to wait. I must make preparations now and I have told Cecil John that he must find the horses and arms right away.'

'But 'alf a mo,' intervened Jenkins. 'I thought you said 'is cupboard was bare.'

'Oh aye.' Jameson's smile was now mirthless. 'The company's cupboard is as empty as a Scotsman's wallet. I understand that Rhodes is going to sell forty thousand of his own chartered shares. They're at rock bottom just now, with all this trouble, so he won't be pleased about that, but we can't afford to wait. So we shall get our mounts and weapons. I only hope they are in time.' He shook his head. 'I also hope that we won't have to use 'em, but that, I fear, is a forlorn hope. Now you will have to excuse me. I must begin the business of organising our men to fight. We want volunteers, and we don't want the Border Police coming in from Bechuanaland.' He smiled wanly. 'This has got to be a company fight, you understand. No Imperials.'

His departure left the little group in silence. Eventually Alice spoke: 'Will you fight, then?'

Fonthill looked at the floor, then met her gaze. 'I will have no alternative—' he began.

'*Of course you will!*' Her anger made her stamp her foot. 'You don't have to go to war just because Rhodes wants his little empire. It's a terrible shame he's had to sell some of his shares, and my heart bleeds for him. But that does not mean that you must risk your life,' she shot a glance over her shoulder, 'and that of 352. If the company wants to fight, then let the bloody company fight!' Her voice softened and took on a more conciliatory tone. 'It's not *your* war, darling.'

Fonthill shook his head. 'I'm afraid it is, my love. Having invested in this territory, I cannot turn my back on the people here. You heard what Jameson said about the rains. Things have gone too far now, and Jenkins and I cannot walk out on the settlers and leave them at the mercy of the Matabele. You saw what Lobengula's impi did to the Mashonas here.' He reached across and seized her hand. 'We couldn't move aside and watch a series of massacres. You must understand that.'

'Oh, I understand all right.' She turned her head away. 'More butcherings – this time of natives by machine guns.' Her voice fell away to no more than a whisper. 'It's too high a price to pay, even for the best farmland in the world.'

Chapter 16

The bitterness that had coloured her reply stayed with Alice that night and through the next day. She received a cable from Cornford in Fleet Street congratulating her on her story of the clash at Fort Victoria and asking her to file further dispatches as and when the crisis escalated. But this did little to ease the agony in her mind and soul. She had agreed with Simon that the four of them should return to Salisbury, which was nearer to their land and to where Jameson had ridden to organise the forces needed to face Lobengula. So her morning was spent in packing their few belongings, but as she did so, her mind was racing.

Her years as a journalist and then with Simon had consigned her to a role as observer and housewife. True, her reportage had been proactive and might even have altered conceptions back home about the campaigns she reported upon, although she doubted it. And as chatelaine of their home in Norfolk, she had been a dutiful and hard-working supervisor of the house, who sometimes helped Simon with the estate. Nevertheless, she had never become involved with things that mattered. As a war correspondent, she had watched and noted, never integral to the events she was describing and about which she often harboured such strong feelings.

In the little wooden house they had rented in Victoria, there was scant privacy, and having packed the last of their meagre belongings, Alice slipped out, climbed on to the ramparts and sat, chin in hand. Below her, native working parties were collecting the dead on wagons and cracking their whips over the oxen to pull them away. It must have been very like this, she pondered, during the great plagues in medieval Britain, when cries of 'Bring out your dead!' echoed throughout the land.

Thus prompted, her mind dredged up memories from the past of so many similar scenes she had observed: the Zulu bodies, rigid in their death postures and stacked in front of the the mealie bags at Rorke's Drift; the dead Pathans, who had had the audacity to defend their country, spread out on the plain before Kandahar; the blazing houses of the bePedi tribe, set afire by Wolseley's troops at Sekukuni; the white-clad Egyptians, poor troops, their scattered corpses strewn across the parapet protecting the guns of El Kebir . . . Alice shook her head. What carnage!

She slapped away a fly that had settled on her dusty riding boots. Boots . . . breeches, shirt, wide-brimmed slouch hat. When was the last time she had worn a dress, for God's sake, or used cosmetics? She spent her time dressed as a man but she did not do a man's work – not *real* work. What had she ever done to try and stop the wars she had reported on so diligently? Nothing, of course. Nothing. And here she was again, observing the beginnings of another conflict and reporting on it. Just damned reporting. Oh, she tried to describe in her dispatches the blunderings and stupidity of the politicians and generals who had created the conflicts she wrote about, but there was no *real* evidence that this affected the course of events. Now it was happening all over again, the relentless, unstoppable march towards war, while she watched, an impotent observer.

But *was* it unstoppable, and was she quite so impotent?

She stayed for another ten minutes considering several courses of action, her eyes watching the disposal of the bodies down below but her brain recording nothing of it. Then, her mind made up, she stood, brushed away the flies and strode back to the hut. She found herself trembling. Was she afraid of the prospect? Dammit, yes!

They set off that afternoon riding as quickly as they could in the heat, watching warily for any sign of remnants of Lobengula's impi who might decide to take revenge on this vulnerable party. But they met no one, except one or two Mashona herdsmen, who waved cheerily at the white people who were freeing them from the Matabele yoke. Alice spoke little and Simon humoured her, realising her distress at the turn of events in this country where she had never really wished to be. But Alice's mind was active. She knew what she had to do, but how, and when?

By the time they reached Salisbury, she had decided upon the answer to the first part of that question, and circumstances provided the answer to the second.

They found the town agog with news of the happenings at Victoria and preparations for war. Rhodes's horses, rifles, machine guns and ammunition were being rushed up from the Cape, and the settlers were flocking to join units to march on the Matabele. They heard that a column was being formed at Victoria and placed under the command of a Captain Allan Wilson, who had earned a reputation for competence when serving in the Cape Mounted Rifles and the Basuto Mounted Police. Jameson himself had hurried off to Tuli in the south to arrange for more volunteers to be enrolled and led by Commandant Pieter Raaf, a Dutch Colonial who had served with distinction in the Zulu War and who was now a magistrate at Tuli. Rumours had it that the High Commissioner of Bechuanaland had moved a contingent of the Bechuanaland Police to the Matabele border in support of the Tuli column, and that King Khama himself had contributed a force of tribesmen to fight in the cause.

More to the point for Alice, however, was the fact that Jameson had left a message for Simon asking for his help in raising a column in Salisbury. Would he move out on to the veldt and 'borrow' as many horses as were suitable from the scattered farms? It would be at least a couple of months before Rhodes's mounts would arrive from the south.

'I shall be gone for at least two weeks, darling,' said Fonthill. 'I will take Jenkins with me, but Mzingeli will stay with you on the farm. There should be no danger there. We are away from things in the north, and in any case, I don't think hostilities will really get moving yet. Some sort of last-minute peace moves are still being made towards Lobengula, I understand, although I doubt if they will come to anything. Anyway, you will be safe enough.'

If Simon was surprised at his wife's ready acceptance of his departure without insisting that he take her with him, he showed no sign. They rode back to their little house on the veldt and parted there, Fonthill having readily agreed that Alice and Mzingeli should keep their horses for the time being.

As soon as Fonthill and Jenkins had disappeared over the swelling grassland, Alice made Mzingeli a cup of tea, strong and black, just as he liked it, sat him down and put to him her proposal.

He listened, his eyes growing larger by the second, then shook his head and said, 'No, Nkosana. Too dangerous.'

Alice sighed, shifted her position on the stool and tried again, but the tracker was obdurate. 'Nkosi don't agree so I don't agree. Sorry, Nkosana.'

Nodding, Alice played her last card. 'I need you very much for this, Mzingeli,' she said. 'I do not know the way and I do not speak the language. I need you also to protect me. But if you will not come with me, then I shall go alone. I am determined. I have to say, though, that I do not know what my husband will say to you when he finds that you have let me go.' She sat back, her face flushed and feeling rather ahamed of herself. There was a long silence while Mzingeli stared at the floor. Then he looked up.

'I go,' he said.

By noon they had set off, each riding a horse – for Alice decided that to take a wagon would slow them down too much – and with spare water bags, one small bivouac tent, blankets and one change of clothing all carried on the back of the sprightliest of mules from the farm. This was one trip, Alice resolved grimly, where a dress would *not* be needed.

As they rode in silence, she felt more and more guilty at using blackmail on Mzingeli. After all, she was probably putting him in more danger than she would be in herself, for there was less chance of a white woman being killed than a member of the Malakala tribe, so despised by the Matabele. She reached across and touched his arm. 'I am sorry, Mzingeli,' she said. 'I have been unfair. I am putting you in danger.'

His features relaxed for a quick second; it was hardly a smile. 'Nkosana strong lady,' he said. 'I once married to strong lady.'

'Ah.' She gave him her best smile. 'Then you know what hell it can be. You will feel sorry for my husband.'

This time he acknowledged her with a brief nod, but his eyes were dancing. Having re-established relations, Alice felt able to ask him: 'How long will it take us to get to Bulawayo?'

'Maybe bit more than two weeks. If we not killed on way.'

'Oh lord, I do hope that things don't get worse before then. If war is declared before we arrive, I will have no hope.'

'Not much hope anyway, Nkosana.' Then, rather surprisingly: 'You leave message for Nkosi? He not like come back and find you gone. He very upset. Not know which way to turn.'

She nodded her head in appreciation. 'It is kind of you to think of it. But yes, I did leave him a note. I have not told him where we have gone because I do not want him to come pounding after us, although,' she pursed her lips, 'I suppose he will guess.'

In fact, the message had been as non-committal as she could make it. It ran:

Dearest Simon,
I just could not sit back any longer without doing something to try and stop this senseless war. Don't worry, I have blackmailed Mzingeli to come with me to look after me (don't blame him). Please don't search for me. We will be back within the month.
I love you.
Alice.

Would he guess that she had gone to Bulawayo to plead with the king? Probably, but she would have a two-week start on him if he decided to follow, which, she concluded glumly, he almost certainly would. By then, she might be on her way back – if, that is, they had not been disembowelled. Ah well. She set her jaw. At least she was at last doing something positive!

Considering that Alice and Mzingeli were riding into the heartland of the enemy, their journey was surprisingly uneventful, although the terrain did not make for easy going. It followed a ridge of high hills that was very heavily wooded, so reducing visibility and causing Alice to worry about sudden ambush. Towards Bulawayo, the ground levelled off somewhat, but it was cut by river valleys, with small kopjes all around. Underfoot, the soil was sandy and grey. Yet they made good progress and met no one until they neared the king's kraal, when they glimpsed many groups of warriors, armed and painted, heading in the same direction. They received puzzled looks, for they had made no attempt at disguise, but they were not accosted nor questioned.

It was nearly dusk as they rode down the familiar hill and passed by the first ring of thorn *zariba*, but Alice decided against attempting to see the king that night. Instead, she pulled her mount round and urged him towards Fairbairn's store, hoping desperately that the Scotsman had not upped and left for the border in the face of the coming hostilities.

She was, then, vastly relieved to see the familiar curl of blue smoke coming from his chimney, in complete disregard of the inflammable thatch all around it.

The Scotsman's jaw sagged when she walked through his door. He took out his pipe. 'Where on earth have you come from, woman? Don't you know that everybody here's talking about murderin' all white folks?'

She smiled. 'Yet you're still here, Mr Fairbairn.'

He waved his pipe stem dismissively through the smoke

haze. 'Och, they'll never turf me out and I'm not going to leave. But where have you come from, and where's your husband?'

She explained. 'I decided to come here to try and talk the king out of going to war. I think he knows that it would be suicide for his people and his country. I am serious, Mr Fairbairn. Someone has got to stop this senseless slide towards more killing. There is just a chance that because I helped to ease the pain of his gout, he might listen to me.' She gestured to Mzingeli, standing diffidently by the door. 'There's just the two of us and we've been riding hard all day. Do you think we might have a seat?'

'What? Oh goodness yes, my dear.' He pushed two old wooden chairs forward. 'Would you like a wee dram? It'll only cost yer two shillings.'

She gave a weary smile. 'Why not? And one for Mzingeli, please. I believe I have four shillings here.' She threw the coins on his counter. The trader poured three small measures and pulled up a chair to join them.

'Lassie,' he said. 'You've got an awful lot of guts, and it's just possible that if you'd arrived, say, a week ago you might have had some chance of success, for surely to God the old boy doesn't want to fight. But something's happened that has pushed peace right out of the window.'

'Oh lord.' Alice passed a weary hand across her brow. 'What is it?'

'You know that Mashonaland – or Rhodesia or whatever the damned place is called now – has got a new high commissioner, appointed by the government in London?'

'Yes.'

'Well, he wrote to Lobengula in one last plea for peace, inviting the king to send three of his most trusted *inDunas* to Cape Town to discuss peace terms down there. The old boy agreed, and dispatched one of his half-brothers and two *inDunas* immediately. James Dawson, one of the traders here – I don't think you met him – went with them to interpret and make sure that they reached the Colony without trouble. I refused to go. Well,' Fairbairn spat on the floor, 'the idiot went off to have a drink when they reached Tuli, leaving the three black fellers in the care of a mine foreman.'

'I don't like the sound of this,' said Alice.

'Nor should you. It just happened that a feller called Gould-Adams had arrived in Tuli with a detachment of the Bechuanaland Police. Gould-Adams had heard that there had been trouble up north and shots had been exchanged, so on learning that Dawson had arrived in Tuli, he presumed that he had escaped from Bulawayo. I don't know what he thought Dawson was doing with three Matabele *inDunas*, but he immediately treated 'em as prisoners of war. One thing led to another, with no one to interpret; the *inDunas* resisted, there was a scuffle and two of the chiefs were shot and killed. The king's half-brother didn't get involved, and when things were sorted out, he was allowed to return to Bulawayo with – you'll never guess.'

'What?'

'A note of apology.'

'Oh, how pathetic – and how typical!'

'He has just returned and told his sad tale. This is the last straw for the king. He is convinced now that all white men are liars and cheats and has declared war. The impis are being called in from across the nation.' He leaned forward. 'Lass, it's no time for you to be interfering, I assure you.'

Silence fell on the little room. Alice stole a glance at Mzingeli, but the tracker refused to catch her eye. He stared straight ahead, expressionless.

'Not exactly propitious, I do agree,' she said at last. Then she drew in a deep breath. 'But I have ridden two hundred damned miles and I am not going back without seeing the king and making one last attempt to stop this killing.'

The trader shook his head sadly. 'It's taking a big risk, you know, for it's not just the king you have to worry about. It's all his *inDunas*, who have been spoiling for a fight for so long. You might not even get as far as his front door before they turn on you.'

'I will just have to risk that I . . . er, I mean *we* will.' She turned her head to the tracker, who was listening silently. 'Will you come these last few yards with me, Mzingeli? You have heard it will be dangerous, but I shall need you to translate.'

The man's face remained expressionless. 'I come.'

Fairbairn nodded in approval. 'Good for you,' he said. 'But, lassie, there's one last thing you should know.' He paused, as though for effect. 'De Sousa is back.'

'Oh no!' Alice put her hand to her face and then withdrew it quickly, as though it was an admission of weakness. 'How long has he been here?'

'About two weeks. He's been pouring poison into the king's ear every day, trying to persuade him to attack and provoke the British. He wants Rhodes to invade, y'see, so that his government can protest to London, perhaps stop the invasion, and then he can take the credit with Lobengula and so take over the mining and other rights that Rhodes has negotiated. At the moment, he won't know you're here, but as he virtually lives at the king's elbow, he will find out soon enough. And lassie, as soon as you leave the kraal, he'll be after you, that's for certain.'

Alice gulped. 'Well, that's one development I hadn't foreseen, I must confess.' Then she shrugged. 'There's not much I can do about it at the moment, so I will worry about him tomorrow.'

'Where are you sleepin' tonight? You won't be gettin' your little hut back, I'm thinking.'

'No, nor will I ask for it. We will sleep as we have on the trek, out of doors – at least, I have a small bivouac tent.'

Fairbairn sucked in his breath. 'No. That will never do. You will find a puff adder slipped under your tent flap just before dawn if you do. No. You must sleep here. I'm just at the back there,' he indicated with his pipe stem, 'and you two can bed down here, in the shop.'

Alice sniffed in a little of the tobacco smoke and coughed. 'That's very kind of you, Mr Fairbairn. Yes, perhaps it would be safer. Thank you very much.'

She slept little during the night and arose well before dawn to make notes about what she would say to the king. It was important, having risked so much to see him, that she should present her case as persuasively as possible. Then she remembered that de Sousa could well be there. Would he shout her down? And once she was out on the veldt, making her way back to Salisbury, having won or lost, would he pursue and kill them both? They would be virtually defenceless out there in the bush. She tried unsuccessfully to prevent a shiver. She would just have to deal with that if and when it occurred.

Alice waited until the sun was well up before setting off down the hill towards the king's inner kraal. As she walked, medicine bag in hand, with Mzingeli at her side, she could not but help noticing an air of surprise and then hostility rising towards her on all sides. When she had made that same journey regularly only five months before, she had been greeted by smiles and waves from the Matabele.

Now, the smiles were scowls and the waves were derisive gestures, with the sharp points of the assegais turned towards them.

'Be careful what you say, Nkosana,' growled Mzingeli. 'Don't be . . . ah . . . hard to king. He different man this time, I think.'

'Thank you. I know what you mean. I will try and be careful.'

As they neared the inner kraal, a howl rose from within it. Their approach had been observed. Immediately, a crowd of natives – warriors in warpaint, women and small children – emerged from the entrance to the thorn fence and surrounded them, shouting and gesticulating. Alice continued to stride forward, however, her gaze fixed ahead, her head held up. She hated herself for feeling fear, yet she knew that the perspiration pouring down the small of her back and staining her shirt was not just caused by the heat of the sun. It was probably the presence of her medicine bag, which she carried like a symbol of authority, that prevented their progress being barred. Was she coming again, as once she had, to work her magic on the king's foot, perhaps at his bidding? The crowd fell back and gave her passage.

Lobengula was holding court out of doors, under the shade of his indaba tree, and the usual smell of goat dung rose to Alice's nostrils as she approached him. The king was sitting on his wooden chair, clutching his assegai. This time, however, there was no air of indolence about him. Stripped to his familiar midriff skirt of monkey tails, his glistening face and body were daubed in slashes of red and white paint and a tall ostrich feather had been thrust into the back of the *isiCoco* ring in his hair. By his side was a large white and black shield, almost as tall as himself. This was a king welcoming

Armageddon, a monarch of war. Except that, endearingly, the sandal on his left foot was not matched by his right, which wore that familiar open-toed carpet slipper. This leader of great impis was still suffering from gout.

The king was surrounded by *inDunas* similarly painted for war. As she neared the great tree, Alice thought she glimpsed a face she knew among the rank and file of the natives watching her. But she could not bring his relevance to mind. Not so with the yellow-uniformed and red-braided man who squatted at the right hand of the king. Gouela was in town, and he was clearly in favour.

Lobengula's jaw dropped when he saw the two approaching, then he scowled and, as they drew near, indicated sharply that they should sit. They squatted on the floor of beaten goat dung.

'Why you come?' asked the king, through Mzingeli. 'You not welcome here.'

'I come from the White Man's Mountain,' said Alice. It was the term the Matabele employed when speaking of Mount Hampden, now Fort Salisbury. 'I come for two reasons. Firstly, I wish to speak to your majesty about this war, and secondly, I hope that perhaps I can be of help to you, briefly, in treating your bad foot.'

Before the king could reply, de Sousa spoke to him quickly in Matabele. The king grunted and turned back to Alice. 'He say you work witchcraft with your box. That why pain returns when you go. And what can you say about war when British soldiers kill my warriors?'

'I do not indulge in magic and I have always told you that my injections' – Mzingeli paused at the difficulty of translating the word – 'would only give you temporary relief. If you want to get rid of gout for good, you must stop drinking the white man's brandy and champagne and eat less meat. Your majesty,' Alice leaned forward to emphasise the force of her words, 'you must not listen to that man. He is evil. He makes slaves of black people and he is a rapist.'

'Humph. I have slaves. My *inDunas* have slaves. Some people not good for anything else. And women like to lie under men. Eh?' He turned to the women among the crowd surrounding him and they all giggled. Some nodded and others, more forward, shouted in acclamation. The king grinned at Alice. 'See?'

Alice realised that the debate was going against her. She swallowed and tried again. 'Your majesty, I have always argued with others – including my husband – that it was not right for the white man's column to invade your country. But you allowed it to do so. The white men are now well established in Mashonaland and I am afraid that you will never get rid of them. All over the world, my people have populated countries like yours and have stayed there—'

The king interrupted. 'Why they want these lands? Why they don't stay in their own country? Why they want my country as well?'

Alice thought quickly. Why indeed? She was uncomfortable in this role of devil's advocate. Better to be honest. 'I do not know the answer to that question. Perhaps it is because we are great traders and roam the world to find new goods, or because we are great farmers who like to bring our modern ways of agriculture to make better use of land everywhere. But that is not the point.'

'What is point, then?' The king's posture had softened somewhat, and when, several times, de Sousa had tried to interrupt, he had gestured to him to be quiet. Lobengula was obviously beginning to enjoy the debate.

'The point is that, in addition to being great traders and farmers, the British are great warriors. Your majesty, I am the daughter of a general, as you know, and I have seen fighting in many parts of the world. Always the British have won.' She began counting on her fingers. 'In Zululand, India, New Zealand, Egypt, Canada . . .'

'I do not know these places.'

'You know Zululand. You know that the Zulus won a victory at Isandlwana, but that the cost of that victory was so great that King Cetswayo said an assegai had been plunged into the bowels of his people. Then the British came again and the Zulus were scattered at Ulundi and the king was forced to flee. The Zulus are fine warriors but they were beaten. I was there. I saw it all. The British now rule Zululand.'

For the first time there was a pause in the confrontation and the onlookers, who had shouted in support of each of the king's responses, fell silent. A look of sadness came into Lobengula's eyes.

'Yes, I know that place,' he said. 'Zulus my ancestors.' He paused again, then leaned forward, and his voice was lower this time, as though begging Alice to understand. 'I try everything with white man. I give English everything they ask for. I let them come into my country to dig holes for their gold and they come and spread everywhere and make homes, not dig. I punish Mashona people because they do not pay tribute, as is custom, so English kill my warriors. I agree one last time to talk peace and send *inDunas* to Cape country. They kill them at Tuli.' He stood and his voice rose. 'The chameleon has struck. It is too late to talk more. No time for talking now. I call in my impis. It is time for war.'

A great roar rose from the crowd as the king finished his peroration by raising his assegai high above his head.

Mzingeli spoke softly to Alice. 'We go now, while we can. Eh?'

But Alice shook her head and looked up at Lobengula in supplication. 'Your majesty, I beg you not to fight the British. I know your warriors are brave and strong, but the British have mighty weapons of war – the new machine guns, cannon and many rifles—'

'Ah.' The king interrupted her again. 'Not like Zulus this time. This time I have rifles and many, many more men than British. This time we throw British out of my country.'

Another roar went up and the people began to ululate, swaying their hips and slowly jogging from one foot to the other. De Sousa had stood, too, and was clapping his hands in time to the rhythm. Then he smiled, turned and said something into Lobengula's ear.

The king relayed it to Alice. 'My friend here offers to take you back to the mountain. Keep you safe on journey. Country not safe for white woman to cross it alone.'

Alice shook her head. 'No. Twice before he has tried to kill me and my husband. He is a murderer and would butcher me and my servant as soon as we were on the veldt.' She thought quickly. How to buy time? 'Your majesty, allow me to treat your foot once more.'

The frown reappeared on Lobengula's features. His uncertainty was obvious. The choice lay between showing his rejection of the white witch and of her people's ways by openly dismissing her, or submitting and gaining some respite, at least, from the pain that nagged at his foot. Eventually he mumbled something very quietly to Mzingeli.

'He say come back when sun is at highest,' translated the tracker.

Alice rose and bowed her head, and she and Mzingeli

walked away, to the derision of the crowd. As they made their way back up the hill, she heard Lobengula shout a command.

'He tell his people not to harm us,' said the tracker.

Alice hardly heard, for her head was spinning. She had travelled two hundred miles all for nothing. Her mission had been a complete failure. It had been a gamble, of course, but she had hoped that the strange half-friendship that had been forged as a result of her ministrations to the royal foot might have gained her a longer hearing. The killing of the *inDunas* at Tuli, of course, had sealed the matter. Now she had put her life and Mzingeli's at risk once again. How to avoid de Sousa on the long ride back to Fort Salisbury?

She put the question to the tracker.

Mzingeli was silent for an unusually long time while he pondered the problem. Eventually he said, 'Don't know, Nkosana. Could go long way back, to Tuli, and ask for help from soldiers there. But Gouela will have trackers with him. They will pick up trail and follow. Kill us before we reach Tuli. Perhaps king will give us men to protect us on way.'

'I doubt it. But I will ask him.'

On her return at noon, the atmosphere inside the king's house was cold, despite the fire that he habitually kept burning. Lobengula hardly spoke, and the pile of empty champagne and brandy bottles seemed to mock Alice as she once again injected him. As she packed her bag, she raised the subject of de Sousa's threat.

'He don't hurt you. I tell him. Now you go. King is grateful for you taking pain from foot. But go back to your own people and tell them that my impis coming to eat them up. Go now.'

Alice bowed, and with Mzingeli made her way back towards Fairbairn's store. The pair were just outside the inner *zariba* when a native appeared from one of the huts and gestured to them.

'What does he want?' asked Alice.

'He say one of *inDunas* has news about your husband.'

Alice paused, a frown on her face. 'What? Simon – oh goodness. He has followed us and been captured. Oh no! Come on, Mzingeli.'

'No, Nkosana. No.' But Alice was already running towards the man and following him down a steep incline into a little copse of trees. The tracker ran after her, and burst into the shade of the thicket to find two assegais at his throat. Alice was struggling in the grasp of a large black warrior of indistinct origin – not a Matabele – while de Sousa, resplendent in gold uniform, nodded in delight at both of them.

'Welcome, Mrs Fonthill,' he said. 'I am sorry you refused my offer of protection because,' he gestured with a cheroot, 'this place can be dangerous, as you see.'

Alice's mouth had suddenly become dry, and it seemed as though her tongue had swollen and made it difficult to speak. 'You will not harm either of us,' she gasped. 'The king has promised us his protection.'

'Ah, but you have said goodbye to the king, and he has other, more pressing matters on his mind than to worry about a silly Englishwoman who has set off across the very dangerous veldt.' He nodded to where a thin, elderly native held a sack well away from his body. It was tied at the neck but something was wriggling inside it.

'This is not exactly puff adder territory, but some of them do get this far north, and this one certainly has, as you can see.' He allowed a thin spiral of smoke to climb into the air.

The realisation of what de Sousa intended made Alice

tremble with a mixture of fright and disgust. She struggled, but the man who held her strengthened his grip. 'Mzingeli . . .' she began. The tracker's eyes were wide and glowing yellow, but with two spearheads at his throat, he could not move.

'Mrs Fonthill!' James Fairbairn's voice rang out clearly from the track above. 'I saw you go down there. The king wants you urgently, I fear. Can you come right away, please? Are you all right?'

Before a hand could be clapped to her mouth, Alice shouted, her voice cracking with relief, 'Yes, Mr Fairbairn. Please hold on to help me up the hill, if you would be so kind. I am coming now.' Then, equally loudly, 'Come, Mzingeli.'

The man holding her looked quizzically at de Sousa, who snarled and made a dismissive gesture with his hand. Alice, her eyes on the sack, grabbed Mzingeli's hand and they both ran out of the thicket to meet the most welcome sight in the world: Fairbairn, pipe clenched in his mouth, coming crabwise down the steep track, his hand extended towards her.

Alice grabbed the trader's hand so tightly that the Scotsman winced. 'Don't worry, lassie,' he said, 'that bluidy man can't hurt you now. I am too close to the king for him to tangle with me.'

The three scrambled up the slope to the track above. 'How did you know . . . ?' began Alice.

'I saw you follow that man down. I knew he was one of the Portuguese's little troop and I smelled trouble. So I came after ye. The king doesn't want you, of course, but he wasn't to know that. Now, don't worry, you'll be safe enough with me.'

'Oh, Mr Fairbairn, we are so grateful.' And she told him about the snake.

Fairbairn wrinkled his nose in disgust. 'Aye. He's a bit handy with the reptiles. I remember how he tried to kill your husband. I'll have my lads take extra precautions around my place.' He gestured towards his store. 'We're nearly there. We'll all have a cup of tea – I'm only charging thruppence a cup now.'

Alice forced a smile. 'Cheap at the price, dear Mr Fairbairn.'

Once inside the store, the three sat together to drink their tea. 'I'm afeared that you've got a problem now, lassie,' mused Fairbairn. 'I know Gouela. He'll stay with the king to show he's not following but he'll send his men after you if you set off. You can stay here if you like.'

Shaking her head, Alice said, 'That's kind of you, Mr Fairbairn, but it would just enrage the king. He has told me to go. No. I suppose we shall have to take our chance out on the veldt.' She squared her shoulders. 'We have guns, after all. We can fight. We will need to buy provisions from you for the journey, and if you will allow us to stay overnight, we will set off before dawn and ride as fast as we can and to hell with them.'

The Scotsman grinned. 'You've got courage, lassie. I will spread the word that you're riding to Tuli. That might send 'em off on the wrong track for a wee while and give you a bit more time. Now, what will you be needing for your trek?'

Later that afternoon, Alice had finished her purchases and was taking a mournful second cup of tea with Mzingeli – 'Have this one on me,' said Fairbairn – when a Matabele and a woman, presumably his wife, came into the store and began speaking quietly to the trader. Alice noticed that the three kept looking at her as they talked, and then the Scotsman walked to his entrance, looked about outside and closed the door.

'Do you ken this man, Mrs Fonthill?' he asked.

'What? Oh, I don't think so.'

'I think he's a friend of yours.'

Alice rose and walked over to the trio. The man was thin and looked silently at the floor as she approached, as did his wife. She remembered glimpsing his face when she entered the inner kraal and walked to face the king. She felt then that she had seen him before but, as now, she could not remember where or when.

'He says you saved his life and he wants to help you now.'

'Why? I don't understand . . .'

Then the Matabele looked into her face and raised his right arm. His hand had been severed at the wrist and only a stump remained.

'Ah. The thief!' Immediately she felt ashamed of herself for so condemning him and involuntarily added, 'I am sorry, forgive me.'

Fairbairn grinned and waggled the pipe between his teeth. 'Don't worry. He can't understand. But he has heard that the Portuguese is planning to send some of his men out after you as soon as you leave tomorrow. And he has a plan, of sorts, to help. He's grateful to you, you see, and so is his wife here.'

'How kind of him to want to help us. But what can he do?' Alice was suddenly conscious that Mzingeli was by her side, listening intently.

Fairbairn nodded to the man, who looked over his shoulder nervously, then, seeing that the door stayed firmly shut, began speaking quickly.

The trader translated. 'He's seen your mule grazing outside and has asked if you have horses. I've explained that you arrived late yesterday and that I've put your horses in my stables just behind the house, where hopefully nobody has seen them. He's happy about that because his plan is this. You will set out after dark tonight, before the moon comes up, leading your horses and leaving by that dried-up watercourse at the back of the store. You will take a less direct course for Fort Salisbury, going due east rather than north-east. It will be difficult for anyone to pick up your spoor among the stones in the donga. At the same time, he and his wife will take your mule and head directly to the fort. They will go as fast as they can to give you time to get away. The idea is that the trackers will follow the spoor of two people and a mule, thinking that it's you two, of course. I have to say it's an ingenious scheme, so it is.'

The trader took out his pipe long enough to send another column of smoke to the ceiling. 'What you've got to do now is to be seen outside the store, ostentatiously loading the mule. I can give you sacks we can stuff for that purpose. You put your real provisions on your horses, of course, keeping them out of sight in the stables. It'll mean you'll have to travel very light, you ken. No tent, for example.'

Alice regarded the two Matabele, who were standing before her diffidently, almost sheepishly, as though they were about to be put on trial. She turned to Mzingeli.

'What do you think?'

The tracker gave his usual pause. 'Could be good way of stealing mule,' he said expressionlessly. 'Man is thief, remember. But if honest, good plan.'

She thought for a moment. 'I am prepared to trust them, Mr Fairbairn. Will you say that I am very grateful and I hope they find the mule useful.' She put out her hand and shook the left hand of the man and then that of his wife. They both allowed themselves to look into her eyes and returned her smile. 'Ah, Mr Fairbairn,' Alice exclaimed. 'I feel I can trust them. Anyway, it seems our only hope. I realise that they are also behaving very courageously. They could well be killed when de Sousa catches up with them.'

The trader nodded. 'You're right. It's damned unusual for a Matabele – let alone his wife – to go out on to the veldt after dark. And as for finding the mule useful, they will if they are left with it after de Sousa's men catch them. I agree with you that they are being very brave. They've got guts.'

The man and his wife left the store carrying several pots and pans – which Alice of course paid for – so giving a reason for their visit to any spying eyes. Half an hour later, Mzingeli began loading the mule, taking his time about it, before leading the animal round to the back of the store.

The night was black when they set out. Alice embraced Fairbairn at the stable entrance, somewhat to his embarrassment, and shook the hands of the two Matabeles before they began leading the mule away to the left as Alice and Mzingeli dipped down into the donga to the right, feeling their way awkwardly on the stones that lined its bottom. Then darkness swallowed them all.

Alice had plotted her course roughly. She had a compass that glowed dimly in the dark, and she planned to walk and then, as soon as the terrain allowed, ride through the night and the following days on a course that took them due east. When she judged it safe, they would turn to the north-north-east and follow a more direct route to Fort Salisbury. It was, she hoped, a course that might even take her into the path of Simon, if, as she fervently prayed, he had deduced on his return that she had gone to Bulawayo and followed her. The thought of that wriggling sack impelled her and they travelled quickly.

On the sixth day after leaving the king's kraal, and when they had broken out of the bush into a stretch of open country, Mzingeli's sharp eyes picked out the tiny figures of two horsemen riding across the high veldt far to the north of them. Cautiously they wheeled their horses round and put them to the gallop towards the riders, keeping low in the saddle. As they neared, the figures turned to meet them, and within minutes, Alice was in the arms of her husband.

Chapter 17

After that first embrace, each clumsily reaching out to the other from their horses, the reunion was not as warm as Alice would have wished, although she had expected nothing less.

'You've been to Bulawayo, of course?' asked Simon, his brow like a low-veldt thundercloud. Their fidgety mounts circled each other as though they too were sparring.

'Yes, I have. I wanted to make one last appeal to Lobengula to hold back his impis.' She tossed her head. 'And I might have succeeded if those fools in Tuli hadn't murdered two of his *inDunas* he was sending on a peace mission.'

'Yes, I heard about that.' Jenkins and Mzingeli had discreetly moved away. Fonthill's face remained set in stone and he spoke quietly but with vehemence. 'Alice, there are times when I think I should throw you across my knee and spank you. You have been thoughtless, foolhardy and downright silly. Things have gone too far for one single person – journalist, politician, woman or man – to have the conceit to think that she could stop this war by arguing. You have put your life at risk and that of Mzingeli, and you have worried me to death. You should be ashamed of yourself.'

Alice flushed. 'I may have been the other things, but I have not been thoughtless. I thought long and hard about what I

347

believed I ought to do before I decided to do it. I am sorry that I had to force Mzingeli to come with me, but I couldn't have reached Bulawayo without him. I am also sorry that I caused you worry, but I knew that if I told you of my intention you would prevent me from going.'

She felt the tears begin to well up and gulped to hold them back. 'As for everything else, I have no regrets. I failed, but I would do it again if there was a chance of success. Simon, for God's sake!' Her voice rose and she stood in her stirrups. 'We are going to war, and hundreds, perhaps thousands of lives are going to be lost because of the ambition of some half-mad millionaire in Cape Town. It was worth risking my life and even that of Mzingeli to try and prevent that.'

Jenkins chose this moment to ride up. He put out his hand, seized that of Alice and gave it a clumsy kiss. 'Thank goodness you've come back safely, Miss Alice,' he said. 'We've both been very worried, look you. You must excuse us all if we're a bit exisp . . . exagg . . .'

'Exasperated?' offered Alice.

'I was just goin' to say that, miss. But anyway, it's lovely to see you without a spear stickin' out of your . . . er . . . chest.'

'Oh dear.' The warmth of Jenkins's words, the genuineness of his welcome and the long-suppressed fear of the snake finally released the tears, and they poured down her face. She reached a hand out to both men and clutched theirs. 'I . . . am . . . so . . . sorry,' she sobbed.

'That's a relief.' Fonthill allowed his frown to disappear. 'I didn't fancy putting you across my knee. You're far too heavy now.'

She aimed a playful blow at him and the tension was released.

'Mzingeli,' called Simon. 'Can you make us all tea?'

'Yes, Nkosi. No milk. Black.'

'Oh very well. Now, Alice, tell me what happened.'

They squatted around a makeshift fire while Mzingeli boiled his billycan and Alice told her story. When it came to de Sousa, Fonthill's jaw dropped in horror. 'My poor love,' he said and took her hand.

Jenkins's face set into a scowl. 'I should 'ave put that shot through 'is 'eart,' he said. 'But I shall get 'im next time.'

'No you won't,' said Simon. 'As I keep saying, he's mine. And we might have a chance yet. If Gouela is in Bulawayo this late in the day, that means he is going to fight with Lobengula. The king said that he was gathering his impis?'

'Yes. We saw groups coming into the kraal from all parts, and Fairbairn told me that a large impi was due to arrive any day from Barotseland. It's probably there by now.'

Fonthill frowned. 'Hmm. Major Patrick Forbes is about a day behind us with his force from Fort Salisbury, and Allan Wilson is coming up to join them from Victoria with a second, slightly larger column. I gather they are hoping to meet up at Iron Mine Hill, just over there,' he jerked his head in the direction from which they had come, 'near Umvuma. We must get back there pretty quickly, because Lobengula will know exactly what's happening in his country and we don't want to be caught out here by an impi trotting in to attack. Pack up and let's mount.'

As they rode, Fonthill reluctantly conceded to Alice that even at this late stage, Rhodes was playing politics. 'This has got to be his war, you see. If he lets the column from Tuli engage with the Matabele, that means that the Imperials are involved, because the Tuli lot have regular troops with them, and Whitehall can dictate terms. So it's a race between the two forces to see who takes on Lobengula first: our settlers from

Salisbury and Victoria or the regulars and policemen from Bechuanaland. If we get there first and beat the king, then Rhodes can make it a company peace and keep out the government back home.'

Alice tossed her head. 'Typical!'

They rode as hard as their horses could go, pausing occasionally to rest them, when Fonthill rose in his stirrups and searched the horizon behind them – they were still in open country – for any sign of a Matabele force coming up to confront the settlers' army. Nothing moved on that plain, however, except for the occasional quick-darting ostrich and guineafowl. Towards dusk, they met the combined forces from Salisbury and Victoria.

'My, they've moved fast,' murmured Fonthill, as the column's outriders rode towards them.

The reason, of course, was that this small army was comprised completely of cavalry, and it presented a fine sight as it moved across the veldt in a jingle of harness, with two columns riding side by side. Rhodes's personal fortune had provided not only the rifles, ammunition and horses, the latter scoured from all parts of Rhodesia and the Cape, but also uniforms for this citizens' militia. Each man wore a jacket – many of them ill-fitting, but who cared about that? – crossed at the chest by a bandolier, with riding breeches, leather leggings, and a broad-brimmed bush hat, pinned up at one side in jaunty colonial style. Underneath virtually every hat stretched a bushy moustache. Rattling along in the middle of the columns were light provision wagons and carts carrying five Maxim machine guns, and bouncing and banging further back were two Hotchkiss seven-pounder cannon. Light on artillery and numbers, yet still a formidable, fast-moving unit.

'How many, d'yer think?' asked Jenkins.

'About seven hundred, now that the two columns have joined together,' said Fonthill, his chin resting on his hand as he watched them approach. 'Mobile, which is good. But not so good if we have to fight in the bush. Horses will be useless there.' He sighed. 'And it's not many men compared with Lobengula's impis.'

''Ow many 'as 'e got, then?'

'Don't know exactly.' Fonthill frowned. 'Between eighteen and twenty thousand, I am told.'

'Blimey. Let's just 'ope they don't all come at once, then.'

Alice drew her horse alongside and shielded her eyes. 'Can you see any press people?'

'Well, they don't stand out. If they're there, they'll be dressed just like the rest.' Fonthill gave a cynical smile. 'They like to think they're soldiers too.'

Alice sniffed.

Riding at the head of the columns were Jameson and his two senior officers, Majors Allan Wilson (newly promoted) and Patrick Forbes, a Sandhurst-trained regular officer who had distinguished himself in brushes with natives in the east and who Jameson had put in overall command of the force. Fonthill and his companions rode forward to meet them.

'Fonthill!' Jameson raised his hat. 'And Mrs Fonthill. Glad to see that you are all reunited.' Alice flushed and wondered what they had been told, but the doctor was introducing his officers.

Wilson and Forbes seemed to be in competition to see who could grow the widest moustache in South Africa. Wilson, perhaps, shaded the contest, for his stretched down and stood out on either side of his chin. He was the younger and much the slimmer of the two, and had come up through the ranks. He carried an air of brisk confidence about the clash to come.

Forbes was heavily built, stolid in demeanour and spoke little.

'Already had a brush with the Matabele,' said Jameson. 'They came at us on our way up from Victoria, before we'd joined Wilson's column. Came out of the bush without warning.' Fonthill marked that the doctor's tone was solemn and utterly without delight at having had the first encounter with the enemy. 'We hardly had time to lift a rifle. We got a few of them, but not many. Alas, Campbell, our ordnance officer, was badly speared in the leg. I had to amputate, but he died the next day. We lost Ted Burnett, too, one of the transport officers with the column. You remember him, Fonthill?'

'Yes, I do. I am so sorry. He was a good fellow.' It quickly occurred to Simon that this was probably the first time that the doctor had had to revert to his original calling and operate on a wounded man after a clash with an enemy force. Would it be the last?

Forbes grunted. 'Not easy to put out pickets in the bush. I'd much rather fight them in the open.'

'If they'll let us.' Fonthill tried to keep the note of warning from his voice. This was not his campaign. Nevertheless . . . 'What are your plans for the campaign, Jameson?'

The doctor removed his spectacles and polished them violently with his handkerchief. 'We are going to sweep round and attack Bulawayo from the north. We will cross the Shangani river and hopefully catch Lobengula napping and capture him, of course.'

Simon frowned. 'If I remember rightly, Doctor, that means you will have to go through some sort of forest called . . .' He turned his head. 'What's it called, Mzingeli?'

'Somabula, Nkosi.'

'Heavy woodland, is it?' The question came from Forbes, whose mouth under his moustache was set in a grim line. He sought the answer from Fonthill, rather than Mzingeli. Was it beneath his dignity to address a native? Simon dismissed the thought. Forbes had campaigned with native troops and would know their worth.

Fonthill diverted the question. 'Mzingeli?'

'Thick, Nkosi. Good place for . . . what is that word?'

'Ambush.'

'Yes.'

'Well, if it's there we shall just have to push through it.' Jameson spoke quickly, as if anxious to get on. He turned to Alice, who had been listening quietly. 'May I ask, Mrs Fonthill, have you come from Bulawayo?'

The two majors swung round in surprise. It was clear that they had no idea why she and the three men with her were riding vulnerably out on the veldt on the brink of war. Alice was not anxious to inform them. 'Yes,' she said.

'And was the place preparing for war?'

'Oh yes. Very much so. Even Lobengula was stripped down and painted. He told me he had called his impis in and I understand that the last of them were due in several days ago.'

'Really. Thank you. In that case, gentlemen, the sooner we get on and tackle them, the better. Oh, by the way, ma'am, there are no journalists with us. I understand, though, that some may be with the Tuli column – if that lot get here in time, of course.'

He gave a grim smile, but Alice did not return it. She was not inclined to join in, however peripherally, with Mr Rhodes's little games. Nevertheless, she was pleased that this was one war that, by the look of it, she could report without competition. She gave a brief nod of acknowledgement and fell back a little as the three officers urged their mounts forward.

Jameson called back over his shoulder, 'You'll stay with us, of course, Fonthill? We would all be glad to have the benefit of your experience.'

'Of course, Doctor.' Fonthill turned to his wife. 'Alice, I would much prefer it if you would continue on to Fort Salisbury. Jenkins and Mzingeli can escort you, and you should reach there in less than a week.' He smiled, persuasively he hoped. 'Jameson will be sending messengers back there to cable Rhodes and you will be well informed. What's more, you can send your own reports to the *Post* from the cable station there without delay.'

Mindful of the worry she had caused him, Alice bit back the derisory response on her lips and instead smiled winningly. 'Thank you, dear,' she said, 'but I would much prefer to stay with the column. So much more comfortable, and I do so like the fresh air.'

Jenkins smothered a grin, but Simon just frowned.

It was quickly decided that it was too late for the troops to advance much further, and Jameson resolved to take advantage of the open nature of the terrain and camp then and there. Fonthill noticed that despite the fact that Forbes was nominally in command, the force of the doctor's personality – or was it his command of Rhodes's wallet? – ensured that he took the main decisions, at least when the enemy was not present. Pickets were pushed out, guards were mounted, campfires were lit and the force settled down for the night.

For five days the two columns advanced, eagerly and yet nervously seeking action but finding none. Their scouts, with whom Fonthill and Jenkins ranged for much of the journey, could find no trace of the Matebele host, even though they rode through bush country that would be ideal for an attack.

It seemed that Lobengula was holding his troops back to defend his capital – perhaps in Somabula Forest.

As the weather worsened, with mist and light rain descending, the British outriders reached the beginning of the forest and halted. It seemed, in fact, not particularly worse in terms of density than any of the more thickly wooded bush country through which they had already ridden, but Fonthill confirmed with Mzingeli that this would be the last and probably the best place for the Matabele to attack before Bulawayo, now only some fifteen miles away.

'What d'yer think, Fonthill?' asked Forbes as Wilson and Jameson joined them at the head of the column.

'Well, in one way it is tempting to push on through the forest during the night,' said Simon. 'The Matabele, like the Zulus, would never dream of launching an attack at night, so we might be able to reach the open ground on the banks of the Shangani on the other side. But I fear that with no moon, and this mist about, we would probably lose our way. The column might break up and we would end up dispersed all over the bloody place.'

He eased himself in the saddle and wiped the damp mist from his face. 'My advice would be that we should camp here for the night, wait until there's decent visibility after dawn and push on. The forest is too big to go round, I understand.'

He shot a sharp glance at Mzingeli, who nodded.

'Oh, we don't want to make a diversion,' exclaimed Jameson. 'I want to get straight on to Bulawayo and have it out with Lobengula as soon as possible. If you agree, Forbes, I think we should do as Fonthill recommends.'

Fonthill stifled a smile. The race against the Imperials was never far from the doctor's mind.

'Quite so. We will make camp and push on in the morning.'

The morning, however, was almost as unpromising for riding through thick woodland as the night would have been, for a thick fog descended on the forest, leaving tendrils of it, like a spider's web, hanging from the tallest of the thorn trees and making the temperature drop by nearly twenty degrees.

'Rains will be here soon,' growled Jameson, wiping his glasses. 'Come on, Forbes. We don't have time to wait about. Let's get on.'

They set off again, their horses stepping delicately through the dripping, shadowy glades and every sound beyond the gloomy greyness of the tree trunks making the outriders twitch their rifles and lick their already moist lips. Fonthill, who rode with Jenkins in the van – Mzingeli had been sent back to stay close to Alice – had no idea how long it took the two columns to pass through the forest, but every minute spent in that fog made him curse the more that his wife was back there in the gloom. If the Matabele came at them here in force, emerging from the undergrowth without warning, dodging and screaming, hurling their throwing spears, then he knew that the little army would be overwhelmed. There would be no time to form a square or create a laager. The warriors would be on them before an order could be given. It would have been much wiser to take another three days, or whatever, and skirt this wet, dripping labyrinth. Damn this childish, dangerous race against the Imperials!

At last they were out of the wood. The country was now more open, although still carrying sufficient timber to provide cover for an attacking force. In the distance could be seen the bulge of the banks bordering the Shangani river. Of the Matabele there was still no sign.

'I don't think they were ever in there waiting,' said Wilson.

'Probably not,' agreed Fonthill. He caught Mzingeli's eye and saw the faint negative shake of the head. He rode over. 'Do you think they were there?' he asked.

'They there,' said the tracker, his face expressionless as usual. 'I heard them and see some. But they go.'

'Why didn't they attack, for goodness' sake? They had us at their mercy.'

Mzingeli sniffed. 'That fog. They think it white man's magic, brought down to stop attack. They frightened in wood – like us. But they go.'

'What? Do you mean they have given in and run back to Bulawayo?'

'No. They attack. Soon, I think.'

Simon rode back and shared Mzingeli's view with Forbes. The big man nodded. 'Probably right,' he said. 'Feel it in me water.' He jerked his head towards the Shangani. 'River will probably be low and the banks high, so we'll have to cut a defile down to get to the water and then lay down brushwood and what-have-you to stop us sinking into the mud. Just as well we haven't got too many wagons. Won't be able to get across today, so . . .'

Wilson had moved away a little to chide a man who had dismounted. Now he returned. 'What's the plan, then, Forbes?' he asked. 'Straight across, eh?'

'No. We'll laager on this bank while we cut a path down and up the other side. Safest. Cross tomorrow.'

The younger man tugged at his moustache and shot a questioning look at Fonthill. 'I would have thought we could easily get across today. There's no sign of the Matabele. We need to press on, you know. What do you say, Fonthill?'

Simon sighed. He had no wish to intervene in what seemed

to be incipient rivalry between the two officers. 'I rather think Major Forbes is right, Wilson,' he said carefully. 'There's still plenty of cover for an attack, and we would be more or less defenceless if they came at us as we were trying to get across in the mud. One more day shouldn't make much difference, I would have thought.'

Wilson gave his cocky grin and indicated where Jameson was spurring his horse on to get a first glimpse of the river. 'I know someone who thinks that a day would make a hell of a difference,' he chortled. 'But you're in command, Forbes, though you may have trouble in convincing the medical department.' He raised a forefinger to the rim of his hat and rode away, to hurry along the last remnants of the columns emerging from the forest.

Jenkins had observed the conversation, although he was just out of earshot. 'What was all that about, then?'

'It was all about whether we should cross the river today. Forbes has decided better not, and I agree.' Fonthill raised himself from the saddle and looked about him. 'I must confess that I don't like this place. Mzingeli feels that the Matabele are out there near us now and are poised to attack.'

'Well,' sighed Jenkins, flicking the moisture from the end of his moustache, 'I wish they would bloody well get on with it. I'm catching pneuman . . . newinia . . .'

'Pneumonia?'

'No. No. Influenza. I can feel it in me bones.'

The two columns redeployed and a rough laager was made from the wagons, carts and cut thorn bushes, curling out in a semicircle from the northern bank of the Shangani. The river itself was wide, sixty yards or more, but not deep, and mud banks thrust up from the water in the centre to glisten in the sunlight, now burning away the last of the morning mist.

From within the protection of the laager, men worked to level down the high banks of the river and then to cut branches and strew them to provide a firmer base for wagons and horses in making the crossing. Forbes sent out patrols on the other side of the river, while work began on the further bank.

The task was completed just before dusk and the camp settled down for the night. Extra guards were mounted at dawn but still the Matabele did not attack.

The crossing began at once, and a very makeshift laager was created on the southern bank. It all took time and it was late afternoon before the two columns had squelched and slipped their way across the deep mud and re-formed on the far side.

'If you think this is bad,' Wilson confided cheerfully to Fonthill and Jenkins, 'just wait a few weeks. This place will be impassable. Once the rains come – and I mean real rain, not this bit of damp – the river will be in full flood. Almost impossible to cross.'

'Crocodiles?' asked Jenkins, his eyes wide.

'Not when the river's in spate. They don't like fast-flowing water and they'll head for high ground. But always keep your eyes open for the beggars.'

'Oh, I'll do that all right, bach. I'll do that.'

'We'll laager for the night on this side and set off again early in the morning,' called Forbes. 'Jameson is anxious to push on, of course.'

Fonthill nodded. The terrain on the south bank was very like that on the north – still suitable for a dawn attack. 'You'll be putting out patrols early tomorrow?'

'Of course.'

'Mind if Jenkins, Mzingeli and I go with them?'

'Of course not. But my feeling is that the Matabele have

retreated to Bulawayo and are going to make a stand just north of there.'

Fonthill nodded. 'You're probably right.' But he was unsure. He pulled Mzingeli to one side. 'I thought you said they would attack on the north bank,' he said, 'once we were out of the forest.'

'No, Nkosi. They frightened of wood and ghosts so rush across the river. Did you not see their marks in mud?'

Fonthill shook his head. 'So they have retreated to Bulawayo after all?'

'No. They come tomorrow. I think they out there.' He indicated the bush with a broad sweep of his hand. 'They come at dawn.'

Jenkins gave a histrionic gulp. 'And you want us to go out early on patrol, bach sir?'

Simon shrugged. 'To be honest, I don't think too highly of these scouts that Forbes is sending out. They're noisy and too sloppy riding in this bush. Not proper soldiers. Perhaps we can stiffen 'em up a bit. Show them how to do it. All right?'

'Very good, sir.'

It was still dark when the three saddled up. The morning was overcast and dampish, with no stars to bid good night to the darkness and no moon to pave the way for the sun. The patrol consisted of twelve troopers, all good farmers, fine horsemen and keen shots, under the command of a sergeant, who had been chairman of their local community outside Fort Salisbury. As they fanned out to pick their way between the trees, Fonthill hung back a little.

'We will stay together,' he said. 'A bullet in your rifle breech but keep the safety catch on. We don't want any accidents in this rotten light. We will stay in the centre and try and keep those two chaps ahead in sight.'

The dawn seemed to be taking its time coming, and very soon they had lost sight of the two troopers ahead of them. To their right, they could hear two of the troopers calling to each other, and to their left, the crackle of broken branches as horses were pushed through the undergrowth. Fonthill frowned. Did they have to advertise their presence so obviously? Ahead, however, there was silence. Riding on slowly, Simon felt the perspiration start to form on his upper lip.

Suddenly the bushes in front parted and a horse came crashing out, its eyes yellow and wide. On its back swayed one of the troopers, an assegai piercing his chest and its blade tip emerging from his back. At the same moment, Jenkins's rifle rang out and a warrior fell on the right, in the act of hurling his spear. Two more came running fast and softly between the trees, and Fonthill aimed quickly and fired, seemingly without effect.

'Back!' he shouted. 'Don't let them get behind us. Back to the laager.' He pulled on his bridle and his horse swung round as a spear hissed by over his right shoulder. 'Ride low,' he screamed.

He became aware that he was riding in the middle of two Matabele who had appeared as if by magic. One of them seized his bridle while the other jabbed at him with a stabbing assegai, catching the edge of his coat with the spearhead and becoming entangled with it. Lashing out wildly with his boot, he raked the spearman's face with his spur and swung the barrel of his rifle into the head of the man holding his bridle, sending him crashing to his knees. His horse surged forward and he heard the crack of Mzingeli's rifle off to his right. Where was Jenkins? 'Three five two!' he yelled.

'Comin'.' The cry came from his left, and Jenkins emerged

from the trees, his head low along his mount's neck and his heels raking its sides. Behind him came a group of natives, all seeming to run almost as fast as Jenkins's horse and sending in its wake a hail of assegais, before they halted, panting. To the right, Mzingeli rode on a parallel course, blood streaming from a cut on his left thigh. Fonthill, clinging on for dear life as his horse took the bit between its teeth, stole a precarious glance over his shoulder. The Matabele had disappeared as quickly as they had appeared. But had they been able to get behind the patrol? He filled his lungs. 'Troopers,' he yelled. 'Back to the laager. Ride for your lives.'

The three horsemen broke out of the brush at the same time and saw ahead of them, in the half-light, the rather pathetic attempt that had been made to form a laager. It was clearly less effective than that drawn up on the other bank the previous evening. A handful of wagons and carts had been pushed together in a rough semicircle, extending from the riverbank. Many gaps remained, however, and as a bugle sounded, Fonthill saw men doubling up to fill them in two ranks, the front kneeling, those behind standing.

'Stand back, we're coming through,' he screamed and led the trio towards the nearest gap. It looked at first as though the line of troopers would not break, but they did so at the last minute, as though in reluctance, and the three galloped through, closely followed by the horse whose rider had been speared. He, alas, had long since fallen from the saddle.

Half tumbling from his mount, Fonthill ran to Mzingeli. 'Not much,' said the tracker. 'Scratch.' Then, with satisfaction: 'I kill him.'

Alice, medical bag in hand, had materialised. Her face was white in the dawn light. 'Are you all right, Simon?' she called, as she knelt down to examine Mzingeli's wound.

'Yes, fine. Look after Mzingeli. Are you all right, 352?'

The Welshman was reloading his Martini-Henry. 'Right as rain, bach sir. But my God, them black fellers frightened the life out of me, comin' out of the trees like that without a sound. Not a nice way to fight, look you. I almost 'ad a spear in me belly before I saw 'em. Like ghosts, they was.'

Fonthill was conscious that men in various stages of undress, all carrying rifles, were doubling up towards the ring of wagons and the line of defenders.

'Here they come.' The shout came from Forbes, revolver in hand, who was standing on a cart to the left of the line. His voice boomed out. 'No one is to fire until I give the order. We will fire in volleys. Front rank first.' A single shot rang out. 'Blast your eyes, that man. I said hold your fire until I give the order. Wait.'

Fonthill and Jenkins ran to join the major. The sun was now beginning to peep over the top of the line of trees some two hundred yards away and the first of its rays shone directly into the eyes of the defenders. 'To hell with that sun,' swore Forbes. Then he shouted, 'Pull your hat brims down. Select your target. Still wait . . .'

Simon shaded his eyes and saw that the line of the bush, some two hundred yards away, had suddenly erupted with a mass of Matabele, who now raised a triumphant yell and began running towards the defenders, their dappled shields seeming to form a phalanx that moved towards them at great speed. He gulped, thrust a cartridge into the breech of his rifle and looked behind him for Alice. She was kneeling just below him, carefully winding a bandage around Mzingeli's thigh. He caught Jenkins's eye; the Welshman winked before nestling his cheek into the stock of his rifle. This was Jenkins doing what he was born to do, with coolness and delight. No fuss. No fright. Lucky devil!

Then: 'Front rank, FIRE!' Simon heard the voice of Wilson, on the right of the half-circle, repeating the order, like an echo, and then he and Jenkins fired together. As the smoke cleared, he saw that the first line of Matabele seemed to have melted away and shields and black bodies were strewn across the earth. But the attack hardly paused in its stride.

'Brave buggers,' muttered Jenkins.

'Front rank, reload.' The voice of Forbes was stentorian and steady, echoed from the right by the higher note of Wilson's. 'Second rank, FIRE! Second rank, reload, Front rank, FIRE!'

Suddenly, a sound that Fonthill had never heard before on any battlefield joined in the awful cacophony. First one Maxim machine gun and then a second began their staccato chattering, causing spurts of dust to rise at the feet of the advancing warriors and then, as the barrels were raised, bringing them down in a great swathe.

'About bloody time,' grunted Forbes. 'They were almost on us. What the hell were those gunners doing?'

But the attack was not finished. From the ranks of the front spearmen appeared a line of riflemen, who knelt and discharged their weapons at the defenders. Fonthill realised with a start of guilt that these were the brand new Martini-Henry rifles that he had struggled to bring up from Kimberley. Then he saw, through the blue smoke, that the sight of each gun was raised to its maximum height and that the bullets were singing past, high over the heads of the defenders.

Forbes turned and grinned. 'They think that the higher they raise the sights, the faster the bullets will go,' he said.

Some spearmen, however, braved the bullets of the defenders – and those of their compatriots behind them – and were able to run close enough to the line of the laager to hurl their assegais. Two troopers kneeling in the front rank in the central gap toppled backwards, trying to pluck the spears from their chests. But this was the high-water mark of the surge forward, and the Matabele turned and ran back out of range.

'Will they come back again, do you think?' The question came from Alice, who, rifle in hand, had joined them.

Fonthill pulled her to him for a quick moment, as much in relief that she was safe as in affection, then said, 'I just don't know. There are so many of them. If they get near enough they could overwhelm us. Stay close, my love.'

It took only some fifteen minutes before the Matabele came again. This time they were led by the riflemen, who ran forward, fired, fumbled to open the breech, inserted another round, fired again then repeated the exercise. This time not all of the bullets sang over the heads of the defenders in the line, but the firing was ragged and on the whole ineffectual, and soon the riflemen were replaced by the more familiar surging mass of spearmen, who swept across the open space, their assegais held aloft and their cowhide shields forward as though to deflect the volleys that crashed out against them again.

The bravery of the warriors was no match for the modern weapons of the defenders, of course, and faced with the terrible fire of the Maxims and rifles at such close range, the Matabele eventually turned and ran back to the cover of the bush. There, some of them stayed to hurl defiance before melting back into the shelter of the trees. They left behind them at least two hundred warriors strewn across the open ground, virtually all of them dead.

Forbes turned to Fonthill. 'Where is my picket?' he growled.

Simon shook his head. 'I doubt if any of them escaped. The Matabele came at us suddenly at very close range out of the bush.' He sighed. 'We only just escaped, and I think we did so because we were riding slowly, carefully and quietly. I am afraid that your lads were making a bit of a noise and rather inviting the attack.'

The major nodded slowly. 'Humph. Just shows what might have happened if they had come at us in that damned forest. Well, you warned us, Fonthill, and I'm damned grateful. Just gave us time to man the ramparts, as it were. Now, let's see what the damage is.'

Jameson and Wilson joined them with the news that in addition to the picket, only two men had been killed and six wounded, including Mzingeli, whose wound did indeed prove to be superficial. To Fonthill's great relief, six of the picket trickled in out of the bush during the course of the morning. They had, it seemed, found that the Matabele had closed in behind them before attacking, and so had simply spurred their horses on and doubled back later.

They did report, however, that they had seen the mass of the Matabele retreating back across more open ground in the direction of Bulawayo.

'Good,' said Jameson. 'That means that we can push on. I am told, Forbes, that there is far less bush that way.' He pointed to the west. 'I suggest that we break up the laager and move on. I doubt whether we shall be attacked again until we near Bulawayo – even if then, that is.'

'I quite agree,' echoed Wilson.

'Very well,' said Forbes. 'But I feel they will attack again. We have given them a bloody nose, but they still have about eighteen thousand warriors to throw at us. They are brave and they won't give up yet.'

'I say,' called Wilson. He pointed out across the scene of battle to where a solitary figure was walking slowly among the dead. 'Who's that?'

'Alice!' snapped Fonthill. 'She could get herself killed.' He leapt over a thorn bush and ran towards her. 'Alice! What are you doing? Come back. There could still be Matabele in the bush.'

She turned, notebook and pencil in hand. 'Oh, I don't think so. They've all gone by the look of it, except these here.' She gestured around her. 'I've counted more than one hundred and fifty dead so far.' She fixed Simon with cold eyes. 'Not much of a battle, was it? I mean – spears against machine guns. More of a massacre, I'd say.'

Fonthill sighed. 'It didn't seem like a massacre when Jenkins, Mzingeli and I were caught out in the bush.'

Alice's expression softened and she put out a hand. 'Yes, sorry, my love. Do you think that this will be the end of it?'

'Forbes doesn't think so and nor do I. I am sure they will make a stand, probably just outside Bulawayo, to stop us from entering the king's kraal. After all, this hasn't exactly been a battle. Lobengula didn't commit many warriors. His army remains intact. It could be a very different story next time.'

Alice ran a desperate hand through her hair. 'Oh God! How long does this nonsense have to continue?'

Simon seized her hand. 'It will continue, Alice, until we have unseated Lobengula and he has been captured. You must resign yourself to that. Come on back now. You remain vulnerable out here.'

Hand in hand, they stepped over the bodies of the dead warriors, already attracting an army of flies, and made their way back to the laager. The wagons and carts were already being harnessed to their horses (no oxen – they would have

367

slowed the advance), tents were being struck and mounts saddled.

'What about these bodies, Doctor?' Alice asked Jameson.

The little man frowned. 'Have to leave them to the jackals, I fear. No time to give them a Christian burial, you see. Not that they would have appreciated that, being heathens.' He gave a mirthless laugh. 'No. Sorry, ma'am. We must press on. I suggest you mount up.'

Within minutes the outriders had cantered out, and shortly afterwards, the two columns re-formed and began to snake towards Bulawayo and the kraal of the King of the Matabele.

Chapter 18

It took them seven more days to approach the capital, during which time, although there were various alarms and scares, there was no sign of Lobengula's retreating impis. Eventually they reached Thabas Induna, the little flat hill that rose some twenty miles north of Bulawayo. Nearby was the source of the Imbembesi river, and Jameson decided that the columns should laager here and water the horses before the last push on to the king's kraal.

The laager was established in comparatively open land, but the passage to the embryonic river was dotted with shrub and trees. Although patrols had reported no evidence of Matabele presence in the vicinity, Forbes decided to send a light escort to supplement the black wranglers taking the horses down to the river, and Fonthill and Jenkins, anxious to attend to their horses, as well as those of Alice and Mzingeli, accompanied them.

The straggling herd had hardly had time to reach the river when the Matabele emerged from the bush. From the moment they burst out from the trees, running fast, shouting and brandishing their assegais and rifles, it was clear that their targets were the horses.

'They are trying to stampede them,' shouted Fonthill. A

small group of Matabele had broken away from the main band and were heading for the horses, waving their arms and screaming. The beasts were now pricking their ears and prancing, their handlers desperately trying to soothe them. Behind the advancing warriors, a screen of natives had emerged and were beginning to direct rifle fire at the escort and the horse wranglers.

Fonthill thrust his foot into his stirrup and struggled to remount. He shouted to the escort, who, milling about and unsure whether to return the Matabele fire or gallop back to the laager, seemed leaderless: 'You men, follow me.' He pointed towards the sprinting Matabele. 'We've got to run them down before they stampede the horses. Come on, quickly.'

Impeded by the need to lead Alice and Mzingeli's horses, neither Fonthill nor Jenkins had a hand free to draw and fire the rifles in their saddle buckets. Instead, they cantered towards the escort, twenty of whom gathered around them.

'Right,' shouted Fonthill. He pointed towards the spearhead of Matabele diagonally to their right. 'Give them a volley and follow me at the gallop. Ready, FIRE!' The noise of the shots made their mounts prance, but a dozen of the running warriors spun and fell. 'Now, hard at them and use your rifles as lances. Stay together. Follow me, GALLOP!'

'Hold tight, bach,' shouted Jenkins, and they were off, heads down, rifles held low like medieval lances, a small but solid mass of cavalry bearing down on the running warriors. It was too much for the Matabele, and they scattered in all directions as the horsemen crashed through them, flying hooves sending tribesmen to the floor and rifles thumping into cowhide shields and sending them spinning away. The fact that he was leading Alice's horse in the charge had unbalanced

Fonthill, never the best of horsemen, and he knew that if he hit one of the warriors he would be unseated. As it was, as they thundered towards the group he realised that he was slipping sideways and about to slide off the saddle. A strong Welsh hand from his right pushed him back again and he regained his balance, to ride through the milling tribesmen unscathed. One horseman was unseated but Jenkins reined in hard, swung round and threw the bridle of Mzingeli's mount to him, and the trooper was able to scramble away to safety.

At the end of their charge, the horsemen reined in, turned and waited for Jenkins and the fallen trooper to rejoin them. Fonthill, perspiration pouring down his face, nodded towards the Welshman. 'Thanks, 352,' he gasped. 'I thought I was gone then.'

Jenkins grinned. 'With respect, bach sir, you really shouldn't lead mad charges when you can't sit on your arse properly on an 'orse.'

Fonthill returned the grin, although there was more relief in his face than amusement. He wiped his face with his hand. 'Yes, well, not exactly the Charge of the Light Brigade, I do agree, but more effective, I would say. Well done, lads. Anyone hurt?'

The question was made more relevant by the singing of bullets winging their way over their heads. The Matabele riflemen had trotted forward and were now kneeling and firing directly at Fonthill's troop. It seemed, however, that the sights on their rifles were still set too high for the firing to be effective. More of a threat were the scores of black spearmen who were now spilling out of the trees and breaking into a run towards them. The group of warriors deputed to stampede the horses seemed to have disappeared, and down by the river, the horse handlers and the rest of the escort were cracking whips, screaming, nudging the lead horses and beginning to turn the mounts away from the water and the Matabele and back towards the laager.

Fonthill gestured towards the running warriors. 'Reload. We'll advance towards those spearmen and put one volley into them. Then let's get out of here quickly and go and help our people gallop the horses back. We will form a screen to protect the rear. Trot forward, now.'

The volley brought down a handful of the attacking warriors but did little to stop the advance of the others, who came on, spears swinging low, pumping strength into their legs, and shields pushed forward. Still they came, appearing out of the trees without break to form a black mass moving very fast across the open ground. Fonthill realised that this was no marauding party, sent out to steal horses and snipe at the edges of the advancing British columns. Lobengula had committed his main impis – probably including his much-famed seven-hundred-strong bodyguard – to overwhelm the white men. As if to underline this, he could hear heavy firing coming from the direction of the laager. He bit his lip. Would there be a laager to return to?

They rode back hard and caught up with the last of the horses, now galloping equally fast. As they broke cover, Simon realised thankfully that the laager was not surrounded and that the escorts were leading the mounts back towards a protected compound, where an opening was being kept for them. Looking behind him, however, he realised that the first of the charging spearmen were breaking out from the bush to complete the ring enclosing the laager.

'Halt,' he shouted. 'Two more volleys before we ride in.'

With impeccable – and surprising – discipline, the little

troop turned round, lined up, fired their volleys and then galloped back into the enclosure.

'Come on,' shouted Fonthill, handing his two horses over to a Kaffir wrangler. 'We must find Alice and then help in the line. I have a feeling that this is the big one.'

Alice was perched between two troopers behind the side board of a wagon, Mzingeli and her rifle by her side but her head down, scribbling furiously in her notebook. 'Make way, lads,' cried Fonthill, and they shouldered themselves in beside her.

'Thank God you're back,' cried Alice, regarding them both, her eyes wide. 'What happened?'

'The captain 'ere decided to charge the 'ole Mattabelly army,' said Jenkins, slipping a round into his rifle. 'So 'e nearly fell off.'

Alice gave a half-smile, but there was little humour in it, more concern. 'Can't be true,' she said. 'My husband is a magnificent rider, and anyway,' she gestured to the front, 'the whole Matabele army is out there, coming our way. Look!'

They followed her gaze. The spacious clearing in which they had camped was black with warriors. This time the attack was not pell-mell but coming seemingly in stages, with riflemen thrusting forward to fire, reload and fire again before the spearmen rushed towards the laager. Once again, however, the firing was wild and the riflemen could be seen fumbling with the Martini-Henry's loading mechanism, some of them dropping their cartridges on the ground and trying to scoop them up again.

This time the laager had been erected more carefully and the Maxims and the two seven-pounder guns mounted strategically, so that the former could sweep the warriors in the lead and the latter send their shells to explode in the rear.

To Fonthill's amazement, he saw that the Matabele riflemen were firing into the smoke and dust on the ground caused by the explosion of the shells. He reached across to tug at Mzingeli's sleeve. 'Why on earth are they doing that?' he asked.

A look of derision stole across the tracker's face. 'They fools,' he said. 'They think that when shell explodes it send out spirits of white men. So they shoot to kill them. Stupid!'

The concentrated firepower of the British was taking a terrible toll. There was no protection in the clearing, nowhere to hide from the volley firing, the sweep of the machine guns, nor the boom of the two cannon. The warriors seemed to be engaged in a dance of death, as they ran forward, jumped high as they were hit and then fell backwards, scattering their rifles, spears and shields before lying still, occasionally moving a limb, like injured beetles.

'Oh, this is brutal,' sighed Alice. 'Why don't they stop and run away?'

But still they came running forward, black waves beating against a hostile shoreline. Some of the spearmen somehow managed to evade the bullets and the shells and reach within a hundred and fifty yards of the laager wall, to throw their assegais in a defiant and futile gesture, only to crumple and join the ranks of the dead behind them.

After letting off two rounds, Fonthill could not bring himself to fire again and merely sat, his arm around Alice, as they watched the slaughter. Jenkins, however, at their side, continued to fire. Then, as he reloaded and lifted his rifle again, he stiffened.

'Hey, bach sir,' he cried, pointing to the edge of the trees. 'It's 'im, ain't it? Look, just there. In the golden suit.'

Fonthill and Alice followed the pointing finger and caught

a flash, nothing more, of a yellow jacket before it disappeared back into the bush.

'De Sousa?' asked Alice, her eyes wide.

'Could be,' answered Simon. 'I couldn't really see.'

'It was 'im all right,' said Jenkins. 'I'm sure of it. Dammit, I was too late in firin'. Now I've missed 'im again, blast 'is eyes.'

Fonthill stared long and hard at the rim of the bush as the Matabele continued to pour out and run across the open ground, but there was no repeat sighting of the yellow uniform. 'Well, it seems that Gouela is now definitely hunting with Lobengula,' he murmured. 'Perhaps we shall yet have a chance of settling scores with him.'

'No,' muttered Alice. 'Please keep away from that awful man.'

At last the waves began to recede and the attacks finally stuttered and died. Simon consulted his watch. He estimated that the battle, if battle it was, had lasted only forty-five minutes. A cheer went up from the defenders in the laager as silence descended on the clearing.

'There must be at least three thousand dead men out there – probably more,' whispered Alice. She turned to her husband. 'What for, darling? Why?'

Fonthill could think of nothing more to say and merely shook his head. Then he raised it and walked to meet Jameson.

'A complete and utter victory, old boy,' said the doctor, his face beaming under the perspiration. 'And I have just heard what you did out there down by the river. If the Matabele had run off our horses we would be at their mercy, for all our firepower. We are all in your debt, Fonthill. Thank you very much.'

Simon shrugged. 'Well, Doctor, you have had your battle. Do you and Forbes and Wilson think it was decisive?' He jerked his head over his shoulder. 'There are enough dead out there, God knows.'

Jameson looked at him sharply. 'Well, my dear fellow, *they* attacked us, if you remember. It had to be done. Brutal, I agree, but necessary surgery.' His voice dropped. 'I hope that your wife was not too shocked by it all. Not good for a lady to be involved in this sort of thing, of course.'

'Oh, she has witnessed much of this in her career. She saw what happened at Rorke's Drift; she was at Ulundi, Kandahar, Sekukuni, El Kebir and Abu Klea, so she has seen more battles than most generals.'

Jameson's jaw dropped. 'Good lord!'

'What do you propose to do now?' Simon asked.

'We will march on Bulawayo, of course. My aim is to put Lobengula into custody. We have given him a hard knock here and I don't think he will attack us again, but we can't have him at liberty. He still has thousands of men under arms and I must get him to make some formal acknowledgement of surrender. We don't want this thing to go on indefinitely.'

'Where is Rhodes?'

'He is riding up from the east. We shall meet him in Bulawayo.'

Jameson took off his hat and fanned his face, then he looked around the laager, where the men were lying in various postures of exhausted relaxation, their weapons at their side. Their jaunty, arrogant air had long since deserted them, together with the smartness of their uniforms. Their hats were stained with black rings of sweat and their brown jackets were bleached by the sun. Leggings were scratched and torn by the thorn bushes and their faces showed relief, not triumph. The acrid smell of cordite lay heavily on the air and flies were beginning to mobilise on the Matabele dead. The edge of the bush offered no threat now, for the cream of Lobengula's impis lay strewn in the dust under the sun and the rest were making their weary way back to the king's kraal.

Jameson swung his head around slowly to take it all in. 'By Jove, Fonthill,' he said, his voice little above a whisper. 'You know, I was never certain we could do it. After all,' he gestured with a dismissive hand, 'this lot were not soldiers. Just farmers really. All volunteers. Oh, they could shoot and defend themselves, but they knew little about military discipline, standing firm under attack and all that sort of thing, and they all remembered Isandlwana, don't forget. Bringing 'em this far in the face of an enemy outnumbering them by twenty-five to one and winning two engagements I have to say is an achievement. Yes, I know it's not over yet, but I feel it is bar a bit of shouting. Eh?' He looked up at Fonthill, rather like a puppy demanding praise.

Fonthill nodded slowly. 'I agree.' He regarded the little doctor with a mixture of admiration and curiosity. He was reluctant to give him the praise he so clearly desired, but he could not help but wonder at how a general practitioner from Edinburgh with no military training and little experience of the African bush, low or high veldt, could turn himself into such a determined leader and logistician. How was Rhodes, slippery, ambitious, driving Rhodes, able to recruit and motivate such men? He sighed. 'Yes, Doctor, I do think it's all over now. But tell me: did you have any strategic reserves you could call on if the columns from the east and the south had been overwhelmed on the march, as could so easily have happened?'

The doctor grinned. 'Not a sausage.' Fonthill thought of

the women and children left unprotected back on their farms in Mashonaland. Then he recalled that Jameson had the reputation of being a compulsive but skilful poker player, a born gambler.

'I see,' he said. Jameson and Rhodes, he reflected, were a well-matched pair.

The column – now a single homogenous unit – laboriously dismantled the laager, inspanned and resumed its advance south towards Bulawayo. Alice continued to scribble intensely, occasionally swearing when she forgot to write in cablese to save the *Morning Post* precious pennies. Mzingeli slipped inscrutably back into his role as tracker, riding with Fonthill and Jenkins to provide meat for the column; the Welshman made no secret of the fact that he was now solely motivated by the thought of reacquainting himself with Fairbairn's liquor stock; while Simon relapsed into contemplation of the future – would Alice agree to keep their holding in Mashonaland, and could their differences over the war and Cecil John Rhodes be reconciled?

For all his defence of the man to Alice, Fonthill still could not make up his own mind about Rhodes. Was he a visionary patriot and a hero of the Empire, in the mould of Clive, Cabot and Wellesley, or a selfish brigand, crushing all opposition in his pursuit of land and glory on the African continent? Back in Fort Salisbury, before setting out, he had heard rumours that the same ambivalence was prevailing back home in political circles. On the whole it was said that the liberals distrusted Rhodes and saw him as a piratical figure, while right-wing politicians applauded the fact that he was accumulating imperial real estate at no cost to the exchequer. In that context, Simon wondered how General Lamb would have regarded the invasion and the subsequent war. At least, he pondered, the original road-building incursion had been bloodless. So perhaps he would be credited with helping to keep Rhodes from invading with all guns blazing. In fact, of course, he had had little opportunity to influence Rhodes. Rhodes was the supreme puppet master, pulling strings from Cape Town that influenced events far, far away. Why, the bloody man had started and conducted a war without even visiting the battlefield!

When they were some seven miles away from Bulawayo, the marching column was startled when they heard a rumble like a roll of thunder and saw a dense cloud of smoke rising to the south. Lobengula had set fire to his kraal, put a match to his store of powder and cartridges and abandoned his capital. There was to be no last-ditch stand against the invading white men.

For the victorious entry into the smoking capital, Jameson, ever the Scot, found from somewhere a pipe major of the Royal Scots Regiment, who led the Mashonaland settlers into the heart of the ruins, where the company's flag was hoisted on the site of the king's inner kraal.

Alice, riding at the head of the column with Fonthill, Jenkins and Mzingeli, just behind the pipe major, Jameson and the two majors, let out a cry of delight when she saw the incongruous figure of Fairbairn sitting on the roof of his store. She dismounted and ran towards him.

'Mr Fairbairn, oh, I am so glad that you have survived,' she cried.

The Scotsman removed his pipe from his mouth. 'So am I, lassie,' he called down. 'So am I. I thought it would be touch and go, but the king, bless him, was a perfect gentleman to me to the end. When he was blowin' up the place, he issued instructions that I was not to be harmed. And nobody touched me.' He grinned, and then sadness descended on his face. 'I don't know what's goin' to happen here now, but one thing's for sure: I shall miss the old devil.'

Alice smiled. 'Do you know, so will I. But where has he gone?'

Fairbairn gestured with his pipe. 'Took his sons, some of his wives and a few thousand of his warriors and trekked up north. Maybe he's tryin' to cross the Zambezi; maybe he just wants to hole up in the bush. It's anybody's guess.'

'One more important question, Mr Fairbairn. Those kind people who helped me to escape, you remember, the man who lost his hand?'

'Oh aye, I remember.'

'What happened to them?'

The Scotsman paused before replying. Then: 'I'm afraid de Sousa's men caught up with them. They were found with their throats cut. Even the mule was killed.' He shook his head. 'I'm sorry, Mrs Fonthill. This is a cruel country, so it is.'

Alice felt tears start into her eyes. She turned to Simon, who had joined her. 'Those two gave their lives so that Mzingeli and I could escape, yet I hardly knew them. I feel so . . . guilty.'

'I'm sorry, Alice.' Simon called up to the Scotsman. 'Mr Fairbairn, I shall ever be in your debt for what you did for my wife. I can't thank you enough.'

Fairbairn waved his pipe. 'Difficult times, Mr Fonthill. Difficult times. We must stand by each other.'

The question of the whereabouts of the king immediately became a burning issue. Alice sent off a trusted young settler back to Salisbury with her cable for the *Morning Post*, which ended with: 'But where is the king? Peace cannot be made until he is found.'

A couple of weeks later, the column from the south arrived. It had seen little serious fighting but had been delayed by the desertion of King Khama's men, who had formed a not insignificant part of the unit. Shortly afterwards, the tall, rather dishevelled figure of Cecil John Rhodes galloped into the home of his old adversary and immediately locked himself into conclave with Jameson.

The explosion that had so singularly marked Lobengula's retreat had torn apart the centre of his kraal, destroying his own house and the huts of his *inDunas* and wives, although, strangely, it had left standing and virtually unsinged the great indaba tree under which he had sat to dispense judgement. It had also left undamaged the other beehive dwellings that stretched out on to the plain and formed the suburbs of the city. These had now become inhabited again as the people of Bulawayo hesitantly returned and realised that the white invaders were not intent on harming them.

Fonthill, Alice, Jenkins and Mzingeli lived in their bivouac tents that had sheltered them on the march. Presuming that the war was now over, Fonthill was anxious to return to Fort Salisbury to see how his farm was faring under the care of Joshua and Ntini, who had been left to tend it, but he found his wife strangely reluctant to leave Bulawayo.

'I am beginning to realise,' she told him, 'that this chapter cannot be closed until the king is found. There has to be a formal peace treaty, with Lobengula signing it, but he has gone off with the remainder of his army up north, it seems. While he is out there with his men he will be perceived to be a threat and I must report what happens to him.' Her grey eyes took on a steely glint. 'I want to be sure that the old boy is not disadvantaged by Rhodes and Jameson any more than is inevitable. I shall be watching them like a hawk.'

Fonthill sighed. A handful of journalists had arrived with the Tuli column, all of them dismayed by the lack of action they had been able to report on the journey north and resentful but resigned that, once again, Alice Griffith of the *Morning Post* had scooped them all. The current attitude amongst them – and, indeed, throughout Fleet Street it seemed – was jingoistic. The King of Matabeleland had to be found and punished for allowing his impis to wash their spears. Simon knew that Alice would be hypersensitive to their reportage and anxious to effect a balance. It was a difficult time for everyone among the smoking debris of Lobengula's 'Place of Man Who Was Killed'.

The day after Rhodes's arrival, Fonthill received a note from the great man asking if he could spare him a minute. He walked to the tent that Jameson had set aside for the Cape premier and found the two men sitting and talking at a single trestle table. Apart from the table and three camp chairs, the tent was completely unfurnished.

'Ah, Fonthill.' Simon smiled at the well-remembered high squeak of a voice and took the hand that was offered to him. The big man was wearing his customary old cricket flannels and, despite the heat, a tweed jacket that had certainly seen better days. Underneath a large black tie that was only loosely knotted, his shirt was open at the throat and his waistcoat gaped to reveal his paunch. The air of an eccentric, bohemian country squire was emphasised by the lock of reddish-grey hair that curled boyishly over his forehead.

'Do sit down,' said Rhodes. 'Jameson has been telling me how very helpful you have been, both on the journey north with the settlers' column and with the fights you've had on the way here. Helpful. Yes, most helpful. Damned helpful.'

Simon shrugged. 'Oh, I did little enough. The doctor here

did a most amazing job in getting these columns together, and Forbes and Wilson did good soldierly work.' He grinned wryly. 'Mind you, that turned out to be not so difficult, given that we had Maxims and the cannon. The Matabele were completely outgunned.'

'Mmm.' Rhodes's protuberant eyes seemed to bore into Fonthill. 'Got your land all right? Started your farm up there? Eh?'

'Yes thank you. We didn't suffer as much as many others in the storm and the rains and we have more or less established it. I want to get back there now, because I haven't seen the place for weeks and I fear I can't stay out in these parts too long. My wife is anxious to get home to Norfolk.'

Rhodes nodded and gave a half-smile. 'Yes, of course. Miss Griffith. I have a feeling, from what I've heard and read in the *Morning Post*, that your good lady is not exactly in tune with what I have been trying to do here in Matabeleland.'

Simon returned the smile. 'I think, indeed, that would be fair to say, sir. I know that, in her role as the *Post*'s correspondent here, she would be grateful to have a word.'

'Of course, of course. I've no complaints. Rough with the smooth, you know. That's what those of us in politics have to do. Take the rough with the smooth.'

'Quite so. How are things progressing with establishing a formal peace?'

Jameson spoke for the first time. 'Ah, that is what we wished to talk to you about, Fonthill. We can't exactly say that things are going well.'

'Indeed not.' Rhodes opened a small humidor on the table and pushed it towards Fonthill. 'Cigar?'

'No thank you, sir.'

'It's the damned Imperials, you see,' said Rhodes, selecting a cigar, snipping off the end and then lighting it with some ceremony. 'Would you believe it, Fonthill, I have been told by the Colonial Office in London that all the negotiations with the king to settle the peace have to be conducted with the high commissioner that the Colonial Office has set up in Salisbury. I mean to say, my dear fellow, I have paid for this damned war myself, and what I haven't paid for my company has. For Whitehall to jump in now and insist that it wants to settle the way this country is to be run in future is not only unfair but a damned cheek.'

He blew out a stream of blue smoke. 'What's laughable about it all is that before we can seal a peace with Lobengula, we have to find him. The High Commissioner and the Colonial Office haven't any idea where he is or how to go about trying to find him. Who has to do that? Why me, of course.' Rhodes leaned across the table. 'Well, I have no intention of letting the bally Imperials mess things up at this late stage. We will find the king and we will settle things with him in an honourable and satisfactory way for all concerned. Jameson here is already working on it.'

Dr Jameson leaned forward, the light reflected in his rimless, circular spectacles. 'Yes. I wrote a letter to the king and sent it off with one of his *inDunas* who stayed behind here and who had a rough idea of where the old rascal has gone. I told him that if he would come back to Bulawayo he would be safe and would receive friendly treatment. Well, I received a reply this very morning.'

He held up a wrinkled piece of paper. 'Most of Lobengula's letters used to be written by Fairbairn, one of the traders here, but this one – according to Fairbairn, who knows the man's hand – seems to have been written by that Portuguese feller that was always causing trouble.'

Fonthill stiffened. 'De Sousa, the man known as Gouela?'

'Yes, that's the chap. He must be with Lobengula. The king says he will come in but he is concerned about what happened to the two *inDunas* who were killed at Tuli. He is also worried about where he could live in Bulawayo, his houses having been burned down.' Jameson sniffed. 'I think he is just playing for time, so I am mounting a patrol to go and bring him in. We are calling it the Shangani Patrol, for we believe Lobengula has gone up that way with the remnants of his army. Nothing too heavy: we shall ask for volunteers and I shall want no more than about three hundred men.'

Fonthill whistled. 'How many are supposed to be with the king?'

Rhodes intervened. 'We don't know accurately,' he said. 'Could be as many as three thousand, but after the hidings these impis have received in recent weeks, we don't expect any real resistance. Three hundred good chaps will do the job well.'

And cheaply, Simon thought to himself. But Jameson was continuing.

'I am putting Forbes in command, of course, with Wilson along as his deputy, but given that the rains are due to break any day now and the bush up there can be pretty thick, Rhodes and I would be most grateful if you, your Welshman and your tracker could go along to lend a hand. Particularly in scouting,' he waved a hand airily, 'and that sort of thing.' He leaned forward again, almost conspiratorially. 'To be frank, I am just a touch concerned about the friction between Forbes and Wilson, and the younger chap can be perhaps a little headstrong. Your experience and knowledge – not to mention the fact that you know the king personally – would be invaluable.'

'I do hope you will say yes, Fonthill,' added Rhodes from behind a curtain of smoke.

Fonthill's mind flashed to two puff adders, a searing pain in his chest, a pockmarked face close to his and the smell of cheap pomade. A chance to settle the score?

'Of course,' he said.

'Splendid,' Rhodes and Jameson responded in chorus. And as though to seal the agreement, a sudden crash of thunder broke over the roof of the tent, and immediately a downpour sounded on the canvas overhead and filled the interior with a noise like a hundred war drums beating. The rains had begun.

Chapter 19

Fonthill's jaw dropped in incredulity. 'Rations for only three days!' he repeated. His horse drooped its head in the sheeting rain and Simon pulled down his hat brim to protect his face. 'That means we will be out of food by tomorrow. Whose stupid planning was that?'

'Can't be helped.' Forbes's face was set in stoical gloom. 'There was little to spare back in Bulawayo and we had no time to go hunting before we set off. Jameson said we could live off the countryside.'

'Not in this weather we can't. Even if we're lucky enough to get one buck, that's not going to feed three hundred men. You know that, Forbes.'

'Yes, well . . . Wilson was in charge of provisioning. We shall just have to go on short commons until this damned rain lifts. I've sent a message back to Bulawayo pleading for more rations.'

The two men, hunched on their mounts, were plodding at the head of the column as they headed northwards. Fonthill stole a glance behind him at the men straggling out behind. Three hundred volunteers had not exactly sprung forward from the ranks when Jameson had sent out his call. The men had been away from their homes for several months already, the lure of loot had receded, for Lobengula had taken his most prized cattle with him, and the prospect of tracking the king into the treacherous bush had little appeal. Every man knew what the rainy season meant: flooded trails, rivers in spate and general misery for travellers. Eventually a force of sorts had been gathered from the three columns, including that from the south, but these were not disciplined troops, and murmurs of discontent were already to be heard as the Shangani Patrol had passed through Inyati, which had been a station of the London Missionary Society. They found that the station had been wrecked and looted and it was clear that Lobengula had a large force with him. No-one knew exactly how far ahead he was, but he was out there somewhere, with a last impi covering his retreat. The uncertainty added to the mud and the unceasing downpour to unsettle the amateur soldiers pursuing him.

'I've had enough of this,' exclaimed Forbes. He held up his hand to halt the column. The wagons are slowing us down terribly in this mud and we shall never catch the old devil at this rate. In any case, I am not at all sure that many of these chaps have got the stomach for a fight. Even if we catch Lobengula, I doubt if we have the spirit to bring him in.'

'What do you intend?'

Forbes stiffened his back so that he sat erect in the saddle, despite the rain lashing directly now into his face. 'I shall send the wagons back to Inyati to form a laager there with about half the men,' he said. 'They will be a fallback base for me and they can have the extra rations that should arrive from Bulawayo. Wilson and I will take the rest of the men – the best of 'em on the freshest horses – ahead in a flying column up to the Shangani to make contact with the Matabele. We will take whatever rations can be spared and it should be easier to hunt with this smaller number. Are you comin' with us, Fonthill?'

'Of course.'

The orders were transmitted, an overnight laager laboriously constructed, and early the next morning the column was split, with the wagons turning round heading south and one hundred and sixty mounted men riding north – heading straight into the steady rain.

Jenkins wiped the water from his moustache. 'I 'ope you don't mind me askin', bach sir, but 'ow are we goin' to bed down at night?'

'No, 352, I don't mind you asking.'

The Welshman let the subsequent silence hang for a moment, as the two rode on with the advance picket. 'Yes,' he said, eventually, 'well now that we've established that you don't mind me askin', like, can you tell me 'ow we're goin' to bed down for the night.'

'On the ground,' Fonthill growled, 'in the wet, in a square, in front of the horses to protect them.'

'Ah, I see. There's cosy then, isn't it? Snugglin' up to the 'orses in the rain. Glad I joined, I am.'

And so the patrol continued heading north, towards the Shangani river. Occasionally, spears were flung anonymously from the bush at the outriders, but no attack was made. The men were particularly vulnerable crossing the river beds, formerly just dried-up dongas but now bubbling with water as brown as cocoa, but Forbes banked on the Matabele sticking to their established tactics of only attacking from the bush. He was also unsure that he was near enough to the king's party to provoke an attack.

'Are we close to 'em yet, Fonthill, do yer think?' he asked one evening, after Simon, Jenkins and Mzingeli had spent the day ranging ahead.

Fonthill shook his head. 'No. I doubt it very much. Mzingeli here is following a faint spoor – faint because of course the damned rain is washing the tracks away. If we were near, the signs would be much clearer. And such a large body of men would leave a swathe of marks in the bush. We will know if we are near the king's rearguard.'

'Humph.'

Once again the men ate cold meat and fruit that night, for no fires could be lit under the continual downpour. Then, after posting guards, they all pulled their horses down, tied their groundsheets up to their own necks and lay down on the soaking ground on the outside of their mounts, facing the bush from which an attack would come, if it came. And once more it did not.

Next morning, however, was marked by a disturbance. Just after the patrol had begun its weary march forward, four men came galloping up from the rear. Fonthill was riding in the van again with Forbes and Wilson, and he saw that the little group was being led by a young officer, and that the man in the rear was covering the two in the middle with his revolver.

'What the hell's this?' growled Forbes.

'Look at this, sir,' said the officer. He handed the major a damp hessian bag, the contents of which were clearly heavy, for the sack hung nearly to the ground. Forbes put his hand in and produced a gold sovereign, then another, and another.

'What on earth . . . ?'

The officer nodded to the two men, whose heads were bent under their sodden hats. 'These two are at the rear looking after the baggage ponies, sir. I went back to check on the rations for the day and found them with this sack. I reckon there could be as much as a thousand gold sovereigns in there. They were dividing them.'

'Sovereigns?' cried Wilson. 'Out here – in a damned sack? Were they just lying about, or what?'

'These two said, of course, exactly that. That they found them lying there. But I caught a glimpse of two Matabele slipping away back into the bush, and by the look of them, they were *inDunas*. More to the point, however, I found this note, scrunched up into a ball and obviously thrown away by these two troopers. I think it had been left by the *inDunas*, with the gold.'

Frowning, Forbes smoothed out the paper and read aloud: '"White men, I am conquered. Take this and go back." He looked up. 'It's signed with a cross and a seal.'

'May I see?' Fonthill stretched out a hand. 'Yes, that's Lobengula's seal. I recognise it.' He shook his head slowly. 'He is trying to buy us off. The poor devil is obviously at his wits' end.'

Wilson face was a study in puzzlement. 'But how would he have such a large amount of gold with him, out here in the bush?'

'It must be part of the gold that Rhodes paid him,' said Fonthill. 'I brought it up to Bulawayo myself, many months ago.' He gave a sad smile. 'He never really had a use for it, you know. This must have been his last throw of the dice.'

Forbes turned to the two men. 'Well, what have you got to say for yourselves, eh?'

The larger of the two men looked up. 'Sure, it's all a misunderstandin', sir,' he said in a strong Irish brogue. 'We was just countin' the money, your honour, to bring it forward to you, so we was.'

'Here, wait a moment.' Fonthill urged his horse forward.

'Don't we know each other?' He reached forward and tilted back the hat brim of both men. 'Well, well, well. Would you believe it.'

'Do you know these two?' demanded Forbes.

'Oh indeed I do. As fine a pair of rogues as you will find in the whole of southern Africa, Major. Their names are Murphy and Laxer, and this is the second time they have tried to steal these sovereigns.'

'Ah, your honour,' Murphy adopted an ingratiating smile, 'it's good to see you again. No, sir, we was not stealin' this time, I promise you. On me holy mother's death bed I promise.'

'They are thieves,' repeated Fonthill. He related the story of the treachery of Murphy and Laxer on his journey to Bulawayo. 'I suppose they joined up in the south in the hope of quick loot. Of all the men in this column, it is ironic that the *inDunas* should have picked out these two to give the money to. I suppose the messengers were frightened to come to the front of the column in case we shot them out of hand.'

'Thank you, Baxter,' said Forbes to the young officer. 'Tie the hands of these two villains, then take two reliable men and ride with them – and the sovereigns – back to Inyati to await trial. You will be responsible for the money and the prisoners. Good work, man. Off you go.'

He turned back to Fonthill. 'It's infuriating that we didn't capture the *inDunas*. They could have told us how near we were to the king and how many men he's got with him. D'yer think it's worth going after 'em now?'

Simon wrinkled his nose. 'I doubt it. This rain is washing everything away, and looking for two men in the bush will be like trying to pick up eels in a riverbed. But we must be reasonably hot on Lobengula's heels, otherwise he wouldn't have thrown his money at us. My advice is to keep pressing on.'

That day proved unusually depressing. The rain had become no worse, but its unvarying intensity was eroding the spirit of the pursuers. None of the horsemen could find a way of sealing their bodies from the water that penetrated every nook and cranny of their oilskins, and moving in the saddle produced a chafing that grew worse with every mile. Many of the horses were now becoming blown, and Forbes was growing increasingly irritable at the pace of the advance. Even worse was his fear that he might be riding into an ambush. Had Lobengula crossed the Shangani, now only a few miles ahead, or was he waiting to attack as the crossing was attempted?

He called Fonthill to him. 'Will you scout on ahead to the river and see if the Matabele have crossed? Rotten job, I know, but I would rather you did it with your two chaps, who can slip through the bush easily, than have a troop go on and blunder and splash about. Come back as soon as you can and report on the state of the river, too.'

It took the three men less than an hour to ride up to the swollen river. Despite the rain, it was clear that a large group of men had made the crossing not so very long before. 'How long, would you say, Mzingeli?' asked Fonthill.

The tracker dismounted. Here the banks of the river were not high, and though they were wooded, the bush was not too thick. Broken branches showed where a wide crossing of the river had been made by many people, and wagon tracks could still be discerned in the mud. Mzingeli shrugged. 'Only yesterday, I think. Many cross. Now on other side.'

'Mount up,' called Fonthill. 'We may have to leave quickly.'

'Blimey,' said Jenkins, squeezing the moisture from his

moustache, 'you're not thinkin' of goin' across now, are you, bach sir? It looks a bit deep to me. Probably full of crocodiles an' all.'

'No. There won't be any crocs in that fast-flowing water, but I don't want the three of us to ride into an impi on the other side. Let's get back while there's plenty of daylight.'

They met the column only two miles or so from the river. Forbes immediately called a halt and held a council of war as Fonthill reported. 'We are pretty certain that Lobengula has crossed, and only yesterday,' he said. 'If you want to go after him, you had better do it soon, because the river is rising all the time. It's about two hundred yards wide. You can make the crossing all right now, but you may have only about twenty-four hours in which to do it.'

Forbes nodded, his face expressionless. 'Any sign of Matabele on the other side?'

'No. But they could be in the bush, of course.'

'Umph. If we cross today and I find we've got about three thousand warriors facing us, I would have my retreat cut off.'

A silence fell on the little gathering, broken by Wilson, who leaned forward eagerly. 'Let me go now with a small patrol,' he said. 'I should be able to make contact with the Matabele and have some idea of their strength and position. I can move quickly if I take the best horses.'

Fonthill looked at the faces of the two men. It was clear that Wilson, younger, less experienced but ambitious, was anxious to have the honour of finding Lobengula. Forbes, himself not without ambition, was obviously also anxious to claim the distinction of catching the king, but he knew that one false move now could jeopardise his whole command. Caution overcame ambition.

'Very well, Wilson. It seems clear that the king's camp is near, just across the Shangani. Take twenty men and establish exactly where it is. But be back by nightfall. Understood?'

'Understood.'

'We will come with you,' said Fonthill.

'No.' Forbes's face was set in granite. 'I may well need you here. We are vulnerable. Off you go, Wilson.'

The young major rode off with his party, which included several officers, and Forbes set about building a laager of thorn bushes to provide some protection for his main force. The rain at last had slackened and Fonthill, Jenkins and Mzingeli settled down around a spluttering fire that the tracker had managed to light and ate their biltong.

'I ain't no general, like,' observed Jenkins, 'but I can't 'elp feelin' that things ain't exactly as we would like' em. What d'you think, bach sir?'

Fonthill nodded gloomily. 'You are right, General Jenkins. Major Forbes has a real problem on his hands. He can't really advance his main force – pathetically small as it is – across the river until he has established where the enemy is and how large it is, but if he leaves it much longer he won't be able to cross and the king will get away again. And if he is caught on the other side without a chance to laager, he will be stuck with the river at his back and no way to retreat or manoeuvre. What do you think, General Mzingeli?'

The tracker munched his biltong. 'Not good, any way.'

The three sat in silence under two clouds: the first, grey and swollen with rain; the second, one of foreboding and almost as real.

Like the rest of the camp they turned in early that night, despondent not only because of the cold and wet but also because Wilson and his men had not returned. Taking this as an indication that the little patrol had been wiped out and that he was about to be attacked, Forbes set extra guards.

But the camp was aroused well before midnight when two men from the advance party rode in, to be followed an hour later by three more. They reported that Wilson had indeed reached Lobengula's camp but was in danger of being cut off by the Matabele guarding the king and had taken up a position in the bush, where he would wait until the main body joined him.

Fonthill and Jenkins arrived just as Forbes had finished questioning the arrivals, with the help of his next most senior officer, Captain Borrow. 'Dammit it all, Fonthill,' exploded the major, 'I told the man to return here before dark. Now he has set himself up right on the enemy's doorstep and as good as ordered me to come and rescue him! Bloody fool.'

'What do you intend to do?'

Forbes looked at each of them in turn, his eyes wide. Simon could not help but sympathise with the man. Soldiering in the colonies, far from home and with no major outbreak of hostilities to offer the chance of distinction, was a dull and slow business, with little real chance of advancement. Forbes had not put a foot wrong so far in this strange campaign. Now he had been offered the seemingly easy but high-profile task of bringing in the recalcitrant rebel king, to put the final touches to his little war under the eyes of the generals back in Whitehall. Yet this small matter of 'clearing up' was proving to be a nightmare, thanks to a thrusting junior officer.

'Well . . .' The major gnawed at his moustache. 'I can't risk crossing the Shangani with my whole force in the dark. We would end up all over the place. I've got few enough men anyway, and we could be under attack here ourselves at any minute.' His voice dropped. He was thinking aloud now. 'But

I will have to send what reinforcements I can to Wilson to help the damned fool get back.' The silence descended again. Then: 'Yes . . . right.' His mind was made up.

'Borrow,' he barked, 'take seventeen troopers right away, cross the Shangani and join Wilson. Tell him I will come to him when I can.' He turned to Fonthill. 'I'd be grateful if you and your two scouts would go with them. If it comes to a scrap, you will be of great help to Wilson, I know. And if you do get near the king, your knowledge of him will come in very handy.'

Simon gulped. It was more an invitation than an order, given Fonthill's civilian status, but it was one that could hardly be refused. Sending just twenty-one men across the Shangani to reinforce the patrol seemed madness. It would mean that Wilson would have too many men to help him patrol, but not enough to reinforce him in fighting a major action. It was neither one thing nor the other. He opened his mouth to protest but thought better of it.

'Very good. We will come with you, Borrow.' He doubled away to bring the glad news to Jenkins and Mzingeli.

''Ow many?' Jenkins's face registered indignation. 'What's 'e doin', makin' up a few 'ands of whist or somethin'?'

The Shangani when they reached it looked menacing by the light of a moon half hiding behind the clouds. Swirling and surging, it was now a dull yellow, and driftwood was being tossed along in the turbulence. The river hissed as it bounced over the wide and comparatively shallow drift. Captain Borrow regarded it with concern.

'May I suggest, Borrow, that we link the horses together?' suggested Fonthill. 'That way the strongest swimmer will help the weakest. Do we have rope?'

Borrow nodded. 'Sergeant,' he called, 'fix a leading rope to my horse. Men, hold your rifles high. Keep the water out of your magazines. Grab the rope and follow me. First six men across, dismount quickly and form a semicircle, rifles at the ready, until we are all across.'

Jenkins, the bravest of the brave in facing an enemy, now showed a face the colour of the moonlight itself. 'I don't like this at all, not at all, bach sir,' he gasped. 'You know I can't swim. An' then there's the crocs. P'raps, look you, I could be a sort of rearguard on this side an' protect you all as you cross . . .'

Fonthill sighed. 'There are no crocs in this racing water,' he said, 'and you are not going to drown, I will see to that. I will be right behind you. Just hold on to the rope. The horse will do the swimming. Give him a kick to keep him going. Here we go. Come on.'

Led by Borrow, a slim man but a good horseman, the little party entered the water. The lead horse, its eyes showing as much yellow as the river itself, tossed its head and baulked, but Borrow skilfully urged it into the water and set the beast swimming. In single file, the patrol followed him, and immediately the weaker horses were swept downstream, but were held by the rope and kept roughly in line – although it was a line that bowed and sagged. It was some two hundred yards further downriver before Borrow was able to reach the far side of the Shangani, but all of his men were able to climb up the bank and reassemble, including a trembling Jenkins.

'Nothin' to it really,' he confided to Mzingeli. 'You see, the 'orses do the swimmin', like. You just sit. It's easy, see.'

One of the messengers from Wilson had volunteered to make the return journey, and he led the party as it picked its way between the trees and bushes in the semi-darkness, for the moon had now disappeared behind the clouds. Every member rode with his heart in his mouth, expecting a shower of assegais to rain in from the darkness on either side, but all was tranquil as the horses trod quietly through the bush. In fact, it was only twenty minutes after leaving the riverbank that a cry of 'Who goes there?' told them they had reached the patrol.

The men were lying behind their prostrate horses in a rough circle in a clearing. Wilson rose and shook hands warmly with Borrow and Fonthill. 'How many have you brought?' he asked.

Barrow smiled. 'Only twenty, I'm afraid.'

For a brief moment Wilson looked dismayed. Then he grinned. 'Oh well. More than enough, I expect.' He gestured over his shoulder. 'We've found the king's camp. It's about half a mile up there. Couldn't attack in the dusk, so we will move in tomorrow at first light.'

Fonthill frowned. 'You won't wait until Forbes arrives with the main party?'

'Good lord, no. We can do the job.'

'How many warriors has the king, then?'

'Oh,' Wilson looked nonchalant, 'not all that many, I think. Couple of hundred perhaps. Maybe more. Fellow we captured thought something like that, but we're not sure, to be honest.'

'And you plan to attack the camp with thirty-odd men?' Fonthill tried to keep the incredulity out of his voice.

'Of course. Get at 'em first thing and take them by surprise. The fact that you got through shows that they have not surrounded us, so they are not anxious for a fight, in my estimation. I know natives, Fonthill. Punch 'em hard and they will fold. Believe me.'

Borrow coughed. 'Fonthill was at Isandlwana *and* Rorke's Drift, sir,' he murmured. 'He may know natives too.'

'Ah yes. Sorry, Fonthill, no condescension intended, old boy. But the Matabele are not the Zulus, you know.'

'Hmm.' Fonthill regarded the great moustache, which somehow looked lugubrious on such a narrow, young face. 'Yet the Matabele showed great courage, don't you think, in attacking us twice on our way to Bulawayo. And this time, we will not be safely laagered.'

Wilson waved a hand. 'Doesn't matter. We've got the firepower. We will move in early, grab the old boy and take him back across the river. They won't have the guts to follow us.'

'Well, it's your decision.' Fonthill tried to sound uncritical. 'I think, however, that Forbes was rather expecting you back last night.'

'Yes, well, I felt that once I had made contact with the enemy, it was my duty not to let go.' He took Fonthill by the elbow and walked him away from Borrow. 'To tell you the truth, Fonthill, Forbes can be a little . . . what shall I say? Cautious, I think is the word. Natural, I suppose, given his age and all that Sandhurst stuff he imbibed when he was young. But I know Africa, y'see, and how to behave here. These Kaffirs don't follow the rules laid down at training college. We have to fight 'em the same way.'

Fonthill looked at him hard. Wilson was confident, almost to the point of cockiness. There was nothing wrong with that in warfare. Better assuredness than hesitation in a commander. But was he being impetuous to the point of foolishness? He had no real idea how many men the king had with him, so better surely to retreat to the river and form a bridgehead on the bank, allowing Forbes and his troopers to cross in the morning and make the attack with a larger force.

As though reading his thoughts, Wilson patted him on the

shoulder, in what seemed a ridiculously avuncular gesture from a younger man. 'We shall have the advantage of surprise tomorrow and should have some fun,' he said. 'Now why don't you try and get some sleep? We shall move just before sun-up.'

'Very well. Ah – just one last point, Wilson. When you approached the king's camp, did you see or pick up any evidence that a Portuguese was with the king? A man they call Gouela?'

Wilson lifted his eyebrows. 'Didn't see the chap because we didn't get that close. But the native we picked up and questioned did say that there was a white man with Lobengula. A feller in some sort of uniform. I didn't pay too much attention, I'm afraid. Obviously not one of us.'

Fonthill smiled. 'Thank you. Good night, Wilson. Good luck tomorrow.'

So de Sousa was still with the king! Perhaps tomorrow would provide the chance for a final reckoning with his enemy. It was a sort of comfort as he faced the prospect of the dawn attack.

In fact, hardly anyone in that small company slept that night. Fonthill's momentary flash of euphoria at the thought of facing de Sousa again was soon replaced by a sense of foreboding. He had two main worries: Alice and Mzingeli. The tracker was a brave man and quite imperturbable in the face of danger, but he was not really a fighter. In addition, of course, this was not his war. Simon had offered him the chance of crossing back across the Shangani before it became virtually impassable, but he had rejected it. 'I stay with you,' he had said. And, knowing his man, that would be that. He must insist that Mzingeli stayed close to him and Jenkins when the attack started.

Alice . . . ah! He stirred uncomfortably on the hard ground. If the battle in this dank semi-forest should prove to be his last, then he wished – oh how he wished! – that his farewell to his wife had been warmer. Her attitude towards Rhodes and Jameson had hardened since the battle at the Imbembesi river and what she called the massacre of the Matabele. She now regarded all of Rhodes's dealings with Lobengula as exercises in dissimulation and deceit, a preface to the inevitable invasion by an army of mercenaries. Fonthill's decision to join the Shangani Patrol to capture the king had been met by her with some ambivalence. She wished him to play no further part in the violence that surrounded the creation of Rhodesia, but his presence on the patrol she hoped would be a kind of guarantee that no harm would come to Lobengula. They had kissed good bye, of course, but her eyes had been cold. It seemed as though she had not forgiven him for his part in Rhodes's negotiations with the king. He sighed and wished he had more confidence in the outcome of tomorrow's assault on the king's camp.

No bugles roused the troopers in the morning. Dawn promised another, wet, miserable day and the men rose from their damp couches without a word. The rain prevented fires from being lit, so everyone chewed cold biltong, drank water, shook the rain from his coat and silently fell into line within minutes of waking.

'Nice day for it, then,' observed Jenkins, slipping a bayonet down next to the Martini-Henry in the rifle bucket hanging by his saddle. As cavalrymen carrying the shorter carbine, the troopers of the patrol had not been issued with bayonets. Somehow, however, Jenkins had procured in Bulawayo two of the long triangular blades issued to the infantry that, fitted to the end of their rifles, made a stabbing weapon just under six feet long. It had proved deadly in the Anglo-Zulu war ten years before, and indeed, the Zulus, so famed for their prowess in hand-to-hand fighting, had come to fear it. Mzingeli had declined to take a bayonet, claiming that it made the Martini-Henry too heavy to use.

'Look.' Fonthill drew Jenkins to one side. 'This is going to be a very tough fight, so we must stick together. In particular we must both keep an eye on Mzingeli. He's a bit old for this sort of thing.'

'Don't feel so sprightly myself, bach sir. But I see what you mean.'

The only man among the thirty-four who lined up that morning who did not seemed possessed by the prevailing air of melancholy was Major Wilson. Even his moustache appeared to bristle with happy expectation as he addressed his troop.

'Now, men,' he said, 'this is our chance to write a glorious footnote to the creation of Rhodesia. It is we who will capture King Lobengula and bring this war formally to an end. We shall be outnumbered, of course, but we have the advantage of firepower, as has been proven over the last few months. So fire quickly and accurately on order and we shall find that the Kaffirs will run, as they always do.'

He paused, as though expecting assent or even a faint cheer, but no sound came from the ranks. 'Right,' he went on. 'Ride until the order comes to dismount. Horses will be taken to the rear. Then we will advance on foot in open order. When we come upon the camp, we will move forward and fire volleys. Myself with Captain Borrow and the sergeant here,' he nodded, 'will run forward and capture the king. There will be no pursuit of the fleeing natives. Any questions? No. Good. Mount.'

'Ah,' muttered Jenkins, 'just like that, eh? No interference from the black fellers, look you. 'Ow very kind of 'em.'

'Come on,' said Fonthill. 'Stay close.'

Somewhere from behind the grey, overcast sky, the sun gave some backlight to the clouds and the patrol set off in the half-light, walking their horses slowly and deliberately through the bush. Jenkins, Mzingeli and Fonthill rode three abreast, with Mzingeli sandwiched in the middle. After approximately half an hour, as the little group approached a giant anthill, Wilson raised his hand and dismounted. A handful of men took the reins of the horses and tethered them at the rear of the hill, as the troopers doubled forward and joined Wilson to form a thin line some fifty yards across. Then, slowly, the line advanced.

Wilson turned. 'I can see the wagons,' he called. 'At the double. Charge!'

Fonthill remembered thinking that a charge without bayonets was somehow toothless when from the bush immediately ahead emerged a row of Matabele riflemen, sweeping out from behind the trees and then being supplemented by others emerging from the side to outflank the charging troopers. The soldiers and the warriors fired at almost the same time, with, it seemed, almost the same results. Captain Borrow and a trooper fell, and three Matabele. The natives were obviously still firing on sights set too high, and the troopers, shooting on the run, could not take steady aim. Nevertheless, the spectacle of a solid line of warriors being reinforced every second as more and more Matabele emerged from the bush was too much for the attackers. The charge petered out, with Major Wilson firing his revolver some twenty yards in front of his men.

The major turned and doubled back. 'Fire in volleys,' he

cried. 'Front rank . . .' His voice died away. There were no front and second ranks; only one wavering line, in danger of being outflanked and gunned down from the side..

Fonthill sensed disaster. 'Quickly, 352,' he said. 'Run along the line and tap the shoulder of every other man.' Then he raised his voice and shouted: 'Every man touched on the shoulder will double back twenty paces and face the enemy. The remainder will fire a volley and then run back through the rear rank and cover it as it retreats.'

Wilson was looking at him in consternation. Jenkins had completed his running and touching task. Fonthill screamed: 'Men touched, run back NOW! Front rank, reload, aim, FIRE! NOW RUN BACK. Rear rank, hold your fire. Now, rear rank, aim, FIRE!'

And so, walking back, Fonthill directed an orderly retreat, with the men running back in turns, covered by the line through which they ran.

Simon had time to shout an apology to Wilson. 'Sorry,' he said. 'Infantry drill for an orderly retreat. Sandhurst stuff, you know. You wouldn't have it in the cavalry. Needed here, though.'

The major neither accepted nor rejected the apology but kept his eyes on the Matabele, who were now pouring out from the king's camp and circling wide through the bush. 'There must be a whole bloody impi here,' he cried. 'They're going to surround us if we're not careful. We need to get to the horses . . .'

'Jenkins,' Fonthill shouted to the Welshman, who was now directing the volley fire. 'Double back with Mzingeli and get the men holding the horses to bring them up. Quickly now.' He turned to Wilson. 'If we can mount up, we may be able to break through them and get to the river.'

'I'm not crossing that damned river.' Wilson's face was white under his tan but his eyes were determined. 'We'll get back to a clearing and make a stand there until Forbes comes across. We can still take the king's camp.'

'Don't be stup—' Fonthill bit back the words and took Jenkins's place in directing the retreat. This time he set the wing men at the end of each line to firing at the warriors who were slipping through the trees on either side. 'Stop them from getting behind us,' he ordered.

One more man had fallen from the Matabele fire, which was still, mercifully, ill-directed. Now, however, Fonthill realised that the main danger was about to come from the spearmen who were trotting out from the bush immediately ahead and threatening to mount a frontal attack. His eyes scanned them desperately. There must be at least a thousand warriors who had debouched from the camp and were intent on engulfing the little band of troopers facing them. So much for a couple of hundred! Yet, respecting the firepower of the white men, the spearmen held back, seemingly relying on their own riflemen to reduce the number of guns facing them.

At that moment, there was a muffled thud of hooves and the mounts arrived, led by Jenkins and Mzingeli on the lead horses. Fonthill looked to Wilson. Would he resume command?

He did. 'A Troop, give covering fire,' he shouted. 'B Troop, mount.' There was a howl from the Matabele as they saw their prey slipping away, and at last the spearmen ran forward, gaining ground rapidly on the troopers, whose horses were prancing and proving difficult to mount. 'A Troop, mount,' screamed Wilson. But it was too late for two troopers, who were speared as, one foot each in their stirrups, they tried to control their skittish mounts.

Fonthill, Jenkins and Mzingeli, riding flat to their horses' necks, were the last to leave the little clearing, thrown spears falling behind them as the derisive cries of the Matabele died away.

'What's 'appenin?' cried Jenkins as they weaved between the trees.

'He's going to make a stand in a clearing near the river. He ought to try and cross it while we have the chance.'

A look of anguish returned to the Welshman's face. 'Oh, I don't know,' he shouted. 'I don't fancy bein' drowned with a spear in me back, look you.'

They caught up with the rest of the patrol in a wide clearing, studded with a few isolated trees and with boulders and large stones scattered about.

Wilson had already dismounted. 'This is our best chance of finding cover,' he said, his breath coming in short gasps. 'I marked it on the way up.' He looked at Fonthill anxiously, as though seeking approval for showing some form of military expertise at last. 'We should be able to hold out here until Forbes crosses over.'

Fonthill looked around. There was little cover for the horses and not much more for the men. If Major Forbes was able to cross the Shangani, all might still not be lost, although he saw no possibility of mounting a realistic attack on Lobengula's camp, given the number of warriors who had obviously accompanied the king on his desperate trek north and who were clearly determined to defend him to the end. A momentary vision of the corpulent old monarch, bouncing on his wagon, desperately trying to avoid his pursuers, flashed across his mind. He felt a pang of sympathy for this Lear-like figure. Was the old boy still riven with gout and wearing his carpet slipper?

Then the first shot hissed across the clearing. 'Put the horses down,' yelled Wilson, 'and get them behind as much cover as you can. Sergeant, give me an ammunition report.' He turned to Fonthill. 'God, they've come up fast.'

'Yes.' Simon gave him a unforgiving smile. 'Just like Zulus.'

It soon became clear that the patrol was surrounded, for bullets were now singing into the clearing from all sides of the bush and men were forced to shelter behind their horses, which became the first casualties. Cries rose as, inevitably, bullets found their mark in human flesh. The troopers, however, were returning fire and their accuracy remained sufficient of a deterrent to prevent that overwhelming charge by spearmen that could spell the end of the defence.

An hour went by without any of the tribesmen in the bush breaking cover, but opposite where Fonthill and his two comrades were sheltering, it became clear that some sort of attack was being prepared. Many plumes could be seen nodding over the thorn bushes, and black figures were flitting between the trees.

'It looks as though they are going to try something,' said Simon. 'Fix bayonets, I think. Mzingeli, fire and then keep low.' He shouted to the troopers on either side: 'I think we are about to be charged. When they come, it will be rapid fire as they advance across the open ground, then, if they still press, use your rifles as clubs—'

He had no time to finish for, with a howl, the Matabele burst from the bush and ran towards them, shields held forward in the traditional offensive mode. It looked as though someone was testing the firepower of the troopers, for only about one hundred of the warriors were deployed in the charge, but they came very fast, their legs pumping and their plumes nodding.

'Brave bastards,' muttered Jenkins, as the defensive line crackled with rifle fire. The troopers fired as fast as they could work the cartridge ejection handles and thumb fresh rounds into the breeches of their rifles, and the .45-calibre slugs tore into the massed ranks of the charging warriors, sending them down in swathes. Yet with the courage that had been displayed in the other battles of the campaign, those behind pressed on, hurling defiance. Given the time taken to reload the single-shot Martini-Henrys, it was inevitable that some of the attackers would somehow escape the fusillade and reach the line of defenders, three of them materialising where Fonthill and Jenkins were kneeling, desperately feeling in their bandoliers for fresh cartridges.

'Bayonets, now!' screamed Fonthill.

He stood, conscious of Jenkins at his side, and parried the thrust from the assegai of the man opposite, the steel of the clashing spearhead and bayonet clanging out over the din of the firing. The warrior pushed forward his shield, seeking to find a way of thrusting around it, and Fonthill caught a glimpse of intense black eyes gleaming at him from a perspiring ebony face. Remembering a technique painfully learned at Isandlwana and Rorke's Drift, he dropped the butt of his rifle and caught it behind the spear pole that stood out at the bottom of the shield, twisting it so that the long shield was pulled round, exposing the warrior's side. With a swift downward movement of the rifle head, he plunged his bayonet between the man's ribs, and twisting it to withdraw it, he heard again the *iklwa*, the sucking noise. The Matabele sank to his knees and then to the ground, blood pouring from his side.

Fonthill had time to look around. Predictably, Jenkins's man was sprawled by the side of his comrade and the

Welshman was wiping blood from his bayonet. 'What about the other one?' asked Simon. Jenkins nodded to the left. There, Mzingeli was calmly reloading his rifle, a tall and very dead warrior sprawled across the rock in front of him.

The tracker nodded. 'Don't like Matabele,' he said. 'They make us slaves.'

'Good man.' The clearing was studded with Matabele bodies. Fonthill stopped counting at thirty. 'I don't think they'll try that again for a while,' he said.

'But they'll come again?' Jenkins's sweat-stained face was set.

'I suppose so, but they will try and reduce our numbers with rifle fire first. That was just to test us. It's going to be a long day.'

As the morning wore on, Wilson wriggled his way towards Fonthill. 'Sorry to get you into all this,' he said. 'I'm afraid it's too late now to think of breaking out en masse and trying to cross the river. We've lost horses and we have too many wounded and I am not going to leave them to be disembowelled.' He gave a weak smile. 'God knows where Forbes is, but perhaps he has no idea of the sort of pickle we are in and is taking his time. Fonthill, your horses are still sound. Do you think you and your two chaps could make a break for it, get across the Shangani and tell Forbes to come on up as quickly as he can? You are scouts and you know the bush better than any of us. Can't order you, of course, and you could well be cut down. But I think you have a fair chance. We will set up a bit of a barrage to make 'em keep their heads down while you mount and set off. What do you say, old chap?'

Fonthill looked at the pinpricks of fire that marked the fact that the Matabele were now well established in the bush all around the clearing. He started as, for a brief second, he thought he saw the flash of a yellow garment. All thoughts of de Sousa had long since dissolved and he deliberately put the Portuguese from his mind now. It was just a question of survival. He looked into Wilson's diffident face. 'Of course,' he said. 'I will put it to the others, but I don't see them refusing.'

Nor did they. 'I go where you go,' said Jenkins, 'but 'ang on to me in that water, please.'

'I come,' said Mzingeli.

The three exchanged their rifles for revolvers – much easier to handle on horseback – spoke a few reassuring words into the ears of their patient mounts, who were lying well protected by stone outbreaks, and tightened their saddle girths. Fonthill crawled across to Wilson. 'How long do you think you can hold out?'

'Depends on the ammunition.' The major forced a smile. 'If it goes on at this rate, I should say that we will all be looking like porcupines with spears in our bellies by nightfall. Unless Forbes can get here, that is. It depends on you, old chap.'

'Right. Good luck.' The two shook hands and Fonthill crawled back to his horse, now scratching restively in the soil with its hooves. Simon took a deep breath, exchanged glances with his two comrades and gave a nod to Wilson, and as the troopers blazed away into the surrounding bush, the three men mounted, kicked in their heels and, heads down, made for the most southerly of the gaps in the trees, to the cheers of the remaining members of the Shangani Patrol.

How they survived the breakout, Fonthill would never know. He was dimly conscious of black figures scattering as they thundered through between the trees. He heard Jenkins's revolver crack to his left and he himself brought down a warrior who attempted to launch his spear at him at close quarters. A spear sped over his right shoulder and thudded into a tree trunk a little ahead of him, and a bullet tore through the sleeve of his jacket. Death, for those few seconds, was all around them. Then they broke through the bush into another clearing and sped across it into the dubious safety of the trees beyond.

Fonthill turned his head. Jenkins was riding well at his side, but Mzingeli was a little way behind, and he saw that blood was trickling down the tracker's arm. He reined in hard and caught the black man's bridle. 'Are you . . .' He tailed off as Mzingeli slumped on to his shoulder.

''Ere.' Jenkins was alongside. He leaned across and lifted the tracker as though he were a feather pillow and deposited him across his own saddle in front of him. 'Take his reins, bach, and follow on,' he yelled, digging in his heels and riding away, one arm holding Mzingeli upright as the tracker's head lolled in time to the beat of the horse's hooves.

They rode this way until they reached the riverbank, where they dismounted and found Mzingeli completely unconscious. A bullet had gone clean through his left shoulder and another had grazed his head.

Jenkins gave an anxious glance at the yellow water. 'It's much 'igher than yesterday,' he said, 'an' I don't think you'll be able to get us both across, bach sir. Best thing to do, I think,' he beamed confidently, 'is for you to take the horses across and go and find Major Forbes. Me an' old Jelly 'ere will creep into the bush and 'ide until you can come back for us with the rest. Makes sense, isn't it?'

'No it bloody well isn't. The Matabele are probably hot on our heels now and they will find you in a second. I shall get you both across . . . somehow.' He looked around desperately.

'Mzingeli is the problem. Is it the shoulder wound, do you think?'

'No. That bullet that grazed 'is 'ead is what's knocked 'im out, I think. 'Ere, 'elp lift 'im down.'

Carefully Jenkins handed the tracker down to Fonthill, who stretched him on the ground and chafed his hands, but the man remained unconscious.

'We can't wait here until he comes round,' said Fonthill. 'The Matabele will be here any minute now. I shall just have to carry him across on my horse and hope that the two of us are not too heavy to prevent it swimming. Can you find something to lash him to me? Ah, unsaddle a horse and tear up the saddle blanket, that should do. I will stuff my shirt into this shoulder wound to try and staunch the bleeding. Quickly now, or they will be on us.'

The two men went to work in feverish haste, but Jenkins had only just thrown off the saddle when a cry made them turn their heads. Two Matabele warriors, their faces fearsomely daubed in ochre and white, throwing spears in their hands, burst out of the bush. Behind them could be heard the distant thud of hoofbeats. For a brief moment the four men regarded each other in a tableau that seemed to be fixed in time. Then, in a blur of action, the first warrior threw a spear at Simon, who was kneeling on the ground. He had just time to roll away so that the shaft buried itself into the soil, but at the same moment Jenkins's revolver barked and the thrower jerked backwards and slumped to the ground. The second man flung his spear at Jenkins, who ducked and fired in the same movement, the bullet penetrating the warrior's shield and hitting him in the chest. The shaft, however, took Jenkins's horse in the throat, so that the beast reared and slipped in the mud, bringing the Welshman down, pinning him under its weight and sending his revolver spinning away. At the same time, Fonthill's horse, eyes wide, stampeded away.

'Bloody 'ell,' shouted the Welshman, 'I can't move. Can you pull me out from under this bloody 'orse?'

'No, he can't.'

The voice came from the edge of the bush, and de Sousa walked his horse forward, his revolver covering both men.

'How convenient,' he said. 'One unconscious, the other pinned under his horse and you, Fonthill, without a weapon.' Perspiration was streaming down de Sousa's face from his gallop through the bush, and his uniform had lost its pristine smartness: stains marked his tunic, his boots were scuffed and he had not shaved for days. The dress sword that usually hung so decoratively by his thigh had now been thrust carelessly through his belt. Life in retreat with Lobengula had clearly not suited him, but his eyes were now gleaming with anticipation and he showed his tongue between his small white teeth.

He dismounted, his revolver carefully covering Fonthill, who remained crouching beside Mzingeli. He made to get up, but de Sousa waved him down. Then the Portuguese slowly transferred the pistol from his right to his left hand and drew the sword from his belt.

'I shall kill the three of you,' he said, 'and I shall take my time about it, I promise you that.' He gestured behind him with his head. 'My men will be here soon and they like a bit of entertainment, so I shall wait until they arrive. In the mean time . . .' He walked towards Mzingeli.

'Even you wouldn't harm a wounded man,' cried Fonthill. He shot a quick glance at Jenkins, but the Welshman, the veins standing out on his neck, was trying without success to push away the dead weight of the horse that lay across his legs.

Simon thought quickly. 'Look,' he said, 'your quarrel is not with these two. There's half of the gold sovereigns that Lobengula left in that bag behind my saddle. Take it and let them go – then you can do what you like with me.'

De Sousa sneered. 'Oh, I'll do what I like with you anyway. And if there *are* sovereigns there, which I doubt, I shall take them. Oh, I am so glad that I saw you ride away, Fonthill, because I could not be sure that you were with this pathetic little party. Now, I will let you watch a little blood-letting before my happy warriors arrive. This sword is not just for decoration, you know. I think we'll begin by finishing off this Kaffir of yours . . .'

Fonthill sprang at him from his crouching position, but his clawing fingers landed in the mud well short of the Portuguese's boots. Instantly de Sousa skipped around and plunged his sword into Simon's calf as he lay spreadeagled. The pain was hot and sharp and Fonthill cried out in agony, clutching his shin to his breast.

'Bastard,' cried Jenkins, panting from his exertions but still firmly wedged under the dead horse.

'Your turn will come in a minute.' De Sousa spoke calmly, then turned back to Fonthill. 'That will stop you running away while I carve you up a little. You could call it unfinished business, I suppose. Yes, I don't think I will wait, after all.' He drew back the sword and Simon closed his eyes.

As a result, he did not see a sweating Jenkins, just able to reach up to the far side of the horse that imprisoned him, fumble in his rifle bucket hanging by the saddle, withdraw his bayonet and hurl it with all his strength at de Sousa's back. The weapon rotated through the air in a silver cartwheel. There was an equal chance of it hitting the Portuguese base or point first. If the former, then it would merely thump into him, causing him to start a pace or two forward, doing no real damage. If the latter . . . As it was, the point of the lunger hit de Sousa firmly in the middle of the back, penetrating tunic, shirt and flesh, not deeply enough to kill, but inflicting a painful wound.

The Portuguese, his eyes staring wildly, staggered towards Fonthill. Instinctively, Simon reached up and pulled the man's tunic so that the two fell back together, de Sousa crashing on to him and expelling the air from his body.

Fonthill heard Jenkins's despairing cry: 'The bayonet, bach. The bayonet, in 'is back.' As the Portuguese put a hand to the ground to push himself away, Simon reached behind his back and his fingers locked on to the blade, now loose from de Sousa's exertions and threatening to fall away. The heavy man's other hand had now reached Fonthill's throat and was beginning to tighten, so that stars floated before Simon's eyes. 'Damn you, English,' croaked the Portuguese. Fonthill made one last effort and slid his left hand around his assailant's back in a desperate embrace, pulling him closer and finding the blade. His two hands now joined together and jerked the bayonet down savagely. He felt the point go cleanly through de Sousa's body and lightly prick his own chest before blackness closed in on him.

He came round to hear Jenkins shouting and feel Mzingeli's hand slapping his face. The tracker had crawled to his side and had somehow pushed the dead de Sousa away.

'Ah, Nkosi,' he gasped. 'Good. You hurt but not dead. Get up. We must move horse off 352 bach and get across river. Matabele coming. I think I hear them.'

'Oh hell, Jelly.' Jenkins's voice was hoarse. 'See to the captain. I'll be all right. Get across while you can.'

'No.' Simon was struggling on to one knee. 'If you can move, Mzingeli, help me up and get me a spear to lean on, can you? Good. Now hand me that sword. Right. Let's insert these under the belly of the horse. That's it. While we try and lift it a little, 352, can you try and struggle out from underneath?'

'Blimey, if you two cripples can do that, I can get out. Right. Try now.'

The two men may have been injured, but the hard life they had led on the veldt had toughened their bodies and given them reserves of strength. Slowly, as they heaved, the dead weight of the horse began to rise. The shaft of the spear snapped, sending the beast crashing down again, but not before Jenkins had extricated both his legs.

'Thank God,' he said. 'Now, where's that peashooter? I can 'ear the Mattabellies comin'. Bach sir, can the two of you get on that 'orse and into the river, while I 'old the devils off?'

'Only if you get on that other—'

His words were cut short as three panting Matabele broke out of the bush. They stood immobile for a second, partly to regain their breath and partly to take in the scene before them. Then they ran forward, stabbing spears held low. Their hesitation gave Jenkins just enough time to pick up his revolver, kneel and fire, bring back the hammer and fire again. The two leading warriors staggered and fell and the third paused, hurled his assegai, then turned and ran back to seek the cover of the bush. Jenkins's third bullet took him squarely in the back.

'Bugger, no more bullets,' cried the Welshman. 'An' no more 'orses.' De Sousa's horse had bolted at the gunfire. Jenkins leapt forward and picked up the Portuguese's revolver. Then he turned and saw a staggering Fonthill pushing Mzingeli up on to the saddle of his horse. 'Get up behind him, bach,' he called. 'I'll cover you.'

'No.' Simon's voice was a croak. 'You're pathetic, 352,

417

being afraid of a bit of water. You get up behind him; you're the only one that has the strength to hold him on. I will hang on to the horse's tail and get across that way. Go on. Get on. That's an order. Look, they're coming through now. Get on, damn you, or it will be too late.'

Jenkins gave a despairing look at the swirling water, then he turned, emptied de Sousa's revolver at the Matabele who were appearing now through the trees and vaulted on to the rump of Mzingeli's horse, clutching the swaying tracker to him to prevent him falling. Then he urged the mount into the water as a hopping Fonthill clutched at the beast's tail.

As the current swept them away, a despairing cry of 'Oh bloody 'ell' merged with the shouts of the Matabele as they rushed to the water's edge, abortively throwing their spears after the disappearing trio.

Chapter 20

Two weeks later, Fonthill sat on the edge of a camp chair in their tent in a Bulawayo that was no longer smoking but still smelled of charred timber, while Alice replaced the dressing on his calf. The crossing of the turbulent Shangani had been perilous and had taken all of half an hour, but had been completed successfully in the end. The yellow water, however, had bequeathed an infection to the open wound in his leg that had delayed their departure from the king's old capital and which was only now responding to treatment.

'Will you please keep still,' commanded Alice.

'I am as still as I can be when you're pulling that damned bandage so tight.'

'It has to be tight to keep the dressing on.' She pulled a face. 'Is it still painful?'

'Only when I laugh.'

'Don't laugh, then.'

'I can't help it. The sight of you on your knees before me is very, very funny. It should happen more often.'

'Oh do be—'

A ridiculously loud cough outside the flap of the tent announced the arrival of Jenkins. 'Come in,' shouted Fonthill. 'Don't knock.'

The Welshman put his head through the opening. 'I did knock, see, but you don't 'ear nothin' on canvas, now do you? Good morning, Miss Alice.'

'Good morning, 352. You would be better at this than me. Do you want to take over?'

'No thank you, miss. I 'ad enough of treatin' the captain up in the north, look you. He ain't a good patient, is 'e?'

'No he is not. What can we do for you?'

Jenkins's eyes lit up. 'I've brought some news. Just come in, it 'as. The old king 'as died – up in the bush there somewhere, miles from anywhere, near that river up north, the Lumpini . . . Lapono . . .'

Fontill sat upright. 'The Limpopo.'

'That's what I said. It seems that no-one knows 'ow he died. Could 'ave been poison, or sickness. 'E wasn't a well man at the end, they say. Oh, an' Mr Rhodes is back in town, I 'ear.'

'Who told you all this, 352?'

'One of the blokes in Dr Jameson's office. One of the Mattabellies 'as come in from north of that river where we 'ad our little swim, like, and says that the king bolted, o' course, when the fightin' started.' His voice dropped as he continued. 'This man was at the fightin' and 'as told 'ow everyone in Captain Wilson's party died. Very tragic it was.'

Fonthill frowned. 'Do you know the details?'

'Nothin' more than that, bach sir.'

Alice and Simon exchanged glances. When Fonthill, Jenkins and Mzingeli had staggered ashore, almost half a mile downriver from where they had first plunged into the water, they had lain exhausted for a while. They could hear gunfire coming from across the river and, full of anxiety for the fate of Wilson and his men, had pushed on, with Simon and Mzingeli on the horse and Jenkins leading it. Eventually, towards dusk, they had come upon Forbes and his command, entrenched behind a laager. There, they learned that Forbes had approached the river early that morning but had been attacked by a force of Matabele. Having lost several men and seven horses, he had decided that the river was too high to cross and had taken his men back.

'I can't risk losing my whole command by having another go,' he told Fonthill. 'Anyway, from what you've told me, we would never get across, and it's too late now in any case.'

Simon had been forced to see the painful logic of Forbes's argument, and eventually the three had accompanied Forbes and his men on their disconsolate march back to Bulawayo. The Shangani Patrol had ended in failure.

'Jenkins,' said Alice, finishing the dressing with a neat bow, 'would you like to make us all coffee while we digest this news.' She looked up at Simon. 'So, now the war is really over . . . or is it?'

Fonthill sighed. 'Oh yes, it must be. Presumably what was left of the impis is still out there, somewhere in the bush. But without Lobengula as a figurehead they will be leaderless, and despite their victory over Wilson and his men, they will have lost so many warriors that I don't see them going to war again. They will just break up and go back to their individual kraals.'

'Will there be any reprisals by Rhodes for the Shangani disaster?'

'I doubt it, but I want to go and see Jameson and Rhodes, now that he is back in Bulawayo.'

'So do I. I will come with you. I have a story to write.'

The rest of the press corps in Bulawayo had returned to the Cape after the flight of the king and the virtual fizzling out of the war. Alice had stayed, of course, because both Simon and Mzingeli were unable to travel. The tracker, in fact, had recovered faster than Fonthill and had now jettisoned the awkward shoulder bandage and sling and was moving freely. The fact that Lobengula's death had been confirmed and that details had emerged of the end of Wilson and his men meant that she could now wrap up her coverage of 'this sordid war' and write her final report.

Sordid or not, the war had given Alice the chance of re-establishing herself as an intrepid and, as it ensued, lucky war correspondent. Her closeness to Fonthill, of course, had given her a succession of exclusive stories, the latest of which had been his account of the Shangani Patrol. Now she would be in a position to scoop her rivals once again with the details of the last battle of Wilson and his men.

They sent a message across to Jameson, asking if he and Rhodes would see them. Normally, Alice suspected, Rhodes would have declined to be interviewed by her, but he could hardly resist meeting and thanking Simon, the hero of the patrol's last days. And he could surely not refuse to see one without the other. She was not above using every trick at her disposal to complete her story.

Acceptance came by return, and as Simon limped across to Jameson's office, established in a rebuilt hut on the site of the king's inner kraal, he could not forbear to warn Alice not to be antagonistic to Rhodes. 'Press him by all means, darling,' he said, 'but you must not thrust your own views on him.'

'Thank you, Simon, but I shall thrust on him anything I wish.'

They found the two men in sombre mood. They both rose to welcome them, however, and shook hands warmly. 'You did splendid work at the Shangani, Fonthill,' said Rhodes, 'and I am only sorry that Forbes couldn't follow up.'

'So am I. I have to say to you both that, frankly, I feel the effort should at least have been made.'

'Well,' Jameson broke in quickly, 'I understand that the river was terribly high. There's a difference between the three of you crossing and taking across more than a hundred men against a hostile far bank. But,' he shrugged, 'I'm afraid it's all too late to argue now.'

Alice opened her notebook. 'I understand, gentlemen,' she said, 'that you have news of how Wilson and his men finally died.'

'Yes, we do indeed, madam.' Rhodes was sitting bolt upright and he looked Alice challengingly in the eye. 'And it is a story that makes us all proud to be English. I hope that you will be able to report it fully.'

'I hope so too,' Alice replied coolly. 'May I have the details, please and the source of your information?'

'Certainly. Certainly. One of the Matabele who was a member of the king's party – not an *inDuna*, you understand, but a minor chieftain from what we have been able to ascertain here in Bulawayo – came in this morning with his family. He wants to return to live here. He fought at the final Shangani battle and then went off with the king, who was trying to make for the Limpopo. He tells us that Lobengula is certainly dead, for he saw his corpse, but he does not know the cause. However, he gave us a graphic account of Wilson's end.'

He coughed. 'Magnificent, if I may say so. He says that the troopers fought on throughout the day, their numbers gradually being reduced by the firing of the Matabele—'

'Ah yes,' interrupted Alice. 'And do you know, Mr Rhodes, from where the Matabele obtained their rifles and ammunition?'

Simon winced, but Rhodes did not flinch.

'I expect, dear lady, that they were part of the consignment that your husband took to Bulawayo, to cement the treaty I had agreed with the king. I regret very much that they were used against British troops, which was, of course, breaking the terms of the treaty, but one must take risks sometimes in these regions if one wishes to progress.'

'I see.' Alice, her head down, was scribbling fast. 'Pray continue. You were saying that Wilson's patrol was reduced by the firing during the day?'

'Indeed.' Rhodes smoothed his moustache. 'They fought off each attack with great bravery as the day progressed until they finally ran out of ammunition. Then . . .' The great man's voice broke. He took a large and none too clean handkerchief from his pocket and blew his nose noisily. Then he wiped his moist eyes. 'Yes, do excuse me. This Matabele said that Wilson – whom he identified because of his large moustaches – and his men shook hands all round, stood and sang one verse of "God Save the Queen", then . . . then . . .' he blew his nose again, 'stood firm and waited for the inevitable as the final charge came. No one survived, of course. They were all speared and then disembowelled as a tribute to them as great warriors. Magnificent. Magnificent. Please do quote me, if you wish.'

A silence fell in the tent as Alice continued to scribble.

'A chapter of errors, I am afraid,' said Fonthill, 'which

doesn't detract from the bravery of them all at the end.'

'What . . . er . . . yes, well, quite.'

'What do you propose to do about the remnants of the king's impi?'

Rhodes made a dismissive gesture. 'We shall send out messengers to say that they may all now return to their kraals without harassment, as long as they promise to forgo further hostile activities. There will be no pursuit of them in the bush. Jameson here will organise for a party to go up to the Shangani and bury the dead.'

'And your plans to expand to the east?'

'Ah, that reminds me. I wrote to you, Fonthill, of course, following the receipt of your treaty with Umtasa, to thank you for your work out there. But let me take this opportunity to thank you again. Jameson here has made contact with the king, but I have to confess that we have met with difficulties with the Portuguese, who of course control the coast. This was to be expected, but the road to the east has necessarily had to take a lower priority to the establishment of our settlements here. This has now been done and—'

Alice looked up from her pad. 'So you are saying, Mr Rhodes, that your aim in invading Matabeleland was always to establish settlements here and in Mashonaland?'

'What?' Rhodes blinked behind his spectacles. 'But of course, madam.'

Alice produced that special sweet smile that so often presaged the killing point. 'But this was not what you told King Lobengula, was it? You only requested mining concessions, surely?'

Rhodes seemed quite unfazed. 'Certainly, and quite genuinely. Unfortunately, the land has proved to be comparatively unproductive so far. But I always also wished to establish good settlers here to spread the values of the English race in a territory that knew only barbarism and cruelty. If the land here seems not to have fulfilled its promise in terms of mineral deposits – and this still remains to be proven – then it is certainly, in the high veldt, good farming territory. It could never have reached its true potential under Lobengula, a feudal despot of the old order.'

Alice put down her pencil. 'I understand, Mr Rhodes, that there are many people in political and other circles back home who do not share your views.'

For the first time Rhodes began to show signs of exasperation. It was clear that a background of buying off his competitors in commerce and a remarkably unchallenged rise to the top in South African politics had not prepared him for debate with a proponent of radical views – and a woman at that.

He leaned forward. 'Then, my dear lady, those people "back home",' he laid heavy emphasis on the words, 'should have done something about what you have called my "invasion".' He took a strong pull of his cigar and waved away the smoke. 'On the contrary, I had approval – unofficial, it is true, but approval all the same – of my actions from government circles and I was allowed to execute my policies at my own expense. In other words, these people back home that you referred to were, on the whole, quite prepared to let me carry on a programme of extension of the British Empire as long as it did not cost the British Government a single penny. It is others, madam, who are guilty of hypocrisy, not I.'

Jameson entered the debate for the first time. 'In dealing with savages, Mrs Fonthill,' he said, 'one cannot be perhaps quite as punctilious as, say, in Europe. One cannot say, "I wish to settle your land," because the king would have said, "No, keep out." That is obvious. So we had to use other means. But let me point out that Mr Rhodes has not been motivated by personal gain. It could well be that there are no minerals to be mined here or in Mashonaland, and as a result, the company of which he is chairman will gain no return on its investment. In addition, he has deployed a considerable portion of his personal fortune in financing this campaign and is unlikely to gain a return on that. His motives have been altruistic: the extension of the British Empire and the spreading of the British way of life.'

Alice opened her mouth to speak, but Jameson held up his hand. 'One more matter. Lobengula's father took this land at spearpoint less than sixty years ago. He introduced slavery and execution on a whim. The king, then, has no more right to it than the good white farmers who are now beginning to work the land following Christian principles.'

Alice wrote something on her pad, underlined it with a flourish and stood. 'Thank you, gentlemen,' she said, her face a little flushed. 'I think I understand your position and I am grateful to you for explaining it to me. I should point out, however, that nothing you have said justifies to my mind the invasion of a land ruled by a man who has a constitutional right to it – you recognised this in your original treaty with Lobengula – and the massacre of his people by machine guns, cannon and modern rifles when they have the audacity to resist your incursion. I fear that this view must be expressed in my final report on this miserable campaign. Good morning.'

She swept out of the hut, leaving behind her a silence as heavy as the blue smoke that hung in the air. Fonthill found himself grinning as he regarded the shocked faces of the others.

'Well, my word.' Rhodes's voice had risen to a squeak. 'You don't share your wife's views, surely, Fonthill?'

'Well, do you know, sir, I rather fear that I do now.' He shifted in his chair and thrust himself upright, wincing at the momentary shaft of pain the movement caused. 'I am certain of one thing, and that is this: many brave men gave their lives for this land. I hope for your sakes that it will be worth it. Good day to you both.'

He hobbled back to their tent to find that Jenkins and Mzingeli had gone hunting and Alice was, predictably, scribbling furiously on a cable pad. She hardly looked up as he entered.

'Now, don't chastise me,' she said. 'I have work to do. I know you don't agree with me, but I had to say all that. I am only supposed to report news for the *Post* and my own opinions, as always, will only be implied. But,' she looked up at him with a triumphant smile, 'I got Rhodes to admit that he invaded to build the empire, not to prospect. That damns him from his own mouth and it's a good story. Now, go away, you Imperialist, and let me write my piece.'

Fonthill bent and kissed her. 'As a matter of fact, I agree with you.'

Alice looked up, her mouth open. 'You do? Good lord!'

'Yes, and I told them so.'

A slow smiled began to spread across Alice's face. 'Simon, you continue to amaze me. I think I am beginning to love you all over again.'

'I should think so. My leg aches. I need attention.'

Then the smile was replaced by a frown. 'But you own land in Mashonaland. You have taken Rhodes's shilling.'

'I know. Listen.' He pulled up the other camp stool. 'I still love the land up there, and I agree with Rhodes and Jameson to the extent that it should be developed and farmed creatively. The Mashonas – or the Matabele, for that matter – will never do that. They are not farmers and never will be. However, I have a proposal for you.'

'Propose away.'

'I would like to give the farm to Mzingeli. He has no roots in the Transvaal, nor a proper home, working for that Boer down there. He would like, I am sure, to be near his father.'

'But is he a farmer? Could he work the land?'

'Actually, he was beginning to do very well, until we took him away to be a soldier, with the result that he got a bullet through his shoulder. No, he will cope, with a bit of help. We will give him a sum of money, which we will invest in the farm, and if he agrees, and I think he will, I will promise to keep an eye on the property for him, visiting him from time to time to help him develop it. Jenkins and I will like the game hunting anyway, and as you know, I love the country. It seems the ideal solution. The land will return to one of its native sons, in a way, and Ntini and Joshua can both work for him. What do you think?'

Alice sat for a moment, deep in thought. 'What do *we* do?' she asked.

'We go back to your beloved Norfolk and give the land there the attention it deserves after our long time away, and still retain a sort of foothold here. But . . .'

'Ah. I knew there would be a but.'

Fonthill frowned. 'Yes. Well, we might as well be completely honest with each other. I can farm happily in Norfolk for a time, but the place runs itself pretty well, and I know that I will get bored after a time – and so will you, not to mention Jenkins.'

Alice sucked her pencil. 'So . . . ?

'I think – no, I am sure – that there will be trouble soon in the Transvaal. The Boers there are still cocky after beating us so completely on Majuba Hill, and the peace agreement afterwards was a cobbled-together mess. To be frank, I sense that Rhodes has got his eye on the province and wouldn't be above stirring up trouble there with the many Britishers who have gone in to work the goldfields on the Rand to justify an invasion.' He smiled sheepishly. 'Jenkins and I know the territory better than most Englishmen – certainly better than most soldiers. With General Lamb as army commander in the Cape, there could be a job for us and a bit of excitement to relieve the . . . er . . . forgive me, my love, but I think the word is *tedium* of life in Norfolk, if and when the call comes.' Then the smile faded and he looked at her anxiously. 'But would you let us go?'

She stood and looked him levelly in the eye. 'Of course, if I could come too.'

Fonthill sighed. 'I knew you would say that. You would want to report it all for the *Post*?'

'Of course.'

'Well, they say all is fair in love and war, and I don't suppose we have run out of either yet.'

Alice stepped forward and put her arms around his neck. Somewhere a dog barked and harnesses creaked as a wagon drove past. 'No, I am sure we haven't,' she whispered into his ear.

They kissed and stood together for a moment, her head on his shoulder, and then she said: 'And I love your idea of giving the farm to Mzingeli. It seems the perfect solution. Put it to them both – for Jenkins must be party to this, as he is to everything – when they return. Now.' She pushed him away and sat down again. 'Go away and let me write.'

'Very well. But go easy on Rhodes and Jameson.'

'Of course I will. Oh . . .' She looked up. 'How do you spell despicable?'

Author's Note

The Matabele War was a virtual sideshow in the great pageant of Victorian colonial wars, attracting comparatively little attention from historians and writers of biographies and autobiographies, probably because it was, on the whole, a piece of private enterprise by Cecil John Rhodes. Nevertheless, it did result in the establishment of a new nation in southern Africa, Rhodesia, and the controversy that surrounded its birth has continued to cling to it, through its split into northern and southern Rhodesia, its unification, its secession from the British Commonwealth and its present reincarnation as Zimbabwe under President Mugabe.

It was also significant in that it represented the high-water mark in the territorial gains that made the British Empire the largest the world had seen. (I discount the bits and pieces of real estate that Britain picked up as a result of the First World War.) For a novelist, however, the war's main attraction must be the clash between its two main protagonists, Rhodes and the Matabele chief King Lobengula. They never met, like those more famous adversaries Wellington and Bonaparte, and Hitler and Churchill, but their vices and virtues stamped themselves on the encounters between Lobengula's impis and Rhodes's army of settlers just as surely as if the two had crossed assegai blade and bayonet personally.

In setting the adventures of Simon Fonthill against the background of the war, I have attempted to relate accurately its twists and turns and also to paint the background to what became a classic conflict between the expansionist march of a great colonial power and the struggle of a barbaric and warlike people to remain independent. The Shangani episode was a tragedy, of course, and among the last of its kind.

As always in the Fonthill novels, I must establish what was fact and what fiction. Simon, Alice, Jenkins and Mzingeli, of course, are fictional characters, as are General Lamb and those two rogues Murphy and Laxer. All of the other main characters, however, very much existed: Beit, King Khama, Fairbairn, Dr Jameson, Chief Umtasa, Captain Borrow and Majors Wilson and Forbes. I did not create Manuel de Sousa, 'Gouela', although I confess to painting him rather more darkly than perhaps even he deserved. De Sousa, a Portuguese agent with a reputation as a rapist and a slaver, was a regular attender at the court of King Lobengula, and he did try to persuade the king to eschew all dealings with Rhodes.

Lobengula did indeed send a bag of golden sovereigns in a pathetic attempt to divert his pursuers, and the two troopers who accepted them from the *inDunas* did try to keep them and were court-martialled. Three men, all scouts, were sent back by Major Wilson to cross the Shangani in an attempt to get Major Forbes to bring aid, and for those who may think that Simon's crossing of the river by holding on to the horse's tail is a little fanciful, then I must refer them to Lieutenant Horace Smith-Dorrien, who escaped the Zulus after

Isandlwana by crossing the Buffalo river in the same way.

Alice's treatment of Lobengula's gout is based on fact, in that Dr Jameson did earn the king's friendship by so treating his ailment in Bulawayo – as well as, it is said, because he could make the king laugh. Rhodes's pursuit of Simon to recruit him to take the gold and arms to the king and to prospect to the east is quite logical, in that he did, in fact, employ many young British adventurers for such tasks – particularly in exploring towards the Portuguese borders to establish contact with the tribes there and to persuade them to sign treaties with his company.

Wherever possible, I have based important conversations on the writings of the participants or those who were present at the time. Rhodes's eulogy to the strengths of British character and his vision of the map of Africa to the north 'covered in red', expressed so forcefully to Fonthill in Cape Town, are taken from his writings. Similarly, Lobengula's colourful analogy of the chameleon (England) and the fly (Matabeleland) was remembered by those who were in his kraal at the time.

Cecil John Rhodes, of course, was a highly complex and controversial character. As I have tried to reflect in the novel, the British Government, the press, the bankers of London, the public of the day – none of them could ever quite make up their mind about him. Was he a capitalistic charlatan or a great man of empire? Amazingly, well over a hundred years later, the jury is still out.

Rhodes attracted opprobrium when – as Fonthill feared – he plotted to send a party of armed men into Kruger's Transvaal under the command of the faithful Dr Jameson to stimulate a rising against the Boer government. This abortive mini-invasion became known as the Jameson Raid, and the good doctor went to jail for leading it. Somehow Rhodes wriggled out of accepting the blame, although he sturdily supported the doctor throughout, and Jameson later became reinstated in society and died an honoured man and servant of empire. He was interred in Rhodesia's Matopo Hills, near to the body of Cecil John Rhodes, the man he had served so well.

The cause of Lobengula's death was never established – he could well have been poisoned, the fate of many African despots. His people wrapped his body in the hides of two newly flayed oxen and buried it in a cave. Rhodes took charge of three of Lobengula's sons, and of their sons, and took them to his home in Cape Town, to be educated and brought up there. One of the boys survived to become one of Rhodes's chief mourners when the great man died in 1902.

The fate of the Shangani Patrol became a cause célèbre back in England. As with Rorke's Drift after the British defeat by the Zulus at Isandlwana, the heroism of the little band – their singing of the national anthem, the formal shaking of hands before they faced the last charge of the Matabele warriors – distracted the public's attention from all that had gone before: the slaughter of the natives by machine guns, modern rifles and cannon. It thrilled the readers of the Victorian newspapers and was what they expected of their heroes. The only things lacking were white pith helmets and red coats.

A memorial to Wilson and his men was erected where they fell, and the remains of their bodies were removed to consecrated ground, to be reinterred later near their memorial in the Matopo Hills, where Rhodes and Jameson were to lie. If the Anglo-Matabele war is little remembered now, the Shangani Patrol lives on in the minds of those lovers of history who respect extreme bravery – particularly when its last moments are acted out with a sense of drama and pathos that even Hollywood would consider too unbelievable to put on the screen.

J.W.
Chilmark
August 2009

Siege of Khartoum

John Wilcox

1884. The eyes of the world are on Khartoum as Queen Victoria's hero General Gordon comes under siege. Hordes of Dervish warriors, loyal to the Mahdi, the Sudanese warlord and Messiah, are baying for British blood. With just a few thousand men and diminishing supplies, Gordon fears Khartoum will fall.

Ex-captain and hardened army scout Simon Fonthill is summoned to Cairo on a vital mission. He must enter the heavily guarded city undetected and make contact with Gordon ahead of the relief force. Failure could mean instant death or slow torture at the hands of the Mahdi's disciples.

Soon Fonthill and his comrade '352' Jenkins are crossing the Nile. But when they're captured by a sadistic Dervish patrol, it seems that, for Fonthill, time has finally run out . . .

Acclaim for John Wilcox's Simon Fonthill novels:

'Grown-up *Boy's Own* stuff, a pacy read' *Sunday Express*

'Full of action and brave deeds. If you are a fan of Simon Scarrow or Wilbur Smith, then this is for you' *Historical Novels Review*

'A hero to match Sharpe or Hornblower . . . Wilcox shows a genius for bringing to light the heat of battle' *Northern Echo*

978 0 7553 4560 1

headline

The Guns of El Kebir

John Wilcox

'Fonthill, if things go wrong, you are dispensable . . . To repeat, you will be on your own.'

1882. Lieutenant General Sir Garnet Wolseley is under pressure. News of an uprising against the British powers in Egypt has reached London, and he must react decisively and forcefully. But there is little time to assemble an army and, for his campaign to succeed, he needs someone on the ground to assess the movements and strength of the Egyptian rebels.

Fresh from a scouting mission in South Africa, former army captain Simon Fonthill is kicking his heels in Brecon. When the request from Wolseley comes, Fonthill and his servant, '352' Jenkins, accept the assignment, fully aware of the dangers they will face in hostile terrain without back up.

But they could never have foreseen the bloodshed that awaits them in the desert at Tel el Kebir . . .

Acclaim for John Wilcox's Simon Fonthill novels:

'Grown-up *Boy's Own* stuff, a pacy read' *Sunday Express*

'Full of action and brave deeds. If you are a fan of Simon Scarrow or Wilbur Smith, then this is for you' *Historical Novels Review*

'A hero to match Sharpe or Hornblower . . . Wilcox shows a genius for bringing to light the heat of battle' *Northern Echo*

978 0 7553 2721 8

headline

Last Stand At Majuba Hill

John Wilcox

'There's nowhere to go, 352. We make a last stand here.'

It is 1881, and General George Pomeroy-Colley, commander of the British forces in Natal, is planning to stamp out a rebellion. He is convinced the Transvaal Boers can pose no serious threat, but he needs reliable information. He calls on former army captain Simon Fonthill.

A veteran of the recent Zulu and Sekukuni campaigns, Fonthill knows to never underestimate an enemy. He and his servant, '352' Jenkins, agree to carry out a covert diplomatic assignment. But the greatest test is yet to come. As the two armies converge on the heights of Majuba Hill, Fonthill and Jenkins are first into the fray. If they are to break the enemy, Colley's men must hold the summit at all costs . . .

Acclaim for John Wilcox's Fonthill series:

'Fast-paced, full of action and brave deeds. If you are a fan of Simon Scarrow or Wilbur Smith, then this is for you' *Historical Novels Review*

'A hero to match Sharpe or Hornblower . . . Wilcox shows a genius for bringing to light the heat of battle' *Northern Echo*

'A rollicking account of a turbulent period in Britain's imperial past' *Good Book Guide*

978 0 7553 2719 5

headline

You can buy any of these other bestselling
Headline titles from your bookshop
or *direct from the publisher*.

FREE P&P AND UK DELIVERY
(Overseas and Ireland £3.50 per book)

The Horns of the Buffalo	John Wilcox	£7.99
The Road to Kandahar	John Wilcox	£7.99
The Diamond Frontier	John Wilcox	£6.99
Last Stand at Majuba Hill	John Wilcox	£6.99
The Guns of El Kebir	John Wilcox	£6.99
Siege of Khartoum	John Wilcox	£7.99

TO ORDER SIMPLY CALL THIS NUMBER

01235 400 414

or visit our website: www.headline.co.uk

Prices and availability subject to change without notice.